The Speed Culture

Amphetamine Use and Abuse in America

Lester Grinspoon, M.D.

and

Peter Hedblom

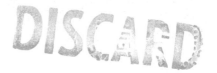
Harvard University Press

Cambridge, Massachusetts

and

London, England

1975

Quotations from *Love Needs Care* by David E. Smith,
M.D., and John Luce, by permission of Little, Brown
and Co.; copyright © 1971 by David E. Smith, M.D.,
and John Luce; copyright © 1969 by John Luce.

Children are the greatest high of all

To David

Preface

This book contains no hastily or casually reached conclusions. It is a result of more than three years of research of hundreds of articles, and careful consideration of innumerable interviews and letters. At one stage the manuscript was almost three times its present length; in part, this is a reflection of the critical importance we attach to the subject of amphetamine abuse.

Our subtitle is not intended to imply that amphetamine abuse affects only the United States. In many areas of the world, particularly in industrialized countries, this problem has become quite serious. Britain, Sweden, Japan, Czechoslovakia, and the Togolese Republic are among the countries that have had to deal with amphetamine abuse. We refer to many of the studies and reports which have emerged from these and other countries, but a detailed consideration of the international situation would require a separate book.

While the book as a whole is addressed to the nonspecialist reader, a few sections — especially those dealing with the psychopharmacology of amphetamines and certain medical aspects and research techniques — are of necessity somewhat technical and perhaps beyond the means or interest of those not trained in pharmacology, biochemistry, or medicine; however, in the interest of providing a reasonably comprehensive picture of current knowledge of the amphetamines, these sections could not be omitted. To our readers who may find them tedious we offer our apologies and the suggestion that they skim over such passages. We believe that even without these sections they will find the book enlightening.

Over the course of the several years it has taken to write this book, we have accumulated varying degrees of indebtedness to a number of people. Among them are Professors William von Eggers Doering, C. Keith Conners, Jack R. Ewalt, and Richard J. Bonnie, and Roger Carpenter, Ogie Strogatz, Susan B. Payne, Betty Lawless, Tom Lewis, Sage Eskesen, Phoebe McGuire, and Betsy Grinspoon. We owe thanks to Susan B. Singer, Linda Twing Shadgett, and Rebecca Shiffman for their invaluable contributions of library research. In addition, we are grateful for the support and encouragement of Dr. William I. Bennett, Editor for Science and Medicine at the Harvard University Press; and we wish to thank his colleague, Ann Louise McLaughlin, for the skill, diligence, and enthusiasm with which she approached her editing task. Special thanks go to June Stillman, who, among other contributions, has assured bibliographic accuracy. We are especially indebted to James B. Bakalar who helped in our struggle to find an acceptable balance between comprehensiveness and comprehensibility; as part of this task he helped us to reduce the manuscript from its original nine hundred pages to its present, we hope manageable, size.

L. G.   P. H.

October 1974

Contents

The Speed Culture

Introduction

Our interest in the amphetamines began several years ago when we became acquainted with a young man whose life has been nearly devastated largely through abuse of these drugs. As an adolescent he exuded self-confidence, and those who knew him never doubted that he would achieve more than ordinary success. His intelligence and capacity for intellectual work, his growing creativity, his interest and skill in athletics, along with an easy charm and an engaging, if somewhat cynical, sense of humor, were expected to open many doors.

Our friend's promise has not yet been fulfilled. Instead of a life of accomplishment and reward, the past thirteen years have been, as he describes, a nightmare:

> Until my senior year in prep school I had been, as far as I or anyone else could see, normal in all respects. I loved athletics, especially football and hockey, did well in scholastic work (I was admitted to one of the best colleges with sophomore standing), liked and felt liked by nearly all my fellow students. Sexually, things also seemed fine. I had an excellent relationship with one girl in particular; we were very close, but this did not isolate either of us from social activities.
>
> But in the spring of that senior year I went through two experiences I was not at all equipped to handle, and without knowing what I was doing I turned to the bottle. The first was the indirect result of a party. Several of my classmates got drunk, and I helped sneak them back into the dormitory. While brushing my teeth shortly afterward, I made some remark to the effect that "you should have seen so-and-so tonight." But I made it within earshot of the head of the student council, who felt it his duty to investigate what had gone on and to report it to the school officials. As a result, I was branded a traitor and was ostracized by all but two or three of my closest friends.
>
> The second unfortunate incident, which occurred during spring vacation in the Caribbean, was my witnessing and trying

1

to help my mother when she had a total psychotic break. The flight back and the next few days at home, where my mother was hysterical (she was finally committed to a mental institution, where she remained until midsummer), were pretty hard to take, for a naive and unworldly eighteen-year-old. Back at school later that spring, I recall having seriously considered suicide—especially after one rainy Sunday visit with my mother, when I returned to school to find my room a shambles, with ink poured all over my class notes and "Judas," "traitor," etc. written on the walls. I was depressed, and I was so ignorant of basic psych that I didn't even know there was a word for how I felt.

I never really managed to work myself out of that initial depression. College came and went in two and a half years; I graduated with honors. I loved it and immersed myself in studies. In the late autumn of my first year I eloped with a girl I'd met there. Unfortunately her parents were strongly opposed to the marriage and put pressure on Alice to leave me. Under the circumstances, it is hardly surprising that my drinking problem firmly established itself.

We somehow managed to hold on to one another through college, and that summer Alice gave birth to our daughter. I wanted to believe we were making some headway, but her parents and my drinking tipped the scales the wrong way, I guess. Christmas was horrible. I was a first-semester graduate student faced with a mountain of final papers and a deeply troubled wife. I would regularly drink myself into a stupor, which would infuriate Alice, and this in turn would lead to more drinking. I knew it was only a matter of time; and shortly after New Year's, Alice told me she had decided on a divorce.

That spring, after Alice's abandonment, I dropped out of graduate school. Spent the next year writing poetry, drinking heavily, and sleeping with as many females as I could possibly manage. It was during the following summer that one of my girlfriends introduced me to my first "drug." (I still refused to contemplate what alcohol was.) I was considerably hungover one morning, and she suggested that I take a couple of her little green pills. (Later, I was to learn that these were Dexamyls: 5 milligrams of dextroamphetamine plus a barbiturate). I took them, and within thirty minutes, not only was my hangover gone, but I felt positively exuberant—better than I had felt in months, possibly years.

That morning stands out as the high point of my drug career. I felt I could do anything; and in fact I did manage to pull together the best day's work so far that summer—working, writing good verse at a fantastic pace during my lunch hour, and—with the bolstering of two more little green pills every three or four hours for the rest of the day—going out on two dates that night, piloting a boat through fog for twenty-five miles to an island and back, and finally retiring, cum original girlfriend, at 4:00 A.M. Then I discovered the second great adventure of this little magic pill: it made sex seem endless, overpowering, soaring beyond description.

I should point out that ordinarily I would have shuddered my way through the morning, perhaps fortifying myself with a few beers or the equivalent in hard liquor at lunch. I then would have stumbled through the afternoon and drunk myself into a quick oblivion by 6:00 P.M. at the latest, with no thought of sex, poetry, or even food.

The next day I didn't allow myself to crash. Before my friend left for her apartment, I asked for and she gave me enough Dexamyls to carry me through the remaining month of summer.

I believe it was Aldous Huxley who wrote that there has been only one addition to the original seven deadly sins, and that one is speed. Sin is not an extremely popular concept among thoughful people today, especially those who work/live in schools. But I think it's just a matter of semantics. Every few decades they change the labels, but like the shrink who is concerned about acting out antisocial erotic fantasies, it all comes to a deep-rooted conviction that some things, words, acts, and even people are just plain bad.

In any case, if Huxley could rank nonchemical speed among the most deadly activities, one wonders what he would think of the speed freak. It seems that the industrial revolution has put us all on an extended speed trip. But then, I am frightened by technology; perhaps because a working IBM is so much like a speedster, stringing beads forever, unless someone pulls out his (its) plug.

I re-entered graduate school that fall, and, deceived by the drug's initial, seemingly positive aspects, I slowly got deeper into speed. My amphetamine-induced self-confidence extended to social interaction in general. Like many people, I am somewhat shy and often unwilling to initiate conversation. With amphetamine I changed from a mild introvert to an outrageous extravert. I would not stop talking or socializing. It was a superficial kind of extraversion, however. The impatience and hastiness generated by the drug made it nearly impossible for me to *listen* to anybody. If I could not occupy center stage, I wasn't interested in being in the play. This attitude gradually drove away all but one of my closest friends.

About this time I discovered that marihuana smoked while under the influence of speed was ten times as pleasurable as grass smoked when otherwise drug-free. It got to the point where my daily consumption consisted of about 100 milligrams of amphetamine, 100 milligrams of a tranquilizer (Librium or Valium), and three or four pipes full of very strong cannabis, usually hashish.

Regarding my drinking habits, speed acted as a crutch,with vastly different short- and long-term effects. The short-term effect was that I was able to function while speeding after having drunk two or three times my normal intake. The drug's long-term effect was to make it much easier for me to cut down on my drinking or to abstain completely, sometimes for weeks. Amphetamines gradually became a total replacement for alcohol, especially when I found that even small amounts of alcohol deadened or took the edge off the speed high.

In the early phase of my drug abuse, I never had great difficulty in procuring speed from doctors. A typical doctor's appointment would run as follows. I'd fabricate a story, usually to the effect that my girlfriend had moved in with my best male friend on the same day that my brother had committed suicide and/or my mother and/or father either had been admitted to a mental hospital or had died in epilepsy. The doctor would listen, express sympathy, sorrow, etc. (how many of those doctors *could* have believed such nonsense!); after which I would inform him that I was (version #1) "starting to drink again, only about a pint a day now, but I'm an alcoholic," or (version #2) "I've had some trouble with alcohol in the past and Eskatrol [a combination of dextroamphetamine and prochlorperazine] has always helped me." The doctor would usually ask about dosage previously taken, duration of medication, etc. Then, in 98 percent of the interviews, he would write a prescription for thirty to one hundred Eskatrols. Generally the doctor noted that five refills were allowed; however, I was occasionally advised that I could get refills as long as I wanted them.

By February of that school year, my amphetamine abuse had established a maniacal cycle of behavior that was continuously repeated. The first phase of the cycle lasted thirty-six hours (though it seemed like minutes), and during it I enjoyed literally everything and anybody. Then would come a twelve-to-fourteen-hour crash, a period of extreme isolation during which I hallucinated regularly. There followed the final phase—one or two days of relatively normal behavior, overshadowed by deep depression and anxiety. At this point I would resume the cycle.

Finally I contacted a graduate student adviser, who lined up an appointment with a local psychologist. I saw him three times weekly, from the middle of March until the end of June. With his assistance, and a maximum of three Libriums per day, I was able to reduce my daily amphetamine dosage to one Eskatrol. But at that point I took a summer job outside of the city; and not long afterward I returned to my booze and pill binges.

I don't know how many times I've decided to get off speed since then. Each time I've delayed the withdrawal until my amphetamine supply was exhausted, and until I've obtained at least a week's narcotizing dose of Librium, or, preferably, Valium (which seemed to make me sleep better), or any barbiturate such as Nembutal. But even with the assistance of these downers, I usually could hold out only for a maximum of one week. Throughout all of these "major crashes," the girl who lived with me through most of my speed experience stood by faithfully, "while the master was hallucinating in the bedroom," as one acquaintance put it.

During these intermittent attempts to free myself from amphetamine, I spent most of my time sleeping. I usually had auditory hallucinations, in which I imagined I was hearing a radio play my favorite songs. Another aspect of my numerous attempts at withdrawal was the effect on sexual urge and activity. After a few months of using downers along with speed I had become, almost without exception, functionally impotent: I could attain orgasm, especially if I was stoned on grass, but I could not get or maintain an erection. However, as soon as I stopped the amphetamine (within a matter of twelve to eighteen hours), I was, in the words of my girlfriend, "a rutting bloody old goat," or "a walking (usually, however, I was prone) erection."

The paranoia was bad. I trusted no one (except, to some degree, my girlfriend), and I was terribly jumpy and suspicious. I also looked like something rejected from hell. My stomach usually gave me a good deal of pain, and I was either constipated or suffering from extreme diarrhea—there was no way to predict beforehand which it would be. The total depression is probably the most outstanding feature, but it was so deep that I cannot fully recall it, and at the time I was unable to verbalize it. In addition, I was usually shaking so badly that I could not hold a fork or spoon—or even a glass at times—so that feeding me was a problem which said dear loyal girlfriend managed to solve by giving me eggnogs through a straw.

But I knew that this misery (which I cannot fully convey to anyone who has not been through it) could be ended in short order. All I had to do was take a few Eskatrols or Dexamyls, and within thirty to forty-five minutes, I would feel as well as I ever had. The problem was that I was so down and out that it was nearly impossible for me to get to a phone to call a doctor for a prescription renewal, much less make arrangements for an office appointment. Once my craving for the stuff had become overpowering, I would resort to forging prescriptions. I stole pads from nearly every doctor I visited. Then I would call a cab and have the driver deliver the phony prescription and return with the magic pills.

I got into trouble only once. A suspicous pharmacist noted that the doctor whose pad and name I had used had died just a week before the date on the prescription, and called the police. That night two narcotics-squad detectives paid me a visit. They were most polite and, I think, favorably impressed. Although the apartment was on the fringe of the city's "slum-drug" area, it was always very clean and neat, thanks again to my young female friend.

I more or less told the detectives the truth, saying that I was sick and was hoping that some amphetamines would help me (I did look as though I had a real case of the flu), because I had to be in shape by the time I returned to school. When the detectives found out that I was in fact an enrolled graduate student, they let me off with a stern warning. I was very lucky; to this day I cannot understand why I was not arrested. In any case, I didn't let that brush deter me for long; after they had been gone an hour, I had a false prescription in the hands of another taxi driver. (This time I called the doctor's office to make sure he was alive.) I often managed to conceal my return to speed from my girlfriend, who accordingly thought that I was finally en route to recovery. But after a few nights when she was alone in bed, or I was unusually talkative, she made the right guess.

Several summers later, around the middle of July, I had an experience with LSD which showed me very graphically that I was killing myself. At the peak of the LSD reaction (I had taken a substantial dose, probably around 8,000 micrograms plus), I looked into a mirror and watched my face turn into that of an old man, and then into a skull. That did it. A week later I was living in a camper van on an orchard many miles south of the city, and I decided to do it cold turkey. I threw away everything but some Bufferin and I tried to carry on, picking fruit from sunup to dusk. Ordinarily as a vacation this would have been an ideal experience; but it was one of the most hellish times of my life.

The first few days were not too bad. My vision seemed affected; I had trouble focusing on objects, saw double, and had severe pains around the eyes and temples. I also felt off-balance; I kept stumbling and walking into corners of buildings and rooms. In addition, I felt very uneasy around all the people on the farm except for one person I had known at school, and in whom I confided what I was trying to do. He wanted to be helpful, but he made one mistake. Thinking that some cannabis would calm me, he got me high one night on strong hashish. I totally freaked out. We were smoking in my camper, and after the first few drafts, everything began to spin. I became panicky and paranoid. My friend helped me to my bunk and brought over a young woman who had some background in nursing and drug-abuse counseling. She gave me a lot of verbal assurance, but it did nothing to stop the mad whirling of objects and thoughts. I contemplated suicide at one point, but was incapable of any planned, consecutive actions. The woman and my friend stayed with me for several hours and, when I seemed to be quieting down, they left.

I made it through that night, and the next day I did manage to go out and pick some fruit; but I kept feeling worse and worse. It was six days since I had gone cold turkey. That night my cousin (whom I know as well as anyone) stopped by, because he had heard somehow I "was having difficulties." I did not recognize him, even when he got out of his car, stood three feet away, and addressed me directly. He might have been a total stranger.

I suppose that my big mistake was in trying to go cold turkey from a daily dosage of twenty Eskatrols, Librium, and Valium, to Bufferin alone. In any event, I could only stick it out another week; then I had to get some help. The only place I could think of, in my mind-wormed condition, was my mother's. I took off in my van, with the whole world seeming to tilt and stretch, and I somehow made the forty-mile drive. When I entered the house, I collapsed on the bed.

Shortly afterward I committed myself to a psychiatric hospital for the treatment of alcoholism and drug dependence. I was regarded as having "adjusted" fairly well ("adjustment" being defined as conformity to the artificial hospital environment). Then I contracted a serious case of bilateral viral pneumonia and was transferred to the city's largest hospital. I remember realizing at one point that all the tubes and needles in the world were not going to do any good unless I wanted to live, and I decided that I did want to live. This attitude must have influenced a turn for the better; my condition improved markedly, and a week later I was back at the psychiatric hospital.

However, I was still weak and I *longed* for some amphetamine, even to the point where I asked a cousin to bring me some. Instead she notified the hospital of my request, and I was punished by being confined to the locked ward for one week. About two weeks after that, the doctors decided that I could spend a day with my family. The visit was a turning point in my stay at the hospital because at home I discovered a small bottle of Dexamyls, about half full and marked "may be refilled three times." I pocketed the pills and told my brother I was going out for a short time. Taking three Dexamyls in order to "prime" myself to lie my way into the full complement of refills, I headed for the drugstore. Whatever it was I said to the druggist, it worked; he gave me the equivalent of three refills, or 180 Dexamyls. Now I was set.

When I returned to the hospital I found it difficult to restrain my euphoria (I had probably taken a total of six to eight pills during my eight hours "outside"), but the staff was completely deceived. My much improved change of mood was attributed to the visit home. Needless to say, from this point on it became increasingly easy to get permission to leave the hospital. After several more weeks, I was allowed to leave for short intervals "to look for a job." Of course the first thing I looked for was a doctor who would prescribe more pills.

Possibly the most alarming behavior generated by my drug abuse was thievery. I broke into a doctor's office three times within a two-month period, and each time I was high on speed. Prior to my use of amphetamines, I had never stolen; if I had been straight, I never would have considered this kind of federal offense against property. On my third break-in, in addition to literally cleaning him out, I took his *Physician's Desk Reference*, which enabled me to identify some of the drugs I had stolen in the previous break-ins. The results of my three nocturnal visits amounted to over 4,600 amphetamines and amphetamine-type drugs, over 2,000 Libriums, about 1,500 Valiums, and an assortment of barbiturates and "non-barbiturate sleeping pills"; I estimated their drug store prescription value as approximately $1,500. I only stopped the raids when, on a fourth attempt, I discovered that the doctor had barred his windows.

It is now over three years since I have used any amphetamines or amphetamine-type drugs and I feel no persistent craving or desire for them. Still there are times, especially if I am overtired or hungry, that I think with fond longing of how much I'd appreciate an Eskatrol. If I could get one at such times, I'm fairly certain I would take it. However, no opportunity has arisen to date, and since the new drug laws have been passed (1971-1972), I have not even considered asking a doctor for a prescription. But my main reason for not asking is not fear of refusal; in approaching well over fifty doctors during a six-year period, I was only once denied free samples or a liberal prescription. Rather, my reason for not asking is fear of what will happen if I ever take speed again.

I don't think I will ever be the person that I would have been, had I never taken speed. This is not all bad; it is possible to apply the hastened thought processes and general hyperactiveness constructively. And I believe I am learning to do this more skillfully every day. But, finally, any possible benefit pales beside the lost wife, friends, time, fun, opportunities, jobs, and money that speed stole from me. I let the thief in, because he seemed so helpful. I found out just in time that he was an indiscriminate killer, and I have been very lucky to get the best medical help.

As we became familiar with the details of our friend's history, we grew increasingly dismayed and began to ask ourselves many questions about the amphetamines. One of us (L.G.) was particularly disturbed because he had prescribed amphetamines over the years and too casually had accepted amphetamine samples from detail men, to pass on to patients, friends, and relatives. We determined to learn as much as we could about the drug and its place in contemporary American society. This book is an attempt to share our knowledge.

The Contemporary Amphetamine Scene

"A Christmas package with a time bomb inside."

The amphetamines, also called "diet pills," "pep pills," "bennies," "dexies," "uppers," or "speed," are a group of synthetic psychoactive drugs pharmacologically classified as nonselective central nervous system (CNS) stimulants, because one of their chief properties is the ability to excite all areas of the nervous system, including the brain. Although research pharmacologists have synthesized hundreds of different amphetamines, amphetamine derivatives, and amphetamine congeners exerting an astounding range of effects on laboratory animals and human beings, only about twenty with distinct structural characteristics are now available to prescribing physicians. These are marketed under more than one hundred different brand names, often in combination with tranquilizers, sedatives, hormones, vitamins, analgesics, alcohol, and other substances. The 1970 United States *legal* production of these twenty amphetamines exceeded 10 billion pills, tablets, and capsules; in 1971 the figure probably exceeded 12 billion.[1]

First introduced as the Benzedrine inhaler in 1932, and several years later in pill form, amphetamine quickly became enormously popular with both the public and the medical profession. By 1946 W.R. Bett asserted that it had thirty-nine "clinical uses," including treatments for epilepsy, postencephalitic Parkinsonism, schizophrenia, alcoholism, barbiturate intoxication and narcosis, excessive anaesthesia administration, morphine and codeine addictions, "nicotinism" (tobacco smoking), behavior problems in children, enuresis, migraine, heart block, the "spasmodic laughter and weeping . . . [and] disturbances of gait" associated with disseminated sclerosis, myasthenia gravis (a chronic and sometimes fatal disease of the nervous system which gravely weakens voluntary muscles), myotonia (muscular rigidity and tonic spasm), head injuries, infantile cerebral palsy, urticaria (hives or nettle rash), Meniere's Syndrome (a chronic, disabling, and painful inner ear disturbance), dysmenorrhea, colic, "irritable colon," irradiation sickness, and hypotension. He also suggested that amphetamines be used as an adjunct to electro-convulsive treatment (ECT or shock treatment), a means of preventing loss of consciousness caused by carotid sinus syndrome, an analgesic, a sexual stimulant, and even for night blindness and "caffeine mania."[2] Bett was just one of the many physicians who considered amphetamines inferior only to a few extraordinary drugs like aspirin in scope, efficacy, and safety.

Today the "accepted" medical indications for the use of amphetamines are very limited, and they have been shown to be both potentially addictive and quite toxic. Nevertheless, many physicians continue to overprescribe them, out of ignorance, carelessness, or a desire to provide patients with immediate solutions to their problems. Furthermore, where drugs are concerned, most of the postgraduate "education" of our doctors is provided by pharmaceutical industry advertising and sales ("detail") men. The industry has an increasingly powerful and well-financed lobby in Washington, amphetamines are a good source of income, and, in the words of the president of one firm, any legal restrictions on amphetamine production would be damaging unless "we have the Holy Grail or something to throw in its place."[3]

Another major problem connected with these drugs has nothing to do with their medical merits: their abuse, mostly by young people, to get high or have fun or even "freak out." And the motives of many older persons who justify dependence on amphetamines on medical grounds differ very little from those of the "speed freak." The first reported misuse of amphetamine in the United States occurred in 1936, while the psychological effects of the drug were being evaluated at the University of Minnesota. Students participating in the experiments passed the word that these new drugs would keep them awake all night for studying or fun. As a result, university physicians treated students who had collapsed, fainted, or suffered from insomnia as a direct result of amphetamine use.[4] Warnings appeared in the national media, but publicity about the dangers of amphetamines did nothing to discourage use. On the contrary, references to "brain," "pep," and "superman" pills aroused curiosity and actually encouraged further experimentation and abuse. The quick and enthusiastic acceptance by the medical profession, which was often accurately represented in popular articles, also reinforced the general impression that this was indeed a wonder drug.

In 1932 the American economic situation was disastrous. More people were out of work than ever before or since; stocks were even lower than during the worst moments of the 1929 panic, and the Gross National Product had been cut in half. Americans spent $10 billion less for food and tobacco than they had in 1929 or would in 1939. Corporations lost $1.2 billion; almost 20,000 businesses went bankrupt, 1,616 banks failed, and 21,000 people killed themselves. Prohibition added to the misery and chaos by creating a well-organized criminal underground set to shift its operations to whatever potentially lucrative drug scientists might invent.

But there were at least two reasons for hope. The Treasury Department's Federal Bureau of Narcotics was preparing to announce that, given enough time and money, it could wipe out the twin devils of heroin and marihuana addiction. And, thanks to Benzedrine, Americans could look forward not only to freedom from blocked and runny noses, but to a euphoria that would let them temporarily forget about their own personal financial depressions. Amphetamines were unique: never before had a powerful psychoactive drug been introduced in such quantities in so short a period of time, and never before had a drug with such a high addictive potential and capability of causing long-term or irreversible physical and psychological damage been so enthusiastically embraced by the medical profession as a panacea or so extravagantly promoted by the drug industry.

Recently, social phenomena similar to those of the 1930s have caused a rise in amphetamine use, although contemporary depression, insofar as it is a reaction to social conditions, results from feelings of helplessness and inadequacy before the onslaught of the superindustrial juggernaut. The speed freak is an outstanding casualty of our technological society, but others, who do not respond by dropping out so completely, alleviate feelings of impotence and inferiority through the use of amphetamines. Unfortunately, this drug is in the words of one journalist, "a Christmas package with a time bomb inside."[5]

Inhalers

Since the 1930s the public has been able to procure these euphoriants in several ways, with little or no assistance or interference from organized medicine, the Food and Drug Administration, or any state and federal drug abuse control organizations or legal authorities. First came inhalers. Although Smith, Kline & French held the patent on the Benzedrine inhaler until 1950, many imitations were marketed without fear of patent-infringement suit because Benzedrine was only one of many easily synthesized and equally stimulating, euphorigenic, and toxic amphetamine congeners and derivatives. By the "end" of the Korean War, at least seven other different inhalers containing large amounts of these drugs could be purchased at drug or grocery stores without prescription. All were very easy to break open, and the techniques of ingestion were limited only by the ingenuity of the abusers. The more observant or experimental quickly discovered that, although dissolving the fillers in alcohol or coffee produced the desired effects, a much stronger kick could be obtained by chewing these bits of cotton, or simply swallowing them whole. Laboratory tests corroborated these lay researchers' findings, and the extent of inhaler abuse was finally documented in the medical literature by the now classic study conducted by R. R. Monroe and H. J. Drell, who published the results of their observations in the United States military prison at Fort Harrison in Indiana shortly after World War II. These physicians wrote that 25.3 percent of about a thousand soldiers had confessed to amphetamine inhaler abuse while "behind the fence," but they stressed that this percentage was, in all likelihood, "deceptively low," because amphetamine intoxication during imprisonment was considered a serious offense and punished severely. The abusers detected included : "only those men who were referred to the [prison] psychiatrist because of bizarre behavior or who became so sick that they voluntarily reported to the medical officer. Because of the urine tests and the threat of punishment most users scrupulously avoided the dispensary [prison hospital].''[6] The 264 prisoners who admitted to abuse of Benzedrine inhalers did so by answering questionnaires. The actual extent of amphetamine abuse within this sample may have exceeded 30 to 40 percent. This was revealed by "several inmates who were forced to seek medical or psychiatric care because of the habituation [and who] were willing to talk freely in exchange for professional care." They claimed that as many as fifteen men in each thirty-five to fifty-man barracks installation were chronic users. Monroe and Drell reported that when they dissolved strips from three different inhalers in various liquids, they found that over three times as much active drug was released in solutions of gastric secretions (probably primarily because of the hydrochloric acid) as in beer, coffee, or tap water. They believed Benzedrine would remain the inhaler of choice, although others might be tried by "an uninformed public."

Just how "uninformed" this "public" actually was when it came to obtaining over-the-counter amphetamine was revealed in 1966, when Army psychiatrists H. R. Greenberg and N. Lustig noted that although: "amphetamine sulfate (Benzedrine) and other such inhalers are not easily obtained through the usual channels without a prescription, at least one inhaler containing a sympathomimetic amine is not only readily available to the general public at this writing, but has been widely advertised through the mass media."[7] This was the Dristan inhaler, containing 250 mg of mephentermine, an amphetamine that has a very close structural similarity to methamphetamine,* but is only about one-third to one-half as potent as amphetamine as a cerebral and metabolic stimulant (and therefore approximately one-sixth to one-fourth times as powerful as methamphetamine). In the course of their work at the United States Army stockade and medical facilities at Fort Lewis, in Tacoma, Washington, Drs. Greenberg and Lustig came across "several individuals who admitted to the misuse of the Dristan inhaler in a fashion similar to Monroe and Drell's subjects." They detailed only four case histories, and mentioned that a fifth prisoner had reported in-

---

*The chemical similarities between amphetamine and methamphetamine (d-desoxyephedrine), and mephentermine are striking. Mephentermine differs from methamphetamine only in that it has a methyl group instead of a hydrogen molecule attached to the alpha carbon of the two-carbon side chain between the phenyl ring and the amino group (see Chapter 2).

gesting the contents of the Wyamine inhaler, "which he had obtained in quantity." But they did point out that:

> All these men told us that the properties of the Dristan inhaler were widely known among delinquent, derelict, or socially marginal populations of the several different urban centers in which they had been raised. One patient had an amused, incredulous "Doesn't everybody know about it?" response to the physician's ignorance. This man (Case 2) had had the widest experience of the four with an addict subculture. He stated: "Some like it 'cause it's a cheap kick when they can't get nothing else, and some just like it. It's an easy thing, you can get it anywhere, in your friendly neighborhood drugstore, man . . . and if you get picked up, so there's an inhaler in your pocket and you got a bad cold, they can't do anything to you for that, can they?"[8]

Greenberg and Lustig charged that there was "an urgent need" for further study "of the Dristan inhaler problem." The manufacturer told these two physicians that after 15 March 1965 the inhaler did not contain a drug of the amphetamine group as the "active nasal decongestant," because after that date "2 aminoheptane base" was substituted for mephentermine. But the authors point out that the 2-aminoheptane-based inhaler was also abused by Monroe and Drell's subjects. Moreover, the change had been made, according to the manufacturer, only in some (presumably northwestern) states.

During 1966, probably as a result of Greenberg and Lustig's report, the relatively innocuous vasoconstrictor propylhexedrine (the active drug contained today in Smith, Kline & French's popular Benzedrex inhaler), which is almost entirely devoid of central nervous system stimulating properties, was substituted for mephentermine in all Dristan inhalers. Nevertheless, mephentermine still could be purchased over-the-counter without a prescription in almost any United States drugstore until over a year after March 1970, when B. M. Angrist and three associates at the New York University Medical Center published a report on three male patients, all under thirty-three years of age, who had separate histories of a total of *twenty-nine* recurrent admissions to Bellevue Psychiatric Hospital with "acute paranoid or paranoid hallucinatory syndromes resulting in disturbed behavior" that were, with six doubtful exceptions, judged to be instances of amphetamine psychosis. All three patients admitted to the abuse of Wyamine inhalers (Wyeth Laboratories). Urine analysis (by gas chromatography) definitely established that mephentermine, and not amphetamine sulfate, methamphetamine, or any other drug was the immediate cause of psychosis in twenty-three instances. Angrist and his associates concuded that the Wyamine inhaler was potentially dangerous and "its availability on the market constitutes a loophole in the current regulations governing stimulant drugs."[9] The Wyamine inhaler was finally discontinued on June 22, 1971, ending a long period of confusion within the pharmaceutical industry. For although some drug companies had been quick to follow Smith, Kline & French's 1949 precedent by removing their own equivalents of the original Benzedrine inhaler from the market voluntarily, many others kept selling amphetamine over-the-counter in inhaler form until 1959, when the Food and Drug Administration banned amphetamines for such use. For reasons that are still unclear, however, the Food and Drug Administration banned only amphetamine and dextroamphetamine, but not methamphetamine (or other, less potent amphetamine congeners like mephentermine). This major loophole was seized upon by many drug firms. Perhaps the most blatant example was the midwestern drug house that marketed its Valo inhaler containing 150 mg of methamphetamine *after* 1959, an inhaler that supplied much of the methamphetamine found in a study of amphetamine traffic in Oklahoma City.[10]

Although the inhalers introduced hundreds of thousands (perhaps millions) of Americans to amphetamine abuse, their abuse assumed major proportions only within prisons and among markedly disturbed or deviant groups, simply because more powerful amphetamine products were so easy to obtain in pill, capsule, or injectible form. Although some state laws forbade the sale of (noninhaler) amphetamines without a doctor's prescription after the passage of the 1938 Pure Food, Drug and Cosmetic Act, this legislation required only that drugs be (1) accurately labeled; (2) manufactured according to certain minimal (and vaguely defined) standards; and (3) shown to be relatively safe (but not necessarily effective). The Act was not strictly enforced, so there were no nationwide controls on nonprescription over-the-counter or mail-order amphetamine sales until the passage of a specific federal law in 1951—and this law still exempted many amphetamine-congener inhalers as prescription items. At least until January 1966, most users and abusers found it easy to procure the pills (or capsules), even if a visit to the doctor was necessary, and they generally preferred this form because it was easier to tell exactly how much amphetamine they had taken.

Armed Forces Abuse

World War II probably gave the greatest impetus to date to legal medically authorized as well as illicit black market abuse of these pills on a worldwide scale. German Panzer troops, according to one source, used methamphetamine to eliminate fatigue and maintain physical endurance. It is at least possible that some of their excesses and atrocities were the result of abuse of amphetamines. This has been corroborated by a German commentator, who noted that "Troops who have been given benzedrine or pervitin [methamphetamine] are very useful in modern battle conditions when used in mass attacks."[11] But the German Army was by no means the only large-scale consumer of amphetamines during World War II: the Japanese used as much or more; and, according to British war statistics, 72 million standard-dose amphetamine tablets were distributed to the British Armed Forces alone. Although the United States Armed Forces did not authorize the issue of amphetamines to servicemen on a regular basis until the Korean conflict, Benzedrine was used extensively by Army Air Corps personnel stationed in England in the 1940s, and it was an open secret that many pilots engaged in a bootlegging operation to supply troops in Africa, Europe, and eventually the Pacific. Amphetamines were also easily obtainable from military medical officers and aides. The amount of Benzedrine supplied to United States servicemen by the British has been estimated at nearly 80 million tablets and pills, and probably another 80 to 100 million were supplied by United States medics. If only 10 percent of American soldiers ever used amphetamines during the war, over 1.5 million men must have returned to this country in 1945 with some firsthand knowledge of their effects. One of the most revealing findings of Monroe and Drell's 1946 study was that only 14.4 percent of the 264 self-admitted Benzedrine-abusing prisoners had taken amphetamine before entering the service; 27.2 percent had been given amphetamine pills by Army medical personnel.[12]

In recent years the Armed Forces have been a breeding ground for the abuse of all kinds of drugs, but especially the amphetamines, which are not only sanctioned but encouraged by military authorities. According to the *Fourth Report by the Select Committee on Crime* in 1971:

Over the past 4 years, the Navy seems to have required more stimulants than any other branch of the services. Their annual, active duty, pill-per-person requirement averaged 21.1 during the years 1966-69. The Air Force has flown almost as high by requiring 17.5 ten milligram doses per person in those years. The Army comes in last, averaging 13.8 doses per person per year. Fortunately purchases are going down, but they are still too high . . .When one considers that preinduction physicals weed out those who are not physically fit for Armed Services, these purchases of amphetamines . . . appear unnecessarily high.[13]

The Committee figures reveal that during four years, 1966 to 1969, the Army consumed more amphetamines than the entire British or American Armed Forces during World War II, and that the total official United States military issue of amphetamines during this brief period came to well over 225 million standard-dose tablets. (These were mostly dextroamphetamine —Dexedrine—which is almost twice as powerful on a milligram basis as the Benzedrine used before 1943.) The publicity about heroin and opium abuse by troops in Southeast Asia has obscured the more serious and widespread problem of amphetamine addiction in the Armed Services. Although the Army instituted a well-publicized (but only moderately effective) detection and detoxification program for soldiers addicted to heroin, it continued to ignore the amphetamine issue, and as late as 1973 was still supplying combat and "advisory" soldiers in Southeast Asia with this dangerous drug as standard equipment. Moreover, during the war amphetamine could be easily purchased over-the-counter without prescription in many Vietnamese towns and cities, and we know at least one American serviceman who re-enlisted for active duty in Vietnam only to continue obtaining this drug at no financial cost. In a September 16, 1971, letter to the editor of the *New England Journal of Medicine*, a physician stated in apparent seriousness that he and his associates were encouraged because they had found that many heroin-abusing Vietnam veterans "have neither required nor used heroin but have taken at least temporarily to the intravenous use of speed."[14]

Increased Use

Most of the country's fears about heroin would be better directed toward amphetamines. Since the end of World War II there has been a considerable rise in the per-capita consumption of legally obtained amphetamine pills, and until very recently public attitudes toward amphetamine abuse ranged from the humorous to the condescendingly tolerant, exemplified by the song "Who Put the Benzedrine in Mrs. Murphy's Ovaltine," popular in early 1946.

In recent years amphetamines have accounted for almost 5 percent of *all* drug prescriptions—including those for nonpsychopharmaceuticals like penicillin—and researchers in California recently reported that, especially among younger age groups, at least one out of every five adults who had taken some drug during the sample year admitted to use of amphetamines.[15] The Food and Drug Administration has no real power to limit the drug industry's advertising claims, and amphetamines continue to be prescribed by physicians for nearly as many different reasons as Bett mentioned in 1946. Only the medical jargon describing the alleged "diseases" has become more sophisticated. By 1958 the annual reported legal United States production of amphetamines was 75,000 pounds, or 3.5 billion tablets—enough to supply every man, woman, and child with about twenty standard (5-15 mg) doses. Less than ten years later, it had risen to over 100,000 pounds—about 8 billion amphetamine tablets—a year, or 25 to 50 pills per person. No one knows exactly how much amphetamine has been legally produced in the United States in the last forty years because many firms (especially small drug companies marketing only amphetamines or amphetamines and one or two other drugs) have refused to reveal production or sales statistics. By 1970, however, the reported legal amphetamine production had risen to over 10 billion tablets, and finally, in 1971, the Justice Department announced severe quotas on legal amphetamine production. Further cuts were continued into 1973. But even if the Justice Department is successful in cutting back amphetamine production to the pre-1958 level, it will still be many times the amount needed for legitimate medical purposes.[16]

The Black Market

One consequence of the overproduction of amphetamines is diversion to illegal traffic. Many published studies on amphetamine use rates ignore this widespread black market distribution system, which continues to thrive despite federal efforts to seal up massive leakages from pharmaceutical companies, wholesalers, druggists, and even doctors' offices. One source of this multimillion-dollar business was the all-night restaurants and gasoline stations catering to long-haul truck drivers, who discovered that amphetamines would allow them to drive for longer periods without rest and to make more trips per week. Some of the early slang names for amphetamines originated among these drivers, who called them "cartwheels," "coast-to-coasts," "West-coast turnarounds," "truck-drivers," and "copilots"—the last term allegedly derived from an accident which occurred because a driver fell asleep, thinking his "assistant," an amphetamine-induced hallucination, would drive.[17] The built-in "mobility" of this early illicit amphetamine distribution system was one of the main reasons for the extraordinary rapidity of its spread: in the middle 1960s it was estimated that the bulk of illicit supplies was being siphoned off from legal production to the black market at some point along the distribution network that ran from basic chemical suppliers to dosage manufacturers to wholesale distributors to retail pharmacists to physicians. One wholesale dealer ("short-line jobber") established his own private drug empire in 1962 by forging thousands of prescriptions and illegally marketing the following amounts of amphetamines: (1) 500,000 amphetamine tablets obtained from a small manufacturer in New Jersey; (2) over 2,000,000 dextroamphetamine pills from Mayrand, Inc., in North Carolina; (3) 3,000,000 amphetamine capsules from firms in Illinois and Pennsylvania; (4) more than 8,000,000 amphetamines from a large Detroit drug house. Not all "diversions" of amphetamines were inside jobs. Until at least 1965 practically anybody could obtain amphetamines by mail from wholesale drug mail-order houses. CBS exposed this situation in 1964, when it presented a report on news producer Jay McMullen's experiment. McMullen had rented an office and mailbox in mid-Manhattan, and set up a bogus "import-export" firm called McMullen Services. Simply by using this name as a letterhead on inexpensive stationery, he obtained from nine drug companies and suppliers more than a million amphetamine and barbiturate pills, tablets, and capsules worth up to half a million dollars on the black market. McMullen's total investment was $600.28.[18]

By the middle of the 1960s the need for controls had become so clear that a bill introduced by Senator Dodd of Connecticut to strengthen the Food and Drug Administration's power to regulate the distribution of amphetamines and barbiturates was near passage. There was wide support from state and federal agencies, and even the Pharmaceutical Manufacturers Association (PMA).

But organized medicine and the drug companies, which had previously refused Dodd access to production and sales records, began to oppose the bill openly. A letter from the American Medical Association complained that it would inhibit the legitimate use of amphetamines (not mentioning the danger to its own advertising revenues) and insisted that "in the United States, at this time, compulsive use of amphetamines and barbiturates constitutes such a small problem that additional legislation to control such abuse does not seem necessary." The PMA now said that any amphetamine abuse problem was due to " 'thrill uses' by those seeking anti-social effects," which could never result in a "compulsive desire"; therefore "the available evidence would indicate that the social abuse of both classes of drugs [amphetamines and barbiturates] is not related to any habituating qualities they might possess."[19] Further opposition came from the two largest organizations of druggists. All these groups used a well-known technique lobbyists use in attacking a reform movement when it has become difficult to deny the existence of an evil: they stalled for time, demanding more research, more convincing proof. Dodd's bill was defeated, but a similar one, effective February 1, 1966, was passed the next year. This law, the Drug Abuse Control Amendments of 1965, required increased record-keeping throughout the system of manufacture, distribution, prescription, and sale. But fines and punishments for violations were not severe, and nothing was done about reducing drug industry profits or eliminating the overproduction of amphetamines by setting quotas, or empowering the Food and Drug Administration to do more than "advise" on "acceptable therapeutic applications."

The controls instituted proved unenforceable and totally

ineffectual in stopping the flow of amphetamines to the black market. Criminal entrepreneurs simply refined their techniques. They discovered it was easy, because of an exemption in the law concerning exports, to have amphetamines shipped to real or imaginary drug houses and "repackagers" in foreign countries and then smuggle or mail them back across the border. According to the 1971 *Fourth Report of the Select Committee on Crime*, United States Customs had reported a 212 percent increase in *seizures* of contraband amphetamines during the previous two years. The Crime Committee reported, for example, that in 1969 Bates Laboratories, a small Chicago drug producer with annual sales of only $1.5 million, had mailed over 15 million amphetamine tablets to a post office box for a nonexistent drugstore in Tijuana, Mexico. On January 19, 1972, the *New York Times* reported that Strasenburgh Prescription Products, the largest United States exporter of amphetamines, had been ordered by the Bureau of Narcotics and Dangerous Drugs to show reason why its export license should not be revoked. "Operation Blackjack," as the Bureau's investigation was called, had revealed that in the previous eighteen months almost a ton of bulk amphetamine resin had been shipped to Strasenburgh's Mexican affiliate, where it was packaged in 25-mg Bifetamina capsules and sold to "drugstores" near the Texas border which were nothing but way-stations for smugglers. According to a spokesman for the Narcotics Bureau, although only one million of these pills had actually been seized, the number smuggled into the United States probably approached forty-five million per year. Strasenburgh's president first denied that his firm was exporting *any* amphetamines to Mexico, but eventually conceded that the charges were true.[20]

There has been widespread and open internal flouting of the legislative controls. In 1966 Abbott Laboratories sold the equivalent of two million doses of methamphetamine in powder form to a Long Island criminal dealer. During 1966 and 1967 two New York amphetamine wholesalers, Sherry-Blank Drug Company and Paramount Surgical Supply, sold about five million amphetamine units to Horn Drug Company in Georgia, without bothering to discover that Horn's license had been revoked in 1965 because of illegal amphetamine sales. In 1968 a South Carolina doctor was arrested after he had sold 32,000

amphetamine capsules to an undercover agent. The owner of a
large pharmacy in Kentucky was apprehended by federal agents
in 1969 for having sold large amounts of amphetamine products
to black-market middlemen and pushers in at least two southern
states. In 1970 a Tennessee grand jury indicted a Massengill
employee on charges of stealing 380,000 amphetamine tablets.
Black-market amphetamines are also obtained by using outdated
prescriptions intended for other persons, printing and forging
prescriptions, stealing prescriptions and supplies from doctors'
offices and hospitals, breaking into drugstores, "conning" whole
lists of doctors in a single day (some sort of record was recently
established by a persuasive young woman who talked seventy
different Manhattan physicians into writing prescriptions for a
total of over 3,500 amphetamines in just four days), and even
raiding veterinary and chicken-farm suppliers.[21] (Most commercial egg-laying chickens are kept awake and producing by
amphetamine; no one has investigated whether or how much of
the drug is passed on to the consumer.) The diversion of
amphetamines is conducted so skillfully, and on such a large
scale, that the illicit price paid is just about the same as that paid
for legally obtained drugs. Since each prescription for
amphetamines now requires a separate visit to a physician—often
costing $15 or more—it is frequently cheaper to buy
amphetamines from nonmedical sources.

Illegal Manufacture

If all legal amphetamine production lines were shut down the
black-market price might remain low, for these drugs are only a
little more difficult to manufacture than alcohol. Illicit
manufacture and sale of "home-cooked" speed seems to have
begun in California in the 1950s. Many servicemen stationed in
Korea mixed cocaine and heroin for intravenous injection; that
was called a "speedball." Then they discovered that
amphetamine was a good substitute for cocaine: it produced
longer-lasting effects and cut their costs in half. Injectible
amphetamine was usually available free from Army medics or
could be stolen from field hospitals; and amphetamine in pill
form, standard battle equipment, could be easily "melted down"
and injected. When returned veterans went to physicians in the
San Francisco Bay area for medical treatment of their mixed

addictions many received injectible amphetamines, because doctors were unaware of the consequences of amphetamine abuse; other physicians simply were willing to profit by writing prescriptions for the drug.[22]

Many persons who received huge amounts of pharmaceutical quality injectible amphetamines (usually Methedrine or Desoxyn) scraped off the identifying label numbers of the ampules, used half of the drug content, refilled the ampules with whatever diluents were available, and sold them on the black market. During the first half of 1962 one observer noted that "the Methedrine business had in three years' time developed into more than a million dollar business at the prevailing black-market prices."[23] The increasing traffic in this kind of illicit speed resulted in a 1963 request from the State Board of Pharmacy and from the California Attorney General's office that the commercial manufacturers of injectible amphetamines discontinue their sale of these ampules to retail pharmacies in California. When the manufacturers complied, clandestine laboratories for mass production of injectible amphetamines began to appear. (According to hippie folklore, the chemist who operated the first "speed kitchen" was the same Owsley who later became famous for the high quality of his distinctively marked LSD tablets.)[24] By 1968 there were between five and ten such laboratories in the Bay area, each supplying about twenty-five to one hundred pounds of illegally produced amphetamines in powder or solution each week. An unknown number of smaller "bathroom" or "kitchen" laboratories, most in Haight-Ashbury, contributed an equal amount. Meanwhile, "formulas" describing the steps from initial procural of the easily purchased amphetamine precursors to synthesis of the final products for injection were being hawked and given away in the Haight. One fifteen-year-old "cook" said she could manufacture speed with only "a vacuum, a big glass, a regular pan, and a heater," plus a hair dryer, amounting to a total investment of less than $20.[25]

Larger speed labs required the outlay of several thousand dollars for equipment before the initial chemicals were purchased and a distribution system established. Because of this expense and because of severe free enterprise competition from the much less expensive and more mobile home laboratories, most large operations received financial backing from "straight" investors y little to do with production, and the drugs passed hands of a few "straight" middlemen entrepreneur before being consigned or sold outright to nickel ($5 or ... ice or 875 mg) or dime ($10 or 1/16 ounce or 1750 mg) "bag" street dealers. The high-level distributor could sell many pounds of illicit speed, costing as little as $25 to $50 per pound to "cook," for a street retail value of as much as $4,000 weekly. Although the street dealers proclaimed that their product was "100% righteous pharmacy speed," it almost invariably contained more diluents than amphetamines. These included lactose, Epsom salts, quinine, baking powder, monosodium glutamate (Accent), photo developer, insecticides, ether—and even strychnine. Many speed freaks actually preferred certain impurities; amphetamine with added ether produced a "heavier flash" or more intense "rush" than pure methamphetamine, which causes a more gentle stimulating effect persisting for a longer time. Another reason "home-cooked" was often preferred to commercially available, legal amphetamine was that most speed freaks quickly developed tolerance to the euphoria-producing effects of the weak 1-percent solutions that could be purchased on prescription in most states (but not California). "Flash speed" in powder form could be dissolved in a very small amount of water, and the thick syrup injected in one gigantic dose.[26]

No one knows how many speed freaks there are in the United States today, because it is as difficult to obtain production and sales statistics from the illegal "kitchen" and "bathroom" laboratories as from the major pharmaceutical firms. A few studies have been conducted, however, and from these it is possible to make rough extrapolations to the national level. In 1964 John Griffith undertook a study of illicit amphetamine use in Oklahoma City (population 300,000). Through interviews with amphetamine peddlers, he arrived at the conservative estimate that 5,000 individual users obtained amphetamine and barbiturates through illegal channels. Use of the numerous commercial-quality amphetamines varied between 80 and 1,000 mg per day. In 1964 (as today), Oklahoma City was not a notorious drug abuse center, and the crime rate in the area was almost exactly at the national average, "so that one, with a degree of caution, might extrapolate results to be representative."[27]

Student Use

San Francisco's Haight-Ashbury was an extreme and conspicuous expression of the phenomenon of enormously increased use of amphetamine among young people in the past decade. Until the early 1960s most psychoactive drug abusers were in their mid-twenties to mid-forties, were socioeconomically deprived, had little education, and were often involved in criminal or semicriminial activities. Today most abusers are under twenty-five and have had the middle class advantages of education and freedom from economic insecurity. Few have criminal records, and many are actively engaged in intellectual and creative work. The typical pre-1960 drug abuser was a narcotics addict; today, he is much more likely to abuse amphetamines, barbiturates, methaqualone, and other legally obtainable drugs.[28]

In considering the use of amphetamines and other psychoactive drugs by students, it is essential to realize that the percentage using drugs varies tremendously from one institution to another. As Kenneth Keniston has pointed out, the widespread public impression of high rates of drug abuse among American college students derives in part from the greater visibility of those colleges where drug use is most common. His basic hypothesis is that the level of psychoactive drug use among college and university students can be correlated with the intellectual climate of the school. In schools where academic or intellectual excellence and personal freedom are stressed, drugs are used more frequently than in schools where social activities and sports absorb most student energies. Within any large college or university drug use is more common among students majoring in the intellectual, humanistic, or "introspective" fields; students of more practical, technical, or "extraverted" subjects like business, economics, engineering, law, and the applied sciences are less likely to take psychoactive drugs. Keniston even says there is some evidence that students who use drugs get higher grades than those who do not.[29]

Ordinarily it is impossible to vindicate or refute the kind of claim Keniston makes, but R. H. Blum and his associates at Stanford conducted a well-planned, carefully executed, and exhaustively analyzed study of student drug use which provides a unique opportunity to evaluate his suggestions—and goes considerably beyond them. The study was initiated in 1962, and most of the interviews and questionnaires were taken during the academic year 1966-1967 on five different Western campuses, by sympathetic interviewers who found the responses to be enthusiastic, open, and candid.

To some extent the Blum study confirmed Keniston's thesis about the relative extent of psychoactive drug use at various kinds of colleges as far as marihuana and hallucinogens are concerned. His guess that drug users tend to get higher grades, however, seems incorrect (see Table 1): Blum found no statistically significant correlations except in the case of alcohol, which is associated with lower grades. He also discovered, not surprisingly, that students who expressed dissatisfaction with their courses and teachers, who had dropped out of college for reasons not related to drugs, or who considered their formal higher education unrelated to the kind of life they wanted to lead were more likely to have used psychoactive drugs. "Idealistic innovators" or "revolutionaries" had a higher rate of drug use than others, but the differences were slight. Those students who had the greatest experience with drugs were least likely to belong to organized groups of any sort, on or off campus.[30] This suggests that the search for self-fulfillment or transcendence through drugs—"putting your head in a different place"—may in fact be

Table 1. Distribution of grade points.

(4 = A; 3 = B; 2 = C; 1 = D)		
	Grade points	
Drug	Non-users	Users
Tobacco	3.0	2.8
Alcohol	3.5	2.8
Amphetamines	2.7	2.8
Sedatives	2.8	2.85
Tranquilizers	2.8	3.0
Marijuana	2.8	2.75
Hallucinogens	2.8	2.9
Opiates	2.6	2.72
Special substances[a]	2.6	2.7

Source: R.H. Blum and Associates, *Drugs II: Students and Drugs* (San Francisco, 1970), p. 78, table 7.

[a]Special substances include materials like glue, gasoline, nitrous oxide (for sniffing), and cough syrups.

an alternative to trying to change the environment, the social institutions, or one's fellow man.

The most important finding of the Blum study may be that Keniston and other investigators concerned mainly with marihuana, "hallucinogens," and opiates have seriously underestimated (or ignored) the extent of amphetamine use at colleges of every socioeconomic composition and intellectual climate. At most schools, as Table 2 shows, reported amphetamine use exceeded the use of marihuana. Most "high-intensity" users (62 percent) had been introduced to amphetamines by physicians; medical sanction and an initial steady supply probably were major influences on the rate of use in this group. Of all users of amphetamines from all sources, only 8 percent reported any difficulty in obtaining the drug.

To follow up their study, the Blum group drew another sample of undergraduates from School I (see Table 2) in the late spring of 1968. It showed a substantial increase in those smoking marihuana (from 21 to 57 percent), using hallucinogens (from 6 to 17 percent), and ingesting and for the first time occasionally injecting amphetamines (from 25 to 35 percent). When the incidence of use of a psychoactive drug reaches half the population of a country, its people usually cease to regard it as "sick" or even deviant behavior, and the drug may cease to be thought of as a drug. That is what has happened with alcohol and nicotine in most countries, and now, as this 10 percent rise in a single year shows, may be about to happen with amphetamine in the United States.

A survey of Ithaca College made by representatives of its own faculty and student body in spring 1968 confirmed Blum's findings on California campuses. Marihuana and amphetamines, in that order, were the most popular of the drugs studied (tobacco and alcohol were not included). Fourteen percent of the males and 7 percent of the females admitted to use of amphetamines, and the actual percentage was probably higher, because 30 percent of the school's students did not respond to the questionnaire and because it was designed to exclude all legal, medically sanctioned consumption of drugs. In the student population at Ithaca there had been an increase from 59 to 133 admitted illegal amphetamine users during the fall of 1967 alone. A curious finding was that only 10 percent of the students thought that use of

Table 2. The extent of drug use at colleges.

Type of college	Used at least one drug	Amphetamines	Marihuana	Tranquilizers	Hallucinogens	Heroin (opiates)
		Drug use (percent of N)				
I. *Private university* Wealthiest families Social science, general, and undecided Largest percentage with no religious affiliation N = 300	60.4	25	21	18	6	1
II. *Catholic university* Middle-income families Social sciences, hard sciences and technical Catholic N = 270	38.3	11	11	11	2	1

III. *Private junior college* Youngest population Nonacademic, vocational N = 201	58.0	26	21	21	7	2
IV. *State college* Oldest sample Arts and humanities Large percentage Jewish and no religious affiliation N = 250	66.3	32	33	28	9	1
V. *State university* Small city in rural area Social sciences, hard sciences, and technical Protestant N = 293 (includes 75 graduate students)	42.5	13	10	19	2	1

Source: R.H. Blum and Associates, *Drugs II: Students and Drugs* (San Francisco, 1970), pp. 31–47, tables 2, 4.

amphetamines and barbiturates should be legalized.[31] This answer to an obviously ill-phrased question seems to mean that most of them wanted legal and medical controls made more stringent. At any rate, they did not have a high regard for amphetamines. Yet most who used amphetamine intended to continue, and by 1970 it had become clear that abuse of the drug was epidemic on many campuses (see Table 3).

A sign of the increasing cultural acceptability of amphetamines is their spread into high schools. Three studies, two in 1967 and one a year later, of San Francisco high schools, found up to 22 percent of the students admitting to the use of amphetamines.[32] Reports from the suburban Boston area show a continuation of these trends. Responding to a 1971 questionnaire, 48 percent of the high school seniors in Woburn, Massachusetts, admitted to illegal use of drugs, and amphetamines were among the most popular. A similar anonymous survey in Quincy found that, although they preferred marihuana, 16 percent of senior high school students had used amphetamines. A follow-up study revealed that 7 percent of the nonusers and 46 percent of the users had taken amphetamines for "medical" reasons in the previous year. A Brookline study produced similar results.[33]

Because of the suspicious attitude of many young people toward research on their use of drugs (partly produced by the absurd but menacing punitive campaign against marihuana), questionnaire surveys are not a reliable source of information. The kind of reaction that decreases their value is seen in this unsolicited comment written by a high school student on one of Blum's questionnaires: "This better not be a God Damned bust. P.S. If it is all my answers are bullshit. P.P.S. You should really show us the conclusions of this corny test."

Obviously our youth culture is drug-oriented to a degree not revealed by investigations. As early as 1967, sixteen of the forty most popular phonograph records contained a more or less open "positive drug message." Of the events of the summer of that year D. E. Smith wrote: "the mind reels at considering the millions influenced directly by friends who had been to the Haight, as well as by often inaccurate pictures represented in the media, and the publications and recordings emerging from the phenomenon. Because of the great turnover of persons directly involved in the Haight during the Summer of 1967, the period was the most

Table 3. Type of drug used by students.

Author, date of publication	Year of study, geographic area	Type of sample, size	Drug tried (percentage)				
			Marihuana	Halluci-nogens	Ampheta-mine	Tranquil-izers	Heroin
Sinnett, et al. 1971	1970 Midwest (Kansas State University)	College, most are drug users N = 33	91	85	73	24	15
Sinnett, Harvey unpublished	1971 Midwest (St. Louis)	Young drug abusers N = 21	100	90	81	43	43
Hinkle 1970	1970 Midwest (Topeka)	Young, most are drug users N = 73	90	79	52	–	14
Anker et al. 1971	– East	College, random sample N = 7030	24	4	11	–	0.4
Gallup Poll 1971	1970 National sample	College, random sample N = ?	42	14	16	–	–

Source: E. Robert Sinnett, K.S. Wampler, and W.M. Harvey, "The Consistency of Patterns of Drug Use (Kansas State University, 1971), table 1.

influential time of the evolution of drug use in America. It is considered by some to have been the most destructive."[34]

And amphetamines were possibly the most destructive of the drugs being abused. In summary, it is clear that medically sanctioned "pushing" in the general culture combined with a high valuation of chemically induced psychological "trips" of all kinds in the adolescent subculture has produced epidemic abuse of amphetamines among young people in the United States.

The following narrative by a young man who was introduced to amphetamine while a student at a small college in the early 1970s illustrates a typical widespread reliance upon the drug.

My experience with amphetamines began during my first year at college. I had gone to boarding school, and although there had been plenty of drugs there, mainly grass, tranquilizers, and psychedelics, almost no one I knew ever used speed for any reason. There was a real fear of getting involved with speed of any kind because of its reputation as a "killer" and because it was understood to be fairly addictive. My impression didn't change, but I soon realized that there were a lot less inhibitions at my new school about using amphetamines, especially if there was a good excuse for it, like a term paper due tomorrow. I was a little shocked to find out that the drug that I had always thought had only bad effects also had some good ones, at least for a hard-pressed student. The other freshmen I knew were reluctant to start using it at first also, but after being exposed to a heavy workload and the distracting countryside for a few months, academic integrity was abandoned in favor of just getting the work done. Speed not only made getting it done much easier; it also made subjects that were dry and boring under any other conditions seem very interesting and important. It turned out that there were other sides to speed than the manic speed rap and the extra physical energy, such as a longer and more intense attention span and the ability to stay up all night reading or typing. Gradually I saw more and more of my friends succumbing to the pattern that had already been established by the upperclassmen as they turned to a couple of tablets of dexedrine when it came down to the wire and they hadn't studied for a big test or they had to get an important paper done. Among the people I knew, it seemed that after a certain point of common understanding it was all right to do speed to get your work done, although there was still a lot of ambivalence about it, and people weren't as willing to take dexedrine or any other amphetamine for any reason as they were to smoke grass or even to trip. Peer group pressure affected people's attitudes toward speed as much as it did with any other drug I've seen people use, which is a very great deal.

By the end of my freshman year, I had been exposed to speed long enough to have lost most of my fear of it. I realized that using amphetamines made for supposedly valid purposes by big companies wasn't going to turn me into a raving speed freak if I used them every so often, and I never even had to see a needle. Taking pills is something I've done all my life for reasons that were always justified in terms of improving my health or well-being, so taking a pill that was speed and not a vitamin was fairly easy to adjust to. And anyway, by that time curiosity had gotten the better of me, and I wanted to know what speed was like more than I was scared by what I had seen it do to people, which wasn't very much, especially compared to what I had expected. After the first experience I had no trouble in feeling the effects of the drug or in adjusting to its use.

I'll describe now as well as I can the effects which the use of speed has had on me, both good and bad (in my own terms of of good and bad). As I said before, I was very glad to discover amphetamines because they provided a new kind of change in mood for me, one that seemed more practical and enjoyable than what other drugs, including alcohol, had provided. Speed has never failed to produce generally the same kind and quality of feeling, one which by its own definition is not dull or boring. That can be nice when school and academic routine becomes very, very repetitive. I'm not making excuses or criticisms, just saying why I did what I did. I get bored pretty easily if I don't have new things to do, and I think of speed now as a kind of vicarious excitement. I found that I would be interested and aroused by things which I had grown very tired of at school, both socially and academically. Speed makes the most routine task, function, or conversation take on a different and more tolerable light. I can talk to people when speeding that I would normally walk past without a word, and this interest in people does not seem at the time to be objective or analytical, rather I really feel involved and sympathetic toward people I usually don't even consider. That feeling alone is enough to justify using speed every now and then, if only to learn something about someone else, or more specifically, to enjoy an encounter that would be a drag any other time. I don't find myself speed rapping to any great extent, or dominating conversations, but I can think of more to say to people that will get them to respond in return. That suggests another important quality about speed that I appreciate—the fact that I can control its outward effects to whatever degree I want. If for some reason it made me talk incessantly without any control, I would probably hate it and not use it. There is also, of course, the added physical energy that results from the artificially induced high and interest and curiosity about things, which allows me to go farther with less motivation than I would usually go. I will make myself find something to do, instead of taking a nap as I would probably do otherwise. And if I don't find anything great to do, I can be more satisfied with what I find than I would be normally. Almost anything, no matter how routine, can be made to seem like a valid activity under amphetamines. The physical and and mental changes seem to be basically the same in terms of impressions and sensations. There is a feeling of warmth, especially in the beginning, that corresponds to a mental impression of well-being, awareness, and interest in the surroundings. My eyes always water at the very beginning for some reason. There is more mental and physical energy, an excess of it in fact, but it doesn't compel you to use it; it's just there if it's needed. A dull activity can be maintained for hours under speed and never seems to be boring. Driving, reading, almost anything becomes, if not enjoyable, at least much more bearable. I feel like I know much more than I could possibly really know about anything in general, although I have no specific idea what that knowledge is about.

I usually wait until I have an excuse to use it, such as a lot of work before I'll use speed. I don't know if that's what most other people feel about it, but I suspect it might be. I don't like to use speed just for fun, usually, because I guess I'm afraid of depending on it too much to keep myself going, instead of using my own initiative, especially at school. Of course, there's another very important negative factor about speed that comes whenever you use it, and that's the crash. Coming off speed, or crashing, is one of the most uncomfortable, if not painful things I've ever gone through. It hasn't been too bad when I only take one dose, but if I continue to speed by taking more pills when the first wears off, when I finally do stop, it causes an intense crash that makes my body feel terrible and is emotionally trying. The crash can last several hours itself, and by that time I usually regret ever taking the speed at all and promise myself never to do it again.

I don't even really know how bad crashing can become, because I've never speeded continuously for long periods of time. People I know that have, go through incredibly bad feelings coming off the drug after a long period of use. The time involved would probably average two days or so. The worst case of crashing that I knew of was a female friend of mine who would speed for long periods and go without sleep several nights in a row. When she finally crashed, she became almost impossible to be around, because her mood would become so bad. She would complain of her teeth hurting, and of losing the feeling in her scalp. She crashed for quite a while after long speed runs and would be totally miserable. The feeling of insanity, even in my case, never seemed very far away. Only a little more intensity, a little more pain, would seem to separate me from losing control over myself. Luckily no one I know ever got really sick, or went crazy. That's probably because they never were speeding for a really long time, and also because most of the amphetamines available at school were of the fairly mild type.

I'll describe the ways I know of to get speed. There aren't that many, at least that I know, at school. It usually comes from sons or daughters of doctors or pharmacists who either sell it directly or to other people who then do the selling. The price was generally twenty-five cents for each pill until it recently went up to fifty because of stricter federal laws. People also may have genuine prescriptions for the drugs and take full advantage of it, selling the prescribed pills instead of using them. Lots of family physicians will oblige if a kid makes a convincing enough case of needing speed. I once went with a friend to his father's drugstore, where we took handfuls of Dex-Amo to use at school. When we got back, it was almost impossible to hold onto, so many people were asking us for some. That will happen to anyone when people find out he has a quantity of speed, and when the campus gets low on speed, rumors will spread far and wide about who has any, no matter how little. Beyond a certain point, though, you have to be someone's friend to ask him for speed if he only has a little left because everyone knows how valuable it is.

People I know don't like to get involved in taking speed for long periods of time or in depending on it to be able to function. For that reason, most people at college, at least, don't use speed indiscriminately. They'll wait until what seems to them to be an emergency comes up; or course, an emergency can be seen in lots of different situations. Usually the excuse would be a need for fast energy to carry out some task that would be impossible otherwise, like a long drive or a long paper. I don't know if kids would let their work go for a long time just to get the chance to speed for a couple of days, but sometimes it did seem that way. And really, I know that I have been a lot more casual about some projects, knowing that if I didn't get them done, I could always speed to do it. When I decided that was possible, it was usually what I would do when it came down to the time the work was due.

Patterns of speed use at my school followed almost exactly the grading periods that were used. Whenever a grade has to be reported to the registrar and to parents, there is a rapid increase in work that makes a big difference in a person's grade, which just naturally causes an increase in the consumption of various kinds of speed on campus. There seems to be a simultaneous shirking of responsibility by everyone involved at times like that—professors pass their grading responsibility on to the students, who pass it on to speed because they can't stand being the last link in the chain of authority. Personally I sympathize with the student's point of view, and I suppose I've proved it by my use of speed to do my work. But really it seems to me that if the work was worth doing, it wouldn't be necessary to use artificial stimulants to complete it. My major complaint is turning class work into a commodity that must be produced by a certain time to be valid. The only way to do that kind of assignment is by artificially induced means, because in all honesty, any personal involvement in it is false and created in a vacuum. I don't want to get very abstract about educational philosophy, really, but I want to tell you what one of my friends once said about speed. He said something like, "I'd like to see most of the people in this college tell their parents at graduation, 'Gee, Mom and Dad, I want you to know I owe my diploma and all my academic success to amphetamines.' " That's probably an exaggeration, but not by much. At crucial times almost anyone would resort to speed, from the best to the worst student. The only difference seemed to be that the good student would actually study while speeding, and the others would "waste" it by running around all night and having a good time. Generally, I'm sure I could say that at my school, users of speed from light to heavy add up to 50 or 60 percent of the students. At any rate, there are no more than thirty percent whom I would believe if they told me they never used speed for any reason. I've known people to speed whom I know would never be seen using grass or acid. Speed at least is "respectable," that is, if you're speeding everyone can assume that you're trying to do your work, instead of just screwing around like you would be if stoned on grass.

My dominant impression is that speed use at colleges, if other schools are anything like mine, is very prevalent, maybe only second to alcohol in popularity. It's thriving on the biggest weakness that academic life has as far as I'm concerned, which is apathy and detachment from reality, however you want to define that word. To feel something, anything rather than the boredom and uninvolvement they feel in relation to school and their work, students use energizing drugs that at least make things seem interesting for as long as they last. I really think it's true that a lot of academic careers, and not just those of dull people, are based on a dependence upon amphetamines. Actually, it's probably the brightest people that I know who find speed most useful, and at times necessary. I don't even see any irony in that anymore. Speed just represents a way of life that I can choose, or not, depending on how desperate I am.

2

Development and Pharmacology

"Any consideration of the pharmacology of the amphetamines which also takes into account the crucial sociological factors and historical antecedents of our current speed problem leads to the somber conclusion that dedicated, hard-working, generous, and kind Gordon A. Alles and his fellow workers unintentionally 'unleashed a Frankensteinian-type monster over which we seemingly have no control.'"

As toxicology preceded pharmacology, drug abuse antedated drug therapy. Primitive man seems to have been more interested in poisons than medicines; even Hippocrates, although he recommended natural salicylates from poplar and willow trees for eye disease and childbirth, considered most drugs useless. (Though when the Greeks wished to dispose of Socrates, they had a most effective herb.) In the case of amphetamine, the historical development has run the other way: pharmacology is reverting to toxicology. In its application to the treatment of a tremendous variety of organic and psychological illnesses, a substance originally synthesized as an inexpensive substitute for ephedrine has become the source of an international drug abuse catastrophe.

Ephedrine, a natural drug obtained from the herb *Ma Huang* (*Ephedra vulgaris*), had been used by Chinese physicians for more than 5,000 years. The (possibly mythical) emperor Shen Nung (2737 B.C.) is supposed to have placed this herb in the medium class of his pharmacopoeia. The Chinese Dispensatory (*Pentsao Kang Mu*), written in 1569 by Shih-Cheng Li, recommended it to lower fever, induce perspiration, and stop coughing. The plant was also used in Russia for respiratory disease and rheumatism and among Indians and Spaniards in the southwestern United States for various ailments including venereal disease.[1]

Ephedrine, the active principle, was isolated in the 1880s but not used until 1924, when K. K. Chen and C. F. Schmidt began to publish the results of their experiments. They pointed out that ephedrine bore a close structural resemblance to epinephrine (adrenaline), the hormone produced by the medulla of the adrenal gland, which had been isolated in 1904 independently by F. Stolz in Germany and H. D. Dakin in England. Because epinephrine dilated the bronchi and was a strong respiratory stimulant, it seemed to hold some promise for the symptomatic treatment of acute asthma attacks. However, it had several serious drawbacks. First, its respiratory stimulating action was transitory, and its administration often resulted in a brief but distinctly unpleasant total inhibition of breathing (apnea). Second, it was unstable, decomposing rapidly on exposure to air, light, or an alkaline solution. Third, the inhaler device had not yet been perfected, and since epinephrine was inactive when taken in pill form, it had to be injected. Fourth, its actions on the human system were not at all specific: it increased cardiac output, systolic blood pressure, and both lactic acid and glucose blood levels, in addition to stimulating respiration. Furthermore, it could cause undesirable reactions ranging from anxiety and dizziness to death by cerebral hemorrhage or cardiac arrhythmia. Chen and Schmidt found ephedrine to be superior to epinephrine because it could be taken in pill form, had a much longer duration of action, produced more pronounced and dependable central effects, and was much less toxic.[2] As a result of this and subsequent research, the medical use of ephedrine increased at such a high rate that it was feared the natural supplies would be exhausted. So the search for an ephedrine substitute began.

Meanwhile, phenylisopropylamine, the volatile base of what became known more than four decades later as Benzedrine, had been synthesized in 1887 by L. Edeleano. He failed to explore its pharmacological properties, and it was not until 1910 that G. Barger and Sir H. H. Dale made the first investigation of the effects on experimental animals of this and a series of related chemical compounds they called "sympathomimetic amines."[3] This descriptive label applies to many other drugs besides those generally referred to as the amphetamines; they are called "sympathomimetic" because their pharmacological actions "mimic" the effects of activation of the "sympathetic" part of the autonomic nervous system. This general subsystem of the nervous system exerts a regulatory effect over most of the involuntary organs of the body—the glands, lungs, heart, liver, and blood vessels—as well as most of the involuntary muscles connected with or controlling the size or rate of activity of these organs. Amine refers to any of a large group of molecules which are derivatives of ammonia (NH-3). The amine component is but one (perhaps the most important) of four distinct molecular components of the basic skeleton of all sympathomimetic substances, naturally occurring or synthetic. All of these four structural moieties are easily manipulated in the laboratory, and even a minor alteration in any one group may result in a drug with significantly different effects.

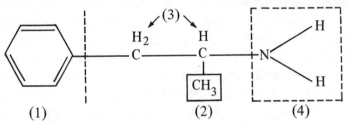

Figure 1   The basic amphetamine skeleton.

Figure 1 represents the basic amphetamine skeleton. Numbers in parentheses indicate the structural moieties critical to amphetamine activity: (1) an unsubstituted phenyl ring; (2) the alpha-methyl group, attached to the alpha carbon; (3) the 2-carbon side chain between the phenyl and amino radicals; (4) the primary amino group. The beta-phenylethylamine arrangement is essential to most of amphetamine's pharmacological and biochemical properties, particularly to its power of releasing norepinephrine from neuronal storage sites and blocking membranal norepinephrine uptake. Substitution of the phenyl ring will eliminate or radically alter its central effects. The alpha-methyl group (2) is also necessary for the effects on norepinephrine; in addition it protects amphetamine from monoamine oxidase (MAO) and confers mild to moderate monoamine oxidase inhibitory (MAOI) activity on the compound. Progressive methylation of either the side chain or the amino group systematically decreases the characteristic actions of amphetamine. Moving the alpha-methyl group to the beta-position eliminates almost all of the central and anorectic effects of the drug.[4]

Although today Barger and Dale's monograph is recognized as a thorough pioneering report on those sympathomimetic amines which are the basic building blocks of all amphetamines, for seventeen years no one in the United States or Britain grasped the implications of their findings. After all, they were comparing the relative potencies of a number of still obscure chemicals with confusingly similar and difficult names and formulas, and mainly describing the effects of these drugs on the peripheral circulation and respiration of decerebrated cats. Although they did suggest that some of these drugs might possess powerful central nervous system (CNS) stimulating properties, the only point that interested the few readers who digested their highly technical paper was that most of these "sympathomimetic amines" had essentially the same "alerting" effects on the *physiological* system of cats (and presumably humans) as epinephrine.

The concept of completely *synthetic* medicines was embryonic in 1910. As Goethe observed, in medicines, as in all art, literature, philosophy, and science, any innovative idea or theory must be compatible with the Zeitgeist, the "current common sense" or "contemporary cultural mentality" of a historical period; otherwise it is rejected out of hand as naive, ridiculous, or irrelevant. This Zeitgeist encompasses all the conventions, technological limitations, and fundamental unexamined assumptions that effectually distinguish between what is and what is not regarded as a discovery or breakthrough. New conceptual frameworks usually follow rather than precede basic innovations; the crucial point is that these frameworks are created from trends and forces originating outside the "systems" or "arenas" which they characterize or delimit.[5]

By the late 1920s the medical Zeitgeist had changed radically. George Piness, head of a research laboratory in Los Angeles, who knew of Edeleano's discovery and Barger and Dale's monograph, suggested that Gordon Alles, one his young research chemists, look for a synthetic amine substitute for ephedrine. Alles concluded in 1927 that the easiest to make, least expensive, and most effective substitute was the original amphetamine synthesized by Edeleano in 1887. Experimenting on himself as well as laboratory animals, he quickly discovered that amphetamine was active whether inhaled or taken orally and that Benzedrine (racemic or dextro-levo-amphetamine) was surpassed by its dextro (right-handed) isomer (eventually marketed as Dexedrine) in power to alleviate fatigue and create euphoric confidence and alertness.[6]

The common occurrence of a major scientific breakthrough by several independent researchers at about the same time is illustrated by the case of amphetamine as well as that of epinephrine. A year before Alles' initial results were published, two Princeton University pharmacologists reported that they had synthesized dextroamphetamine, although there is some doubt whether their product was pure. Eight years before Alles began his work, a Japanese pharmacologist, A. Ogata, had synthesized an amphetamine compound which he called d-phenylisopropyl-methylamine hydrochloride or d-desoxyephedrine hydrochloride, and which more recently gained considerable notoriety under its simpler, nonproprietary name methamphetamine. (In 1968 the Burroughs Wellcome Company, manufacturer of "Methedrine," discontinued its United States production of what is still one of the most popular names for methamphetamine—especially among users and abusers who abbreviate it to "Meth.") A few years later a German pharmacologist, H. Emde, elucidated the chemical structure of ephedrine by experimenting with rearrangements of Ogata's original compound, and demonstrated that ephedrine itself could be simply and inexpensively synthesized.[7] Thus, ironically, by the time Alles established that amphetamine was an effective ephedrine substitute, there was no longer any need for one. But by 1932 it had become apparent that these new synthetic sympathomimetic amines, although they produced many of the same peripheral effects as ephedrine and epinephrine (such as elevation of blood pressure and pulse rate, a slight relaxation of bronchial and sometimes intestinal muscles, and an excitation of other smooth muscles and certain sweat and salivary glands), were much more potent as central nervous system stimulants. This unique property has become the psychopharmacological criterion for distinguishing between drugs generally referred to as amphetatmines (or amphetamine "congeners" and "derivatives") and other sympathomimetic amines. Dextroamphetamine is about twice as potent a central nervous system stimulant as Benzedrine (dextro-levo-amphetamine or dl-amphetamine), and methamphetamine is intermediate in this respect.* On the other hand, methamphetamine and, to a lesser degree, dextroamphetamine (d-amphetamine) exert fewer peripheral effects than Benzedrine.

---

*The dextro isomer is three to four times as potent as the levo isomer in eliciting excitation of the central nervous system, whereas the *l* isomer is slightly more potent than the *d* isomer in its cardiovascular stimulating (or at times paradoxically slowing) actions.

A Medicine Is Born

Shortly after Alles' experiments were reported, F. P. Nabenhauer, chief chemist at the Smith, Kline & French laboratories, made the discoveries that led to the production of the Benzedrine inhaling device, and Alles transferred his patents to that drug manufacturer. The company convinced the medical establishment that amphetamine was a truly unique drug with potential therapeutic applications extending far beyond the uses for an ephedrine substitute, and the Council on Pharmacy and Chemistry of the American Medical Association approved Benzedrine in pill form on December 18, 1937. The AMA Council recognized amphetamine tablets as effective in the treatment of narcolepsy (a rare disease characterized by "dream-sleep attacks" of short duration) and also postencephalitic Parkinsonism. It stated further that Benzedrine was "useful" in the treatment of "certain depressive psychopathic conditions," but that only persons "under the strict supervision of a physician" should take amphetamine in order to capture "a sense of increased energy or capacity for work, or a feeling of exhilaration."[8] The five articles in the medical literature referred to as justifications for the sanctioning of amphetamine as a "pick-me-up" (the AMA's phrase) involved fewer than 150 experimental subjects. Only one of the five studies was well-controlled, with some attempt to compare an amphetamine-treated with a (much smaller) placebo-administered group; the other reports were anecdotal and highly subjective, and the authors of all five denied or ignored the possibility of adverse effects. If these articles were submitted to the *Journal of the American Medical Association* today, it is hard to believe that they would be accepted for publication or that, if they were, they would be officially cited as "evidence" for the safety or efficacy of a relatively unknown drug in the treatment of narcolepsy, Parkinsonism, and depression.[9]

By 1943, over half of Smith, Kline & French's Benzedrine sales went to fill prescriptions written for people who wanted to lose weight, obtain a temporary "lift," or stay awake for extended periods. Benzedrine had also become popular in the treatment of alcoholics, and it was the only antidepressant available to psychiatrists. Few users fully appreciated its cardiovascular and other sympathomimetic adverse "side effects," though executives at Smith, Kline & French undoubtedly were aware of these dangers. The manufacturers also probably knew that, although dextroamphetamine was twice as powerful a euphoriant as Benzedrine on a milligram basis, it was less physically toxic in any immediately obvious way. Smith, Kline & French may have feared that other firms might contest its legal right to market the dextro isomer solely on the basis of its Benzedrine patent and recognized the possibility that a foreign drug company might introduce Americans to either dextroamphetamine or methamphetamine, which had appeared on the British market in 1940. Accordingly, the "new" dextro isomer of Benzedrine was patented and marketed as Dexedrine.

Racemic amphetamine (Amphate, Bar-Dex, Benzedrine, Dietamine, Monophos, Nobese, Profetamine, Racephen, Raphetamine and so forth) and dextroamphetamine (sold under more than forty-four brand names) remain the most frequently prescribed amphetamines, but today there are at least twenty other closely related drugs in over one hundred brand-name preparations on American pharmacy shelves. Many represent very minor structural and pharmacological variations. For example, although methamphetamine hydrochloride is marketed under more than thirty different brand names, a few drug companies also offer the same basic drug as the dextro isomer (Fetamin and Span-RD) or the saccharate (Amphaplex and Obetrol). Dextroamphetamine is sometimes made available as the hyrdrochloride (Amodex), the tannate (Synatan), or the di-basic phosphate (Phetobose) instead of the more usual sulfate. Levoamphetamine sulfate (Ad-Nil) is merely the levo isomer of Benzedrine, and both Amodril and Cydril are the closely related succinate of levoamphetamine.

Drug Combinations

In attempting to produce an "ideal" anorectic (appetite-inhibiting) preparation, the drug industry has also exploited the need to counteract the anxiety-producing and irritability-provoking effects of unadulterated amphetamine products. Firms have marketed many compounds containing sometimes highly addictive barbiturates (such as amobarbital, butabarbital, pentobarbital, and phenobarbital) and "minor" tranquilizers (mainly meprobamate, whose best-known brand names are Miltown and Equanil). They have been, at least in terms of sales, extraordinarily successful. Dieting housewives and others to whom these compounds have been prescribed have discovered that they, and many other combinations of depressants and amphetamines ingested simultaneously, create a "synergistic" $(1+1=3)$ effect; they feel both more euphoric (amphetamine effect) and more relaxed (depressant drug effect) than they would if they took either drug by itself. In this way hundreds of thousands of Americans have drifted into dual dependencies that sometimes become addictions.

In 1962 two British physicians conducted a controlled, double-blind* experiment in which 300 mg of a barbiturate, 15 mg of amphetamine sulphate (Benzedrine), these two drugs combined, and identical "dummy" lactose placebo tablets were administered to four groups of medical students. The mixture of the barbiturate and the amphetamine was significantly more potent in eliciting euphoria, elation, and excitation than either of the two active drugs taken singly. The combination tablets also led to fewer reports of "haziness," "jitteriness," or unpleasant "autonomic effects," as well as a marked diminution in loss of skills measured by simple mental and motor performance tests, as compared with either amphetamine or cyclobarbitone.[10] Numerous other studies have demonstrated that nearly all sedatives, tranquilizers, and depressant drugs potentiate the stimulating mental, psychological and even physiological effects of amphetamines in this little-understood synergistic reaction and simultaneously reduce amphetamine-induced nervousness, anxiety, and tension.[11] A teenage male oral amphetamine abuser recounted his own discovery of this phenomenon:

> I was usin' during the day twenty, twenty-five [Benzedrine or Dexedrine 5-mg tablets]. It's not like uh—I think that you have

---

*Because drug testing is a situation of human interaction in which participants are affected by their knowledge of and attitudes about what is occurring, double-blind technique was devised. This procedure, rarely employed until thirty years ago, tries to insure that neither the administrators of the drugs nor the recipients know who is receiving active substance(s) and who is receiving inert placebo(s). It is difficult to maintain complete double-blindness: administering personnel may be tempted to peek at the code prematurely; patients usually know that the chance that they have been given a particular type of psychoactive drug is at least 50-50; and often attending nurses or staff technicians who recognize the "side-effects" of drugs suggest their nature to recipients by chance remarks or even facial expressions.

to use more of these things to stay high than any kind of drug except for maybe heroin, I don't know you take in ten and maybe three hours later you need another ten, y'know? And you start losin' weight 'cause you're not- eatin'. I've lost fifteen pounds in a week—from takin' these things y'know? And then I found a better way like, uh—you can get high, the same kind of high if you take maybe six Benzedrine and one and a half cibas which is Doridens [the trade name for glutethimide, described by the manufacturer as a "rapid-acting sedative" indicated in the treatment of insomnia and for day-time and preoperative sedation] y'know? And that's uh—it gives you a high almost like Benzedrine—like takin' Benzedrine, y'know, it's an "up" high. But uh—

SF [interviewer]: How did you learn this?

John: Well, see, after a while on a say you take, you wake up and you take Dexedrine after a couple of hours you get this feelin' like ya can't sit down, you can't stand up, y'know, like you sit down, you want to stand up—it's like an indecision thing—you don't know what you want to do. Say you might be thinking what you want to do that night or somepin and you think "Oh," uh. "I think I want to go to a dance," and then you think about that for a couple of seconds and then you say, "Naw, naw, that's no good," and then you think that you want to go to the movies and it seems great for a second, a good idea and then you think, about it for a second and say, "Aw, that stinks too." So then I would say, "Oh—this high is killing me," y'know and so a friend of mine told me to get rid of it, y'know, this feelin', ya take these cibas and that takes it away. So I took two cibas and then it took away that high that indecision feelin' and then it just brought back a nice high again. Like y'know, talkin' and feelin' nice and walkin' aroun', and all . . . And uh—I thought I would jus' try it that way by maybe takin' six or seven Benzedrine and one of these things y'know. And it worked—so instead—I cut myself down on Benzedrine from about thirty a day to about ten a day with two of these cibas. [12]

This kind of drug mixing has never been confined to addicts or other obviously delinquent or deviant types. Huge numbers of Americans have exercised the power to manipulate their affective and cognitive states in what they consider desirable directions, "balancing" amphetamines against tranquilizers, sleeping pills, barbiturates, and liquor. Perhaps the most dubious "advance" on the part of the pharmaceutical industry in this area of "up-down" preparations has been the introduction of prolonged action compounds. In this category belong the "spansules," "extentabs," "gradumet tablets," "Strasionic exchange" capsules, and pills with other catchy trademark (copyrighted) names. Most contain amphetamines and the more addictive varieties of depressant drug (especially barbiturates and meprobamate). The slow-release effect greatly increases the already high danger of addiction to both ingredient drugs, as well as the risk of sometimes irreversible physiological and psychological damage. Laboratory investigations using experimental animals have established that lasting adverse drug reactions, including addiction, are difficult to produce if medications are administered only once a day. To experience the full addictive impact of psychoactive drugs, one must ordinarily take them several times a day; otherwise the organism is able to recover from the relatively brief period of intoxication. But the prolonged action preparations produce persisting (up to fourteen hours after a single capsule in some cases, according to one manufacturer's advertisements) amphetamine (or barbiturate) effects, so that people who think they are being cautious because they take only one (or two) amphetamine "spansules" every morning are being deceived—or deceiving themselves.

Derivatives

Besides these obvious amphetamine congeners there is a vast reservoir of other amphetamine derivatives. Two of these, methylphenidate (Ritalin and Ritonic) and pipradol (Alertonic), have been extensively promoted, and drug houses have misled doctors and the public about their close pharmacological relation to amphetamine in their advertising and prescribing information. Ritalin until recently was described by Ciba as "mild stimulant and antidepressant, which brightens mood and improves performance, usually without producing hyperexcitability or depressive rebound."[13] Medical journal advertisements have suggested more specifically that these stimulants are "non-amphetamines," because they supposedly do not cause any decrease in appetite, and (it is still claimed) tolerance does not develop. But no controlled laboratory or clinical experiments have yet been conducted to prove these claims. As a matter of fact, Swedish experience with Ritalin shows that it is highly addictive and strongly toxic, and suggests that it is anorectic at sufficiently high doses. The Swedes have also demonstrated that pipradol has the same high abuse potential as other amphetamines. Although it is not as powerful a CNS stimulant as other amphetamines on a milligram basis, the spectrum of its actions and properties is almost the same, as could have been predicted from its chemical structure.[14]

At least nine other closely related compounds have been found to produce many of the stimulating and euphorigenic effects of the amphetamines: reactivan, prolintane, thozlinone, cypenamine, zylofuramine, Mg-pemoline, Sch-5472, Al-1095, and 84 F/1983. These represent only a tiny fraction of one set of possible rearrangements of basic amphetamine and from the names it appears that at least three of them are still new, and very likely the objects of intensive research. The drug industry may well turn to these if the federal government continues to move toward the imposition of strict quotas on legal amphetamine production in what appears to be a trend toward outright prohibition. According to J. H. Biel, methylphenidate, pipradol, and the other nine closely related drugs now stockpiled in drug houses were directly derived from amphetamine by forcing the "free-swinging" aminoalkyl side chain into a heterocyclic ring system, while preserving the basic beta-phenethylamine skeleton.[15]

On the other hand, one cannot always be sure that a compound will exhibit the typical amphetaminelike stimulating properties even if its chemical structure is closely related to that of basic amphetamine. As Figure 2 reveals, phenylpropanolamine is almost exactly the same chemical compound as amphetamine.

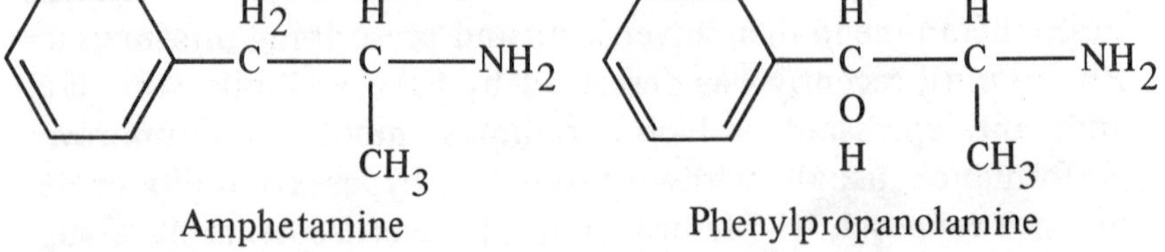

Amphetamine   Phenylpropanolamine

Figure 2.

The only difference is that phenylpropanolamine has an OH group substituted for an H at the beta carbon of the side chain between the phenyl ring and the primary amino group. This seemingly insignificant structural difference completely deprives phenylpropanolamine of any central nervous system stimulating effects. Although it is available (as Odrinex) from at least one company (Fox Pharmaceuticals) as an over-the-counter non-prescription "reducing tablet," several groups of researchers, in particular one led by J. F. Fazekas, have demonstrated that it has no more effect on appetite than a placebo.[16] Other drugs like cocaine that have chemical structures quite unlike the basic amphetamine skeleton are in fact potent central nervous system stimulants.

In short, mere inspection or superficial analysis of structure is a poor method for predicting amphetaminelike properties, although a compound with the amphetamine skeleton is *likely* to exert some of the same effects as the generally recognized amphetamines. This lack of any definitive structural criteria has caused a tremendous amount of confusion, and manufacturers have often taken advantage of this confusion to make claims for the safety and efficacy of their "nonamphetamine" compounds that are close to blatant lies. Drug companies probably will continue to produce increasingly sophisticated and disguised amphetamines, and these "new" drugs undoubtedly will be greeted with initial enthusiasm by the medical establishment until it is recognized that any drug with amphetaminelike CNS stimulating properties almost invariably is just as toxic, potentially addictive, and therapeutically limited as Benzedrine or Dexedrine.

Psychedelic Amphetamines

In 1962 T. C. McCormick observed that "no other group of drugs can affect or change personality traits to a greater degree than the amphetamines."[17] This was written before LSD was known outside a few research centers and about two years before it became available on the street and college campuses. Until 1967 most knowledgeable pharmacologists, physicians, and drug users might have expanded his claim to include LSD, but in the last six years a whole new spectrum of psychedelic amphetamines has re-established the validity of McCormick's statement. Most amphetamines, including the most commonly used varieties, may produce hallucinations at sufficiently high dosage, but there are two basic groups whose main interest lies in their hallucinogenic or psychedelic properties.

Clinically speaking, an hallucination is a perception, or, more accurately, an *apparent* perception, of an object, person, place, or even memory, which has no analogue, no causative equivalent, no source, in the external, "real" world that we all must assume we share and must believe is revealed to us through our perceptions. A *true* hallucination is completely spontaneous: there is no discoverable relation between anything in the immediate or recent environment and what is "seen." A person with a perceptual disorder may experience a true visual, auditory, or even tactile hallucination; but in nearly all reports of drug-induced "hallucinations" there has been a stimulus of some sort as the basis, the starting point, the primer, or the material. Similarly, the term "psychotomimetic," popular in scientific and medical reports for a few years, was first employed because some researchers thought that the drugs so distinguished actually "mimicked" psychoses. However, it is now clear that there are important differences between clinical cases of endogenous psychosis and states induced by drugs. "Psychedelic" has been used because it carries no connotations of mental illness; other terms include "psychodysleptics," "pseudohallucinogens," "illusinogens," "mysticomimetics," "phantasticants," "psychoticants," "schizogens," and "psychotomystics." "Hallucinogen" will probably continue to be used most frequently to denote chemicals that induce conditions approximating true hallucinations.

Chemically the two groups of amphetamine derivatives with hallucinogenic properties are designated as (A) methoxyamphetamines and (B) methoxymethylenedioxyamphetamines. The (A) group is derived from basic amphetamine by the addition of various combinations of H and OCH-3 moieties to the benzene ring of the simple amphetamine skeleton; the (B) group are basic amphetamine derivatives with a second ring (the so-called "five-member heterocyclic ring") attached to the skeletal benzene ring. The pharmacological basis for the hallucinatory properties of these psychedelic amphetamine derivatives remains a matter of dispute. J. H. Biel points out that the progressive methoxylation of the skeletal benzene (phenyl) ring apparently destroys the capacity of amphetamines to inhibit neuronal reuptake of norepinephrine or to release it from its "binding sites" in brain cells. "Thus, unlike [basic] amphetamine, these drugs presumably exert their characteristic effects by direct receptor interaction rather than through an intermediate neurotransmitter."[18] On the other hand, A. T. Shulgin has suggested a different hypothesis based on:

> observations that dopamine can be hydroxylated in the 6-position in certain *in vivo* experiments. This results in 2,4,5-trihydroxyphenethylamine which is the exact substitution pattern found in TMA-2. If one recognizes the known capacity of the intact organism to methylate this trihydroxy material, and the demonstrated ability within the human to demethylate materials such as mescaline, it is possible that there may be a metabolic intersection between exogenous psychotomimetics and endogenous neurohumors.[19]

The twenty compounds which have been studied in man are listed in Table 4. The M.U. number indicates the psychedelic potency of each compound as compared to mescaline on a milligram basis. Mescaline, or 3,4, 5-trimethoxyphenylethylamine, the active principle of the peyote plant, is itself a sympathomimetic amine related in structure to both epinephrine and the hallucinogenic amphetamines. On a milligram for milligram basis, LSD is by far the most potent of all the hallucinogens, since it produces noticeable effects at doses below 0.1 mg. However, it is available (only illegally to most people in this country) in units of *micro*grams ranging from 250 to 1,000 and higher, whereas STP is often sold on the street in units of 20 to 900 mg and higher—that is, up to three hundred times the minimal hallucinogenic dosage. On a pill or unit basis, as available in the illicit drug marketplace, STP must therefore be judged more powerful than even LSD.

STP. The most interesting and thoroughly studied of these compounds are DOM (STP), MDA, and MMDA. DOM, or 2, 5-dimethoxy-4-methylamphetamine was first synthesized by Alexander T. Shulgin during the mid-1960s. The formula got into the hands of the legendary Owsley, who had already made a fortune on LSD. DOM was an ideal product for him, because it is difficult to synthesize and requires pharmacological expertise as well as expensive laboratory equipment. Owsley renamed the drug STP after the popular American oil additive, "Scientifically Treated Petroleum," and advertised it as "making your motor run smoother and lubricating your head." The *San Francisco Oracle* and the *Berkeley Barb* gave the acronym a different

Table 4.   Twenty compounds studied in man.

Methoxylated Amphetamines (methoxyamphetamines with one ring, open chain structure)		Methylenedioxy Amphetamines (methoxymethylenedioxy-amphetamines, having a 2-ring structure with 5-member heterocyclic ring attached to the benzene ring)	
M.U.[a]	Abbreviation	M.U.[a]	Abbreviation
2	4MA	ca. 1	MDA
2.2	TMA	3	MMDA
17	TMA-2	12+	MMDA-2
2	TMA-3	3	MMDA-3
4	TMA-4	10+	MMDA-3a
10	TMA-5	12	DMMDA
13	TMA-6	5	DMMDA-2
(dimethoxyamphetamines)			
1	2, 3-DMA		
8	2, 5-DMA		
5	2, 4-DMA		
1	3, 4-DMA		
50–100+	DOET		
50–100	DOM ("STP")		

Source: S.H. Snyder, E. Richelson, H. Weingartner, and L.A. Faillace, "Psychotropic Methoxyamphetamines: Structure and Activity in Man," in E. Costa and S. Garattini, eds., *International Symposium on Amphetamines and Related Compounds: Proceedings of the Mario Negri Institute for Pharmacological Research, Milan, Italy* (New York, 1970), pp. 905–928.

[a]The Mescaline Unit (M.U.) figure represents the intensity of the psychedelic reaction in factoral comparison with effects produced by a standard hallucinogenic dose (roughly 300 mg) of mescaline. Snyder et al. define it as "the effective dose of mescaline divided by the effective dose of the compound evaluated," with "effective dose" as "the minimally detectable dose in humans or ED_{50} in animals."

interpretation, praising the drug as a legal substitute for LSD which produced "three days of Serenity, Tranquility, and Peace." In June 1967 more than five thousand STP tablets of varying dosages were distributed to young people gathered in Golden Gate Park to celebrate the summer solstice. (According to one of Owsley's intimate associates, who prefers to remain anonymous, the average dose per pill was supposed to be 15 mg, but the last few hundred tablets produced on this occasion ranged from totally inert ingredients to 250+ mg of pure STP, because of a rare error in Owsley's "quality controls.") Fortunately, Dr. D. E. Smith and other workers at the Haight-Ashbury Clinic were already alerted to the possibility of an "epidemic of STP reactions," because they had observed and treated several severe cases of STP poisoning. They had also learned that chlorpromazine, or Thorazine, which usually ameliorates even the worst LSD trip, only aggravated and prolonged the STP experience. Accordingly, they used only supportive therapy and minor tranquilizers for the few patients whom they were at all equipped to treat—most needed intensive physical care immediately—when the flood of panicky and wildly hallucinating victims began to appear at their clinic on the night of June 21. Thanks largely to the efforts of the Haight-Ashbury Clinic doctors and their assistants, who printed and distributed thousands of posters warning of the dangers of STP and cautioning against combined self-medication with Thorazine or other phenothiazines, STP had all but disappeared from the Haight by the end of the summer. It reappeared on November 11 as the "pink wedge," a tablet alleged to contain 1,500 micrograms of the purest LSD, but actually consisting of 250 micrograms of poor quality LSD and an incredible *900* milligrams (over three hundred times the minimum hallucinogenic dose) of STP. Again warnings were issued by Smith and his coworkers, but by this time STP had "turned the Haight around," and "speed" had displaced LSD and marihuana as the preferred drug among the denizens of this center of our drug subculture.[20]

At about the time the "pink wedge" (which was to be followed by eight more STP wedges, capsules, and tablets in the Haight before 1967 was over) began circulating, the first brief report on the effects of STP in humans appeared in *Science*. S. H. Snyder and his associates tested STP at dosages ranging from 2 to 14 mg on twenty-one normal young male and female volunteers. They found that even 2-mg doses caused moderate euphoria and significant alterations in perception, and that amounts above 3 mg caused "pronounced hallucinogenic effects lasting about eight hours and similar to those produced by hallucinogenic doses of lysergic acid diethylamide, mescaline, and psilocybin." One subject, who received only 3.2 mg, described the following experiences, which lasted more than ten hours: "I started staring at the orange sherbet which was beautiful, brilliant orange, falling disorganizedly like a whirlpool . . . Later, I began shrinking, and water in the glass on the table was getting bigger and moving toward me, coming to envelop me . . . I was really scared . . . I saw a witch doctor, then a horse on the wall . . . Then the ceiling started moving up and down and was purple and yellow . . . I felt I was losing control."[21] The Snyder group found no STP-chlorpromazine synergism (observing only that three subjects who received simultaneous oral doses of 200-mg chlorpromazine and 10-14-mg STP experienced mere lethargy and moderately attenuated hallucinations), but this may have been because their STP dosages were so much lower than the 250- to 900-mg tablets and "wedges" then being distributed in San Francisco. Today STP is almost universally shunned, although it is available sporadically as "super acid" or "organic mescaline."

MDA. Nowadays MDA is especially prized as a safe, smooth psychedelic experience, although very few people have ever had access to the pure, "uncut" drug. It seems that at least two different kinds of "MDA" are circulating on the streets and among college students. First, there is MMDA (3-methoxy-4,5-methylenedioxyamphetamine), an amphetamine derivative which can be synthesized but is usually extracted by simple steam distillation in low (about 4 percent) concentrations from nutmeg, or, more accurately, from the psychoactive element elemicin (3,4,5-trimethoxyallylbenzene) myristicin, or "Myristica Oil," in nutmeg. MMDA is about three times as potent a hallucinogen as mescaline on a milligram basis, but even "pure" MMDA is often avoided because of contamination by toxins from the original nutmeg that can produce a distinctly unpleasant physical and psychic state persisting two days or longer. Second, there is genuine MDA (3,4-methylenedioxyamphetamine), which, like MMDA, is a "double ring" amphetamine derivative. MDA was first synthesized by G. A. Alles in 1932, more than ten years before A. Hofmann discovered that LSD-25 had psychoactive properties, and twenty-two years before Aldous Huxley published his classic account of his first experience with mescaline. But MDA is even more difficult to manufacture than STP and so did not become at all popular until some supplies were "leaked" from unpublicized Defense Department testings in the late 1960s. People who have taken substantial doses of uncut MDA can understand why the Defense Department would be especially interested in a drug that is sometimes referred to with wistful

longing as the "Love and Harmony Groove Pill," or si
"Love." This extraordinary chemical produces very ιυw
subjective alterations at dose levels under approximately 400 mg.
(This figure may vary from person to person; practically no
controlled clinical evaluations of the effects of MDA on normal
people have been conducted or, if so, they have not been reported
in the medical literature.) However, if sufficient amounts (usually
from 400 to 600 mg) are ingested, the user experiences a "dream
state" almost entirely devoid of any typical amphetaminelike
psychological or physiological "side effects." Furthermore, when
taken at medium doses, MDA rarely produces the feelings of
"profound insight or religious significance so characteristic of the
indolic psychotomimetics [such as LSD or psilocybin] or of the
methoxylated amphetamines [STP, TMA-2, and so forth]."[22] The
following excerpt is from Alles' account of what seems to have
been the earliest (1932) use of MDA. Bear in mind that he took a-
bout half the minimum hallucinogenic dose and had not previously taken any psychedelic drug or read any "description of
any hallucinatory phenomena [resulting] from the taking of any
compound, or [any] . . . description of hallucinatory phenomena
that result from pathological effects, so that I was entirely on my
own resources in observing what was happening":

> I took . . . 36 mg. During the following two hours, I observed
> no noticeable change in blood pressure or heart rate, and sub-
> jectively, I felt nothing comparable to the effects of ampheta-
> mine within the same period of time. Consequently, I raised the
> dosage and proceeded to take, after two hours, a dosage of . . .
> 90 mg additionally. Within a few minutes, I realized that a no-
> table subjective response was going to result; I began to feel
> quite different promptly. Within 20 minutes . . . I became sub-
> jectively attentive . . .
>
> Forty-five minutes after the second dosage . . . when I was
> seated in a room by myself, not smoking, and where there was
> no possible source of smoke rings, an abundance of curling
> gray smoke rings was readily observed in the environment
> whenever a relaxed approach to subjective observation was
> used. Visually, these had complete reality; and it seemed quite
> unnecessary to test their properties because it was surely known
> and fully appreciated that the source . . . could not be external
> to the body.

When I concentrated my attention on the details of the curling gray forms . . . they melted away. Then, when I relaxed again, the smoke rings were there. I was as certain they were really there as I am now sure that my head is on top of my body. . . . When I heard footsteps, I looked out into the corridor and found no one there. I repeated this a number of times. Somehow, I felt that this was not a hallucinatory phenomenon, and that I was hearing actual walking. Then I finally realized that . . . the sounds must be coming through the window. (I was on the sixth floor of the medical office building at that time.) I looked out and saw people walking along the sidewalk. That was not sufficient correlation, so I sat down and waited until I heard definite footsteps. Then I looked out and saw that a person was passing. After doing this three or four times, I realized that there was a one to one correspondence between my hearing footsteps and the passing of a person on the street below.

. . . This was not an increase in auditory perception, or not entirely so. At that time, I tested the distance at which I could hear the ticking of a watch, and . . . [later, under nondrug conditions] . . . found it was only a little less acute . . . Apparently the change lay in the differentiation in the perception of different sounds. But if I had not persisted in looking for the source of the footsteps, I would have remained under the impression that I was having auditory hallucinations.

Alles went on to describe his persistence as deriving from a sort of "double consciousness," a strong feeling that his observing self was physically "detached" from his functioning self "to a place above and to the right rearward." He also described in some detail what he considered a related phenomenon "that may have a relationship to understanding the mechanism of this changed [MDA-induced] awareness":

I had long been accustomed, after taking vasoconstrictor substances, to feel vasoconstriction . . . in my finger tips, through the change in circulation. I found that now, too, I had a qualitatively different sensation in my finger tips. Then, as I tried stronger stimulation of the finger ends, I experienced a peculiar phenomenon that I had never noticed before; nor have I noted it since, under any conditions. If you watch as you touch a table top with your finger, you will notice that the time when you hit it, as determined visually, and the time when you feel it are in essential coincidence. However, under this drug, I found that I first hit the table and then felt it; the feeling was a very definitely delayed phenomenon. I experimented with this for a half hour or more, and it was very clear that the time I saw my finger tip hit and the time I felt it were not simultaneous.[23]

Taken at higher (800- to 1,200+ -mg) doses, MDA produces a profoundly altered subjective state. Although most reports are anecdotal, it appears that the individual (1) is infused with a conviction of the oneness of all things, organic and inorganic; (2) feels marked "peaceful" euphoria; and (3) retains the "double consciousness" mentioned by Alles. Because of this last fact, it is usually possible for someone using massive dosages of MDA to ascertain the "external reality" or objective validity of what appear to be visual and auditory hallucinations, and the MDA experimenter often discovers, like Alles, that he is amazingly able to hear and differentiate sounds ordinarily blotted out by foreground static. Alles' pioneering observations that his "vision at a considerable distance"—he mentions three or four city blocks—"was remarkable in clarity of detail" and that he was able to "make out very minute details of things" at such distances and later confirm their accuracy by close inspection have also been at least tentatively confirmed by anecdotal reports. No "bad trips" or "bummers" have been reported with uncut MDA, even at doses approximately ten times the amount Alles took. However, no one (except perhaps for a very small and close-mouthed circle of Defense Department researchers and their employers) seems to know what the effects of massive doses of MDA on large groups of soldiers or civilians might be. "Chemical warfare" or "drug pacification" by MDA would probably suppress the fighting instincts of soldiers (or civilians) and make them expansively warm, friendly, and concerned for the welfare of their "enemies." They would probably be so absorbed in the astounding and enjoyable effects of the drug on their perceptions that they would be interested only in exploring their new "capabilities." Shulgin has suggested that the additional capacity of MDA to increase "apparently valid memory recall, coupled with [the user's] capability of maintaining to some extent normal behavior through voluntary visual contact with the surroundings," might make it useful in psychotherapy.[24] With LSD and most other psychedelics, including these amphetamine derivatives as well as basic amphetamine or methamphetamine taken at hallucinatory dosages, the individual almost invariably retains a hyperacute memory for all—or at any rate the most significant—aspects of his experience. This memory persistence may be related to the so-called "flashback" phenomenon reported to occur after LSD use.

Unfortunately, the same mentality that classifies cannabis, LSD, and heroin together as "Schedule I" substances, which have no legitimate medical or psychiatric—much less religious or merely pleasurable—uses, has made it difficult to conduct controlled clinical evaluations of the potential applications of drugs like MDA. Most "evaluations" of this and related drugs will probably continue to be conducted on the streets (often under the worst imaginable conditions of set and setting and without adequate dosage guides or quality controls), or they will be instituted by the FDA at the insistence of the Drug Enforcement Administration or the Justice Department in order to "prove" high abuse potential.

Many other hallucinogenic amphetamines may be synthesized by "kitchen" and "bathroom" chemists. When we consider Table 4, noting that MDA and MMDA are among the three least potent of the seven methylenedioxyamphetamines so far tested, we can begin to envision the possibility of a synthetic amphetamine derivative psychedelic so much more powerful than mescaline—or even LSD—on a milligram basis that comparisons will be made in terms of "A(mphetamine) U(nits)" instead of "M(escaline) U(nits)." At any rate, we may expect to see a manyfold increase in the use of new synthetic psychedelics in the next few years.

An equally serious although less immediately obvious problem derives from a combination of two factors. First, the tremendous simplicity, ease of manipulation, and chemical affinity or "receptivity" of the basic amphetamine skeleton makes it an exceedingly profitable venture for legitimate drug companies as well as illicit manufacturers to overproduce not only amphetamine, dextroamphetamine, and methamphetamine, but also drugs like Ritalin (methylphenidate) or even amphetaminelike drugs in the experimental stage. There is no limit to the range or variety of "new" and not very subtly disguised amphetamines which pharmacologists, whether officially licensed or strictly amateur, could—and may—produce in the next few years. Second, this potential flood of amphetamine products represents a grave social as well as health danger, because our present legalistic system of drug abuse controls has primarily evolved into a de facto prohibitionary machinery, with a minimum of attention or effective effort directed at any of the root causes of drug abuse in general, or amphetamine abuse in particular. This approach is largely responsible for the paucity of resources invested in detoxifying and humanely rehabilitating addicts and abusers, and for the absence of any rational program to prevent drug abuse in this country on anything but the smallest scale. Indeed, any consideration of the pharmacology of the amphetamines which also takes into account the crucial sociological factors and historical antecedents of our current speed problem leads to the somber conclusion that dedicated, hard-working, generous, and kind Gordon A. Alles and his fellow workers unintentionally "unleashed a Frankensteinian-type monster over which we seemingly have no control."[25]

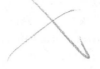

Effect on Mood and Performance

"Fatigue is the natural protective device the body uses to indicate that an activity cannot safely be continued. By masking fatigue, amphetamine jeopardizes the athlete's—or the student's, soldier's, or truckdriver's—health."

The amphetamine user almost always considers the excitation of the central nervous system it produces a pleasant experience, at least in the beginning, and often he has a feeling of increased efficiency, perseverance, endurance, and overall competence. "Drug-induced euphoria" is a vague phrase that gives many different kinds of experience a single label and implies falsely that each psychoactive drug has some reliable, uniform effect on mental state. Whether a person will interpret the effect of a drug like marihuana, LSD, or an opiate, especially the first few times he takes it, as euphoria or pleasure depends very much on set and setting and other complex psychological and social conditions.

Early experiences with amphetamines, on the other hand, are almost inevitably described as enjoyable. The first observation in medical literature on the euphoric properties of amphetamine was made by two English research physicians, who reported in May 1936 that they had observed unexpected feelings of confidence, elation, and well-being in patients they were routinely studying for psychologically caused variations in blood pressure. Amphetamines made them feel happier, brighter, more energetic, and free from care and worry. In September of the same year one of these researchers published the first medical journal article suggesting the use of amphetamine "in the therapy of manic-depressive insanity" in order to provide the patient with "a demonstration of a possibility of recovery."[1] A. Myerson in 1936 may have been the first American physician to recommend Benzedrine for "amelioration of mood" in "neurotic persons."[2]

The vast literature on amphetamines begins with a report by

M. H. Nathanson, a Los Angeles physician who studied their subjective effects in normal persons in a fairly well controlled (but not double-blind) investigation during the Depression. Fifty-five young hospital workers were each given 20 mg of Benzedrine; a similar group of twenty-five healthy volunteers got placebos. In the control group, 84 percent reported that they had perceived absolutely no "drug" effects at all. All fifty-five of the amphetamine-treated group experienced some reaction and in 87 percent (forty-seven) of the cases the intensity of the response was at least moderate. The most frequently reported effect was a strong "sense of well being and a feeling of exhilaration," described in detail by 67 percent. This euphoria seems to have been closely related to the next most common (62 percent) effect, "lessened fatigue" in "reaction to work." Some of the expressions used were:

> "increased energy, felt as if I could not get places fast enough"; "usually tired at dinner time, resumed work after dinner and continued until 10 P. M. and no fatigue"; "I have done things today I usually dislike but which I rather enjoyed doing today"; "the last hour and a half of work is usually an effort, today I felt fine"; "did not have my usual lethargic period after lunch"; "sense of well being, nothing seemed impossible of accomplishment"; "I wanted to stop and talk to everybody I met"; "I felt unusually friendly toward other people"; "my spirits have been high all day, felt bubbling inside"; "this is a few days before the menstrual period and in the last two days I had my usual premenstrual depression; today this was all gone"; "I was able to organize my work quickly and efficiently"; "my mind felt clear all day."[3]

Other research has confirmed Nathanson's findings. In a 1938 study in Denmark, Poul Bahnsen and two coworkers gave either 20 mg (men) or 10 mg (women) of Mecodrin, a Scandinavian brand name for Benzedrine, to one hundred normal subjects. Both the amphetamine-treated group and a control group completed three questionnaires on the day they took their initial doses. They filled out the first early in the morning, before the pills were taken, in order to determine whether any nondrug biasing factors might make them feel "indisposed or particularly well disposed." The afternoon questionnaire attempted to determine how amphetamine had influenced the subjects' attitudes toward work or "emotional life," and also to note the presence of "organic sensations." They completed the third questionnaire on the morning after the day they took the pills; it was designed primarily to determine the effects of the drug on sleep, and also whether and to what degree the subjects had enjoyed the amphetamine experience.

The Bahnsen researchers were impressed by the large number of subjects who said that amphetamines increased their "desire for work in general" or made them feel that it was easier to "get started," or to "perform a task." Respondents indicated enhanced general well-being, good humor, loquaciousness, excitement, and exhilaration. Very few reported any sensations of anxiety and fear, although some mentioned "organic symptoms" of varying intensity, including increased muscle tension, dry mouth, "heat" or "cold waves," palpitations, headache, diminished appetite, tremor of the hands, and weakness in the knees. A majority of the subjects, including those who reported impaired sleep, considered the experience distinctly enjoyable and wanted to take amphetamine again. Of the seventy-three subjects who reported perceptible effects, only three felt "such thoroughly unpleasant effects that it . . . influenced their attitude toward work in a negative direction."[4]

A 1955 study by Lasagna, von Felsinger, and Beecher reveals the difference in immediate attractiveness between amphetamine and the opiates. The group tested reactions to morphine, heroin, a barbiturate (pentobarbital), amphetamine, and a placebo (saline solution) through interviews and self-scoring questionnaires. The drugs were administered intravenously (pentobarbital) or subcutaneously (all other drugs) under double-blind conditions. The dosages given twenty normal and healthy medical student volunteers were as follows: all received 1 ml of sodium chloride (placebo) solution per 70 kg body weight and, at a different time, 20 mg of amphetamine sulfate; half also successively received 0.05 gm pentobarbital sodium, 2 mg heroin hydrochloride, and 8 mg morphine phosphate, and the other half received twice as much of each of these three drugs.

Heroin and morphine had little appeal. The volunteers who took the lower dose of heroin reported only neutral and (a few) dysphoric reactions. Of the eleven who took the higher dose, seven found it unpleasant and only two pleasant (though not so enjoyable as amphetamine). Reactions to morphine were even more marked: six of the eleven who received the higher dose considered it the most unpleasant medication in the series, and only two (both had taken the lower dose) found the experience enjoyable as a whole, although a few others reported transient pleasant feelings. In a questionnaire rating of mood effects, heroin and morphine received high scores for dysphoria (-9 and -16 respectively; 0 was neutral). Only four subjects wanted to take heroin again and only two morphine. Here are some of their comments:

J.C. (4 mg heroin per 70 kg body weight): Very shortly I felt quite dizzy and my calm and happy disposition when I came in soon disappeared. I felt rather sad, melancholy, rather nauseated throughout. It was hard to concentrate but I could not relax. All in all a rather unpleasant experience.

I.I. (4 mg heroin per 70 kg body weight):The major effects began almost immediately and consisted of dizziness and inability to concentrate. This decrease in ability to focus on a problem and analyze it adequately led to a period of distress and then irritation.

D.S. (2 mg heroin per 70 kg body weight): I lost interest or at least the ability to concentrate. My mind wandered freely and I had to force myself to stay awake. I felt a slight heaviness in my head. No emotional changes, but the whole experience was mildly unpleasant.

F.C. (15 mg morphine per 70 kg body weight): Just after medication was given, I began to feel a bit nauseous and a dizziness in my head. Stomach feels uncomfortable. I have to squint to keep my eyes open and from burning. Can't concentrate. Feel generally uncomfortable and shaky. Mouth dry. I feel tired and grouchy.

P.L. (15 mg morphine per 70 kg body weight): Eyes and head heavy. A little nausea. I got the shakes about 10 to 12 minutes after the injection. Heart is beating a little harder. If effect went any further it would be very irritating and would no doubt give me the humps and might make me throw up.

M.P. (15 mg morphine per 70 kg body weight): The first effect was a tightening of the jaw region. Then a slight tingling sensation of the body and a slight feeling of relaxation and serenity. Mind does not seem to be too effectual. I have not enough motivation to concentrate and read anything difficult. Would rather lie back and relax. Later, a slight feeling of nausea, with loss of feeling of optimism. Very dizzy. Feel lousy and sleepy.

H.M. (15 mg morphine per 70 kg body weight): Numb and slightly dizzy. Reading very slowly. My senses feel dulled, and there's a numbness in my head. Late effect was a diffuse itchiness. Urge to act as if drunk. Feeling that I've been doped. Numbness finally gave way to a mild "high" feeling. Pleasant sense of well-being like that experienced in first experiment (pentobarbital).

T.M. (8 mg morphine per 70 kg body weight): There isn't any good feeling from this drug, only a pressure on the head and back of neck, and a feeling that my pulse and respiration are faster than usual.

P.T. (8 mg morphine per 70 kg body weight): Felt sleepy after about ten minutes, with a slight moodiness, on the blue side. Didn't feel like talking or seeing anyone. Got quite sleepy and dozed off for 10 minutes. Had trouble concentrating.

The authors concluded:

Our data thus indicate that morphine and heroin, in the described situation and doses, were not pleasant drugs to the majority of subjects. We cannot confirm the frequently quoted statement that nausea and vomiting after morphine are "not associated with the usual unpleasant emotional reactions" . . .

Such findings are in keeping with usual clinical experience, although not in accord with the statements in nearly all textbooks of pharmacology. The use of morphine for relief of pain is rarely followed by true euphoria. Out of 386 doses of morphine (10 mg.) administered to 150 patients after operation in recent analgesic studies in this laboratory, on only 14 occasions did the patients (either by statements on questioning or by their appearance) suggest any reaction that might conceivably be called euphoric . . .

Of interest to us was the similarity between morphine and heroin in our data, beyond the difference in actual weight of drug required to produce a given effect. The results with heroin did not justify its reputation as a great stimulant or as a producer of intense euphoria.[5]

The reaction to amphetamine was quite different. Thirteen of the twenty subjects found it the most enjoyable, and two others the second most enjoyable. Of the five who disliked it, one found *all* the drugs except pentobarbital unpleasant, and another disliked the secondary effects but not the initial experience. On the rating scale amphetamine received +21 for euphoria, and it was the only drug judged to improve mental functioning. Fourteen of the volunteers wanted to take it again. Some of their remarks were:

J.C.: The most striking effect occurred very soon after medication. Suddenly my body felt light and I became very happy, indeed, exhilarated. This new state filled me with excitement and joy. A delightful drug!

P.L.: An "all-over" good feeling. I felt capable of doing almost any task (within reason; at least I felt I could make a darned good try at accomplishing almost any task), and I felt confident of my abilities, not only for the present time, but also for the future . . . The drug is a good "pick-me-up."

H.M.: The medication took no effect for perhaps ten minutes. Then I began to feel a deep sense of well-being come over me and a feeling of control over myself and confidence and power. I feel similar to when I'm playing the piano at my best . . . a feeling of exhilaration and satisfaction, not unlike the feeling that accompanies sexual satisfaction. All feelings of inadequacy or depression that I've felt at other times seem remote and trivial.

The authors comment: "Although amphetamine is generally acknowledged to be capable of inducing euphoria, we were surprised at the intensity of this response to the drug. The descriptions of our normal subjects after receiving amphetamine were closer to the usual textbook and literary descriptions of the euphoric effects of opiates than were the reactions to morphine or heroin."[6]

This point is worth emphasizing. The traditional lore about heroin, passed along by ill-informed rumor, exaggerated literary descriptions, and even medical and pharmacological texts, is that its power to produce euphoria is so great that a single dose can lead to lifelong addiction. Researchers who have taken the trouble to observe the actual effects of opiates or try them themselves know that this is absurd. Many have concluded that in a healthy person heroin not only fails to cause euphoria but is unpleasant. Even those who eventually become addicted usually have to learn to like heroin or morphine.

Origin of the Pleasurable Effect

The physiological basis for the euphoric and energizing effect of amphetamine is little understood. One approach is the hypothesis of a "pleasure" or "reward" center in the brain. Rats with an electrode implanted at a certain point in the hypothalamus may press a treadle to switch on electrical stimulation up to 1,800 times an hour without stopping for twelve hours or more, often going without food, water, or sleep.[7] This site seems to lie in the center of a cluster of brain areas that monitor (and perhaps even actuate) signals of thirst, hunger, temperature regulation, elimination, sex, aggression, and so on. It appears that "circuits" of some kind, analogous to feeder lines, run from the "pleasure center" to, for instance, the hunger and sexual sites, and that this pleasure perception focal point effectively determines when a person has, for example, "eaten enough" by regulating some adjacent brain "appestat." Thus, the "pleasure center" of the hypothalamus comes into play when other drive-regulating sites are activated and controls the duration or intensity of satisfaction-seeking behavior.

As one writer phrased it, "the finding of 'pleasure sites,' where stimulation produced no particular action but only evident gratification, prompted some speculation that animals and men were indeed pure hedonists . . . striving only for the excitement of these regions of the hypothalamus."[8] There are many objections to the pleasure-center explanation for human behavior in general and drug effects in particular. The hypothalamus, central in the experience of emotion, cannot function in isolation.[9] Although it seems to be of particular importance with regard to more primitive drives or needs, most human organizing, integrating, and generally "expressive" or emotional behavior involves or is mediated through central and higher regions of the cerebral cortex. The pleasure sites seem associated mainly with eating and sex—which account for only a small part of life. There is strong evidence that amphetamine stimulates most regions of the brain; although the hypothalamus may mediate the amphetamine "lift," in men as well as animals, perception of the effect as a "lift" requires stimulation of the cortex.

A more promising line of research is the study of EEG (electro-encephalograph) tracings, that is, recordings of the electrical signals produced by brain activity. Research into the interactions of catecholamines (neurohormones like norepinephrine and dopamine) reveals little about the sites (as opposed to the modes) of drug actions, and examination of EEG studies can help us evaluate various theories suggested by neurochemistry. When an individual is drug-free, well-rested, in good physical health, and under no psychic stress, his EEG yields a predictable, roughly orderly pattern of voltage changes. Its most easily distinguished frequency, the alpha wave, is generated in the occipital lobe of the cortex and predominates when one is physically resting and fully alert, but with eyes closed. When one reacts to a particular stimulus, the alpha wave is replaced by higher frequency waves at lower voltages, which can be described as "highly desynchronized and irregular low-voltage fast activity."[10] M. Fink noted that during the last twenty years there have been many studies of the effects of various drugs on the "normal" EEG, but few systematic or quantitative ones. Most of these studies, especially in human beings, have assayed single drugs in noncomparative, loosely controlled experiments at low dosage levels, and the authors tend to describe changes in the EEG in vague or inconsistent language: "Changes in the EEG were referred to as 'normal' or 'abnormal,' or were given descriptors such as synchronization and desynchronization. Chronic studies were rarely undertaken. The technical issues of electrode placement, amplifier characteristics, and recording methods were rarely defined." Fink does believe, however, that "psychoactive drugs have specific EEG 'signatures,' even in scalp recordings, and that the patterns reflect differences in the chemical effects of drugs. Furthermore, these patterns are sufficiently consistent in their relation to behavior to support a theory of the association of EEG and behavior."[11]

The effects of amphetamine on EEG tracings have been studied. In 1953 P. B. Bradley and J. Elkes noted that massive doses (3 to 5 mg per kg of body weight) of basic (dl-)amphetamine (Benzedrine) administered by mouth to fully conscious healthy cats produced low amplitude, diffuse, fast (15-30 c/s) activity throughout the brain. (According to Leake and some early investigators, EEG changes after amphetamine occurred *only* in the mid-brain, particularly the "reticular activating system," including the hypothalamus). Bradley and Elkes noted that the cats became more attentive, and sometimes excited. Their data seem to support the hypothesis that amphetamine stimulation of higher brain regions—even of cats—is as important as mid-brain inter-actions in causing behavior changes.[12] In fact, in 1955 the Russian I. I. Baryshnikov confirmed the earlier speculation of his colleague B. K. Faddeyeva that the amphetamine derivatives 1,1-diphenyl-2-aminopropane (structurally and pharmacolog-ically almost identical with Benzedrine) and 1-phenyl-2-nicotiny-laminopropane (a simple nicotinic acid amphetamine congener available in western Europe as Phenatin) caused a direct stimula-tion of the cerebral cortex of human beings readily discernible on EEG recordings.[13]

Three American studies conducted in 1942 and 1943 are even more important. M. A. Rubin and his coworkers reported an in-crease in the percentage of time when alpha waves were predominant in normal persons given amphetamine. These find-ings were replicated by F. A. Gibbs and G. L. Maltby, who also observed a shift toward higher frequencies throughout the EEG spectrum. And D. B. Lindsley and C. E. Henry, studying the ef-fects of amphetamine on the EEG's of a small group of children with behavior problems, showed, for nearly all, a reduction in (presumably) abnormal brain impulse from the frontal regions, along with an increase in frequency and a decrease in amplitude of the "normal" alpha rhythm.[14] This apparent effect on the alpha waves may be a clue to the euphoria produced by ampheta-mine, for it is now well established that alpha-wave fluctuations are closely correlated with immediate manifestations of a diffuse, highly pleasurable state of *relaxed* enhanced awareness.

Fatigue

A common rationalization of students, truck drivers, soldiers, and businessmen is that amphetamine staves off normal fatigue and enables them to work efficiently for days with little sleep or food. Studies, as well as everyday experience, confirm this to a certain extent. In 1938 J. E. Barmack had subjects fill out bore-dom and fatigue self-rating scales after each of eight 15-minute work periods during which they added six-place numbers. They were given either 10 mg amphetamine or a placebo fifteen to forty minutes before beginning. The subjects treated with amphetamine felt considerably less boredom, fatigue, and irritation. The following year Barmack obtained similar results with a slightly higher (15 mg) dose. In this experiment the effects of 60 mg of ephedrine hydrochloride were, unlike those of the amphetamine, exceedingly variable and unreliable. In 1950 H. F. Adler reported that 5 mg of methamphetamine was roughly equivalent to 10 mg of d-amphetamine in reducing unpleasant or undesirable symptoms reported at simulated altitudes of 15,000 to 18,000 feet. During World War II researchers in many countries consistently reported that the use of amphetamines resulted in the amelioration of fatigue after heavy or tedious physical or mental labor.[15]

This phenomenon was the subject of a series of experiments in the middle 1950s at the USAF School of Aviation Medicine. Because they had doubts about "concepts of psychological fatigue which regard work decrement as symptomatic of cumulative task aversion and failure to maintain proper attitudes," R. B. Payne and G. T. Hauty analyzed the relation between attitude toward a task and performance on that task. They used the USAF SAM Multidimensional Pursuit Test, a simulated airplane cockpit built for aviation cadet training, which required that the subject monitor and compensate four dial pointers which drifted erratically in either direction from a zero point. Keeping the continuously fluctuating pointers at the null position by constant readjustments of a joy stick, two rudder pedals, and a throttle lever was usually considered just as demanding and tedious as it sounds, and the investigators had already established that work decrement is apparent after an hour—two at the most. They allowed their eighty volunteers to practice long enough to get past the basic learning to a substantial level of skill, then assigned them randomly to three groups. The twenty members of the first group, told simply that the investigators wanted to find out how well they could perform for a four-hour period, were encouraged to do "the very best" they could, since "you will be giving us information that will help us deal with important practical problems." With the second group of twenty more emphasis was placed on elaborating this "theme at length, stressing the similarity between the task and the real flight, the necessity for alertness, and the important role played by S [Subject] in helping the Air Force solve one of its most important problems." The third group of forty (all presumably—although this was not specifically stated—drug "naive") were given no such instructions, but were divided into five clusters of eight subjects receiving respectively the following "pharmacological treatments": (1) 5 mg of dextroamphetamine; (2) 20 mg of a caffeine derivative; (3) a "depressant" (0.65 mg of hyoscine hydrobromide mixed with 50 mg of diphenhydramine hydrochloride); (4) a lactose placebo; or (5) no drug at all (control group). At the end of the "flight testing," all eighty men were administered a brief questionnaire "designed primarily to elicit information about their covert dispositions as they reviewed the experience from which they had just emerged," but which also asked each respondent to answer specific questions about fatigue in eight body locations. Amphetamine proved superior to pep talks or other drugs. It not only prevented any decline in performance over the four-hour period (a decline especially marked in the subgroup treated with the depressant mixture), but actually raised average performances above the levels reached during the introductory practice period. Payne and Hauty concluded that, although mood or "task disposition," as well as performance, improved under the effect of amphetamine, "the way in which the drugs achieve their effect on performance . . . [is] *not* through the motivational properties of the subjective dispositions they create, as some have suggested." They proposed that the improved performance was caused by the drugs' "presence in the body fluids which bathe or penetrate the nerve cells mediating task performance," or, less vaguely, by "their capacity to inhibit the enzyme, amine oxidase, which normally alters certain enzymes in the brain to form aldehydes that depress tissue respiration."[16]

Payne and Hauty then set out to determine the comparative efficacy of various drug preparations, in terms of "mitigation of work decrement" resulting from fatigue, using a "reward" or "success" signal (a bell which rang or a light which flashed when the subject had accurately adjusted any one of the four pointers to the null position). The general procedure was almost the same as in their earlier investigations, but now the simulated cockpit work period was lengthened to seven hours, though half of the subjects were told at the outset that they would be expected to work for only four hours. As anticipated, dextroamphetamine strongly counteracted the usual decline in performance for the full seven hours. The most interesting findings, however, were on the value of amphetamines relative to nondrug anti-fatigue measures. First, the group who had been told that they were participating in a four-hour experiment consistently performed much more accurately throughout the full seven hours of testing than those who had been told the actual time involved at the beginning. Second, the subjects who had received no drugs but whose performance was monitored or rewarded maintained much higher levels of proficiency that those given no such clues or rewards. This relative lack of decline in task proficiency was especially noticeable among subjects who heard a bell each time they made a correct adjustment. Hauty and Payne explained this as a result of a reduction of "visual load," but they might also have ascribed it to simple novelty or lessening of boredom. In fact, although the Dexedrine-treated subjects maintained their initial levels of performance better than any other group, this investigation supported the general hypothesis that simple task fatigue and boredom can be substantially diminished if (1) the individual is supplied with feedback on how well he is doing; (2) the task involves some novelty, challenge, excitement, or intrinsic meaning; and (3) he is allowed to shift to new (even if closely related or almost identical) tasks at regular intervals. The importance of variation was indicated by the finding that there was no carry-over or transfer of diminished efficiency to a terminal task which demanded that the subjects respond to randomly presented pairs of red and green lights in a cockpit situation very similar to that of the original test.[17]

In their next report Payne and Hauty presented more precise differentiations between the effects of feedback and pharmacological treatments. Trying to distinguish between "motivational (or incentive) failure" and "organizational (or directive) impairment," they divided their subjects into three major groups of forty-eight. Group T received directive feedback through a graded series of visual signals illuminating the dials. Group M were provided with motivational (incentive) feedback by pegboards which indicated scores. Volunteers in the third group (D) were given substantially the same drugs used in the earlier experiments. The resulting data showed that the directive feedback given to group T was especially effective in immediately *raising* and then sustaining performance levels during the entire four-hour testing period. As Figure 3 demonstrates, the subjects treated with 5 mg

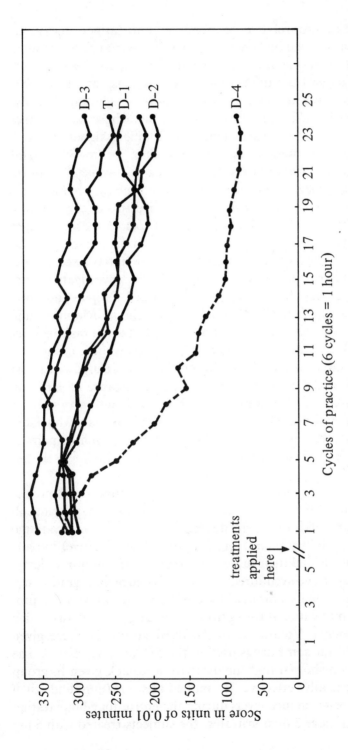

Source: adapted from R.B. Payne and G.T. Hauty, 'Effect of psychological feedback upon work decrement, *J. Exp. Psychol.* 58 (1955), 346. Copyright by the American Psychological Association; used by permission.

Figure 3   The effect of directive feedback and drugs on performance.

of dextroamphetamine (D-3) showed a slightly higher average level of proficiency than group T, although not so high an initial level; whereas the subjects who received only motivating feedback did relatively poorly. But even they performed much better than those given the depressant drug combination (D-4), and significantly better than the control (D-1) or the placebo-treated subjects (D-2). Payne and Hauty concluded, however, that dextroamphetamine sulfate was amazingly effective in minimizing work decrement, whereas the immediate increment in task proficiency induced by "directive feedback" signals was not maintained during the final performance stages. They even claimed that no conditions or combination of conditions existed under which directive feedback had postponed work decrement.[18]

What is perhaps the most important conclusion of the Payne and Hauty studies—that the effect of amphetamine in "work decrement" is *not* mediated by any change in attitude toward the task—has been challenged by a number of reports that insist on the importance of enhanced interest, confidence, and initiative in producing improvement in standard psychological and psychomotor tests. These reports often conclude that any amphetamine-caused performance improvement can be equalled or exceeded by fairly simple changes in situation and environment.

In 1947 Dr. D. R. Davis, head of the Medical Research Council of Applied Psychology at Cambridge University, summarized the results of investigations carried out by a medical branch of the RAF during and after World War II, as well as his own laboratory's extensive research into the relations between the psychomotor effects of amphetamines and fatigue phenomena in air crew as well as civilians. His excellent review is especially valuable because of the scope of the experimental data it incorporates, and also because Davis was aware of the dangers in extrapolating from laboratory statistics to conclusions about drug effects on persons engaged in normal day-to-day work and recreation. He emphasized that in almost all of the clinical and laboratory explorations of amphetamines the subjects had been assigned specific tasks and narrowly limited tests which were bound to result in (positively) biased data, because they were almost invariably designed, albeit unintentionally, to "provide subjects with scope for their energies and allow a considerable degree of success." He pointed out that in more complex tasks the amphetamines often produced *less* efficient performance. This was especially true when the subjects had to discriminate between simultaneously presented stimuli calling for segregated manual responses or had to decide on the most efficient sequence of responses. Even the most mechanistic testings sometimes revealed not only "unfavorable" amphetamine effects on performance but also generalized disorganization of behavior, manifested in "impulsive and inappropriate activity," as well as irritability and restlessness. Although the administration of amphetamine often increased the rate of response, it also increased the number of errors. Davis noted that "an increase in speed with only a small [perceptible] loss of accuracy may be regarded as a favourable effect in a test situation in the laboratory, but would not be so regarded if the subject were driving a car in everyday circumstances." In the same way, increased attentiveness or persistence resulting in higher scores on laboratory tests is not always beneficial outside the laboratory. Here he described one of his research colleagues, "left to his own devices after a dose of amphetamine, [who] spent a morning preparing with great thoroughness a grandiose research-plan, of which he would never find time to carry out even a quarter."

Davis was convinced that amphetamine-produced improvements in test performance were related to the greater interest subjects took in them rather than any increase in capacity, and that such improvements could be produced by other means which increased interest. He thought the benefits claimed for amphetamines could be produced without drugs "by training and other measures which lead to good morale," thereby incurring no danger of impaired judgment, and especially none of dependence or addiction.*

Examining the rationale for giving amphetamines to air crews on long flights, Davis observed that "fatigue" was a vague term which had slowed the solution of many practical problems; he suggested dispensing with it, and asking instead "under what precise conditions errors occur." First he described the "cockpit

---

*William Burroughs, who has had personal experience with a wide range of psychoactive drugs, says that "Anything that can be accomplished by chemical means can also be accomplished by other means, given sufficient knowledge of the processes involved. Recent experiments show that . . . Any trip you want will soon be available without drugs" ("Playboy Panel: The Drug Revolution," *Playboy* [February 1970], p. 64).

experiments." These were conducted in a stationary flight-simulating apparatus, usually referred to as the "Cambridge Cockpit," similar to the USAF SAM Multidimensional Pursuit Test training device. Almost every aviator who worked in the Cockpit exhibited a disintegration of skills and an increase in the frequency of errors after a brief initial "instrument flying-exercise." His findings were that many highly trained, completely drug-free air force personnel experienced a distinct "disorganization of skill" in the "experimental analogue of flying," not primarily because of fatigue resulting from prolongation of the test situation, but because of the anxiety provoked by isolation, confinement and intense psychomotor coordination demands. Davis believed his experiments

> indicated that, in the case of the cockpit-test, anxiety was due to the difficulty experienced by predisposed subjects in attaining a satisfying standard of performance. The machine was very unstable, and excessive activity was penalized heavily. These characteristics made some subjects feel insecure, particularly if they aspired to a high standard of accuracy. It was concluded that the general conditions of disorganization of skill are factors in the environment which signify danger and evoke in the subject anticipatory tension, the subject not having the means of removing the danger and thereby relieving the tension.[19]

After citing two series of experiments, conducted during World War II by the British RAF, and confirming his position, Davis reaffirmed that both "incriminated stress and the resultant anxiety, rather than the prolongation of work and fatigue, as the conditions under which errors are made. Many of the arguments, by which the use of amphetamine by aircrew is justified, are therefore irrelevant."

Davis' results suggest that fatigue or work decrement applies primarily to simple, often laboratory-instituted tasks, and has little relevance to complex emotional and intellectual demands made on someone like a military airplane pilot. The case for improving performance by amphetamine seems to be shown only in situations of boring, repetitive, prolonged, and simple labor. Amphetamine often fails to improve performance on simple psychomotor tests of non-fatigued subjects, as an interesting study conducted by Conan Kornetsky of the NIMH shows. Kornetsky used a simple "multiple stimulus-response apparatus," consisting of a panel of ten signal lights situated above ten numbered buttons (also referred to as a "subject panel"), designed to measure "a variety of types of behavior while always evoking the same motor response on the part of the subject." It was constructed to allow the experimenter to pair any stimulus light with any button and to program the flashing of the lights in any sequence. In his carefully controlled, double-blind, comparative experiment, an unfortunately small (five males and three females) group of "normal" young (eighteen to twenty-two years old) volunteers were given three different drugs (meprobamate, 800 and 1600 mg; phenobarbital, 60 and 120 mg; dextroamphetamine, 5 and 15 mg), as well as placebos, over a period of fifteen days. Neither 5 nor 15 mg of dextroamphetamine had any "beneficial" performance-improving effects on two tests of response time ("simple" and "choice" reaction) or on a single test of simple learning. Somewhat surprisingly, it also failed to decrease either simple or choice reaction time; both 5 and 15 mg of dextroamphetamine caused an increase in the number of errors—even compared with the sedative-depressant phenobarbital at 60 mg (on the simple reaction time test only).[20]

The following year Kornetsky and his colleagues reported on a similar series of investigations prompted by their consideration of Eysenck's findings which seemed to indicate that psychomotor performance was facilitated by dextroamphetamine when prolonged continuous work was required on a simple but boring psychomotor coordination task. The Kornetsky group interpreted these findings as suggesting "that this drug will improve performance only if the individual is functioning below his potential level when the drug is given." Accordingly, they designed a complex experimental sequence to assess the facilitative effects of dextroamphetamine on nineteen healthy, "normal" young volunteers (six males and thirteen females between eighteen and twenty-five) who had been deprived of sleep for seventy-two hours. (These subjects served as their own controls.) The first three testings were identical with those used in the Eysenck investigation: determination of (1) simple, and (2) choice reaction times, and (3) simple learning speed and accuracy. Kornetsky used a multiple stimulus-response instrument panel for testing. Each subject was also given a modified Digit-Symbol Substitution

Test (DSST) adapted from the Wechsler Adult Intelligence Scale (WAIS), and fifteen of them took two ten-minute Continuous Performance Tests (CPT).

Sleep deprivation up to forty-four hours significantly impaired performance on the two reaction-time testings as well as on the DSST and the CPT for all subjects. After sixty-eight hours without any sleep every volunteer exhibited moderate to extreme deterioration on all five tests and tasks; 10 mg of dextroamphetamine administered after forty-four hours of sleeplessness improved their subjects' performances on reaction-time testings and the DSST but had no effect on their CPT scores or their scores on the simple learning test. After sixty-eight hours of continuous sleep deprivation another 15 mg of amphetamine produced significant improvement on all tests except simple learning, but no subject's performance was restored to base line (pre-sleep-deprivation) levels.

It was suggested that prolonged sleep loss resulted in "momentary lapses in performance which increase in frequency as sleep deprivation progresses." These "lapses"—elsewhere described as microsleep periods generally lasting less than ten seconds, during which the subject is "in an eyes-closed resting state"—did not have a strong negative effect on performance when the subjects were able to control the display of stimuli and hence the rate at which they had to respond, although their efficiency and speed (but not necessarily accuracy) were lowered. On the other hand, when subjects could not control the time of appearance or the duration of the stimulus display, their performance fell off markedly, and amphetamine only partially restored a few relatively simple functionings to normal levels.[21]

Stress

By far the most extensive and painstaking exploration of the effects of amphetamines and other drugs on performance under stress is the 1966 monograph by P. M Hurst and M. F. Weidner with its detailed analyses of three different sets of experiments designed to "investigate possible drug enhancement of cognitive performance in nonfatigued humans" in stressful situations. Its working hypothesis was that *drug enhancement of cognitive performance is achieved through mitigation of disturbing influences, rather than through direct facilitation of cognitive processes.*[22]

Because Hurst and Weidner believed that the "stress" in most earlier similar studies on amphetamine effects resulted from an extraneous "stressor"—for example, electric shock or some kind of "background static" emanating from the task-environment or the general task conditions—it was necessary to devise tasks in which the stress-component was *inherent*, not externally imposed. J. G. Miller's concept of "information input overload" was basic to their approach. Miller observed that studies on sensory deprivation had shown that information input *underload* often resulted in highly specific "pathological function of the nervous system and abnormal behavior," and suggested that analogous phenomena occurred under the "reverse condition" of, for example, "prolonged daily pressure to make many rapid-fire decisions," or "the many blatant and competing sources of information—radio, television, movies, magazines, and newspapers—[which] contribute to the increased tension said to characterize our age."[23]

Hurst and Weidner wrote:

> Certain task parameters—e.g., high input pacing in the presence of certain perceptual and/or decision-making demands —appear to induce a type of stress in the human operator. Many operational tasks involve these parameters. The occurrence of a "dropoff" phenomenon, a sharp decrement in the information transfer rate when input rate exceeds a critical value, has been demonstrated in the laboratory by various investigators.[24]

They gave two possible interpretations for these findings: (1) decreased performance caused by stress was the result of "input queuing, due to channel-capacity limitations in the organism" resulting in losses of usable information "during short-term storage while awaiting processing"; or (2) the decrease was the result of psychological or "emotional" factors interfering with optimal functioning "of the human data-processing machine." If the first hypothesis was correct, amphetamine would possess almost no power to prevent or reverse performance losses, and in fact these drugs had shown little ability to increase short-term storage capacity in non-fatigued subjects. Although there was some evidence that amphetamine lowered "disjunctive reaction time" (the time between a stimulus and the response to it), the effect was very small "in the absence of fatigue or oxygen deprivation." Therefore, Hurst and Weidner conjectured that amphetamines selectively blocked "the emotional component of task-induced stress" or "panic" through a specific " 'anti-stress' component."

In their first experiment it was postulated that 10 mg of dextroamphetamine sulfate (Dexedrine) would exert stimulant and antistress effects; that 10 mg of methylphenidate hydrochloride (Ritalin) would act as a "pure" stimulant, lacking any anxiety-alleviating properties; that 10 mg chlordiazepoxide hydrochloride (Librium) would exert antistress effects; and, finally, that the placebo would produce no changes. Sixty-three Pennsylvania State University students were recruited for a "psychological experiment" offering a chance to earn ten dollars. The main measuring device was the "Paced Sequential Memory Task" (PSMT). This consisted of a sequence of "member" words (like "pine," "tin," and "polo") interspersed with "class" words (like "tree," "metal," and "sport"). Whenever a "class" word was presented, the subject was required to recall the most recently presented "member" word that belonged to it. The PSMT allows for systematic manipulation of the so-called "storage load," the amount of information a person has available at conscious or preconscious levels. It also involves "concurrent storage and retrieval operations, [so that] it was presumed to have a certain degree of intrinsic stressfulness," *not* superimposed by any threatening attitudes or instructions from the investigators or by the environment or the situation.[25]

Drug-induced mood changes were measured at regular intervals throughout the three-hour experimental sessions by self-ratings on a version of the Nowlis Mood Adjective Check List (ACL). The postulated antistress effect was measured by negative "anxiety" and positive "elation" scores, while the purely stimulant effects of the various drugs were determined by negative "fatigue" and postitive "vigor" scores. Three major hypotheses were tested. The first was that amphetamine-treated subjects would excel nondrugged students in performance under high stress as well as low stress circumstances. This hypothesis was partly substantiated: amphetamine-treated subjects scored about eight percentage points higher than placebo recipients on the first performance test (40 minutes after ingestion of the medications); those receiving Ritalin scored slightly better than the controls (57.18 percent as opposed to 55.50 percent) or the students given Librium (54.83 percent, the lowest mean score at this testing). However, on the second performance test, administered 95 minutes after the drugs or placebos, no significant differences were found between the placebo and any of the drug groups. "Thus, during the second test d-amphetamine generally lost its statistical superiority over the other drug conditions . . . both d-amphetamine and chlordiazepoxide yielded relatively better results early in the session, and . . . *virtually all of d-amphetamine's overall superiority derived from the 'high stress' condition."* Hurst and Weidner noted that this "fading" was quite unexpected, particularly in view of "the widespread belief that amphetamines are most effective (or *only* effective) when performance has been degraded by fatigue, monotony, etc.," and they ascribed it to the overwhelming importance of the antistress factor.[26]

Their second major hypothesis was that increased stress would improve the performance of the Librium and Dexedrine groups relative to the Ritalin or placebo groups, on the supposition that both of the former drugs, but neither methylphenidate nor the placebo, had specific stress-alleviating or stress-mitigating properties. This hypothesis was not confirmed to any statistically significant extent, although performance score changes were in the expected directions. The final hypothesis was that "lengthened exposure to the test task will improve the performance of methylphenidate [Ritalin] groups relative to chlordiazepoxide [Librium] or no drug." Once again, although the results were vaguely in the "predicted direction," the hypothesis was statistically unconfirmed. The findings on mood, too, were noteworthy: while dextroamphetamine yielded significantly higher scores on the "vigor" index and lower scores for "fatigue," it *increased* both the frequency and the intensity of reports of "anxiety." Hurst and Weidner attributed this to "sympathomimetic components which could outweigh any increases in assurance, self-confidence, etc. that may be produced by these drugs."

In their summary, the authors stressed that the slight superiority of dextroamphetamine (at least during the first hour or so of the testing), especially under high stress conditions, "tended to contradict the viewpoint that cognitive performance enhancement by amphetamines is dependent upon the prior existence of fatigue or boredom." In order to verify this apparent discrepancy with most of the earlier literature, they designed a second experiment, testing the reactions of one hundred thirty-six students (none of whom had participated in the original tests) to 10 mg dextroamphetamine, a combination of 10 mg dextroamphetamine with 50 mg secobarbital, another combination of 10 mg dextroamphetamine and 10 mg of chlordiazepoxide (Librium), and a placebo. These mixtures of amphetamine—in one case with a popular barbiturate and in another with one of the most widely prescribed tranquilizers—were used to "explore the further possibility that cognitive performance under stress might be further improved," in some synergistic manner. The same test procedure used in the first experiment was followed, with the addition of a "boldness" factor to the adjective self-rating checklist, as well as new time perception and performance self-judgment tests. To the surprise of Hurst and Weidner, and regardless of the "SL" (storage load) imposed, *none* of the medications or placebos produced any reliable or statistically significant performance-enhancing effects. Nor could they discover any relation of drug effects to stress levels or confirm the earlier suggestion that performance effects from d-amphetamine were stronger early in the test sequence. The findings on the time perception test were as expected: amphetamine tended to speed up slightly the subjective passage of time. But the results of the performance self-judgment analyses were entirely unexpected. The amphetamine groups showed a stronger tendency to underestimate their scores than any of the others. However, all groups underestimated performance to some extent, so the amphetamine-treated subjects' self-evaluations may indicate the drug's characteristic propensity to exaggerate thought processes, habits, attitudes, and basic judgment, causing overattribution of meaning or significance to any given perceived difficulty in the task.[27]

Because of the many discrepancies between their initial and follow-up studies, Hurst and Weidner set up a third experiment, with five major goals: (1) to confirm or refute the hypothesis that amphetamine enhances performance in nonfatigued normal subjects, employing a more powerful experimental design; (2) to explore any differential effects of 10-mg versus 15-mg doses of dextroamphetamine; (3) "to determine the interaction of drug effects with pacing variations in the PSMT (storage load had previously been manipulated, but input pacing had not)"; (4) to compare the PSMT results with results obtained from a "supplementary non-paced task that imposes no short-term storage requirements"; and (5) to determine the effects of 100 mg secobarbital (the "hypnotic" or sleep-inducing dosage for most subjects) on performance and mood, and compare these results with those obtained for amphetamines.

A new group of students (forty males and eight females) was recruited for treatment with the following drugs and dosages: (1) dextroamphetamine sulfate, 10 mg (D-10); (2) dextroamphetamine sulfate, 15 mg (D-15); (3) sodium secobarbital, 100 mg (S); (4) placebo capsules, identical in appearance (P). A fifth group (ND) was given neither active medications nor placebos. The researchers decided to "pace" the PSMT inputs at two-against three-second intervals "to permit independent within-subject assessments of rate effects and serial effects." All sequences had a constant storage load of 4.8, the highest in any of the three testings. The PSMT pacing variations explored the possibility that the primarily psychostimulant amphetamines might exert "some facilitative effect upon data-processing ability that is independent of the mitigation of emotional stress." A one-hour arithmetic test (involving addition and subtraction of columns of signed numbers) was administered to "introduce new parametric variations (as absence of pacing and storage requirements) and to determine whether the enhancement effects reported by Holliday could be obtained with non-sleep deprived subjects."[28]

Dextroamphetamine at the 15-mg dose caused a slight but statistically significant improvement on PSMT scores and at the 10-mg dose a statistically insignificant gain. Secobarbital exerted a marked and highly significant negative effect compared to all other drugs or placebo or no-drug. The apparent superiority of 15 mg of dextroamphetamine could not be accounted for strictly in terms of numbers of answers attempted (increasing willingness to guess) because subjects receiving both the 10- and 15-mg doses had not only more correct recalls but also slightly higher ratios of correct to incorrect recalls. According to the authors, "the drug treatment effects were independent of input rate, reaching comparable levels of significance with both rates during all five sessions." Observed drug effects on arithmetic performance generally paralleled those obtained from the PSMT. On the other hand, 10 mg of dextroamphetamine caused a reduction in accuracy scores as compared with all groups except the one receiving secobarbital, and 15 mg resulted in more errors than the placebo and about the same number as no drug treatment. In fact, in the final session, the subjects receiving 15 mg did worse in terms of accuracy than any other group except the nondrug subjects. After two and a half hours of testing, even subjects given a hypnotic dose of secobarbital, as well as those who received placebos or no drugs at all, were as accurate as those given 10 mg of amphetamine and markedly more accurate than those who had taken 15 mg.

Hurst and Weidner maintained that their first hypothesis (that 15 mg of dextroamphetamine would improve total PSMT performance relative to 10 mg of the same drug, 100 mg of secobarbital, placebo, or no drug, regardless of input rate) was definitely confirmed. The second hypothesis (that 10 mg of dextroamphetamine would exert a mild overall enhancement of performance, slightly less than 15 mg, but more than secobarbital or no drug-placebo) could not be confirmed. The third hypothesis (that increased storage loads and hence increased stress would result in a dose-related curve of performance enhancement with 10 and 15 mg of dextroamphetamine), required further testing. Although 15 mg produced a sharper rise than any other treatment (or placebo and no-drug conditions) between the first two 14-minute intervals of the PSMT, it failed to improve—or even maintain—its relative position thereafter, so it was impossible to demonstrate that even this higher dose genuinely mitigated work decrement caused by fatigue or boredom. In fact, the results of Experiment I, in which the only significant improvements occurred about 80 minutes after drug ingestion, suggested that the primary facilitative effects did not involve any "stabilization" of decline resulting from performing a monotonous task over a substantial (more than 60-90 minutes) period. "Thus there is no satisfactory explanation for these intra-period differences." The fourth hypothesis was that dextroamphetamine would exert a genuine anti-stress effect—in particular, on the PSMT. According to Hurst and Weidner, "The anti-stress viewpoint was moderately successful in predicting *inter*-period comparisons." That is, after repeated weekly exposure to the PSMT and amphetamines, performance enhancement by either 10 or 15 mg decreased asymptotically toward placebo levels: "Thus increased practice with the PSMT seems to have precluded continued enhancement by d-amphetamine."[29]

Intelligence

For tasks involving more than simple monitoring, memorizing, or arithmetic operations, amphetamine does not seem to aid performance. In 1936 a report in *Lancet* by W. Sargant and J. M. Blackburn caused a sensation, because the authors claimed an average increase of 8.7 percent in I.Q. scores as determined by the Cattell test among a group of forty-eight patients at Maudsley Hospital after the administration of 20 mg of Benzedrine. But, J. E. Barmack pointed out, "certain deficiencies in procedure appear to be sufficiently serious to question the validity" of the inference that Benzedrine had a favorable effect on intelligence test performance. The problem was that the control group showed *no* increase in scores on the same test readministered within a twenty-four hour period, which was, "in the view of the literature on the subject . . . most unusual." Although Barmack did not attempt to explain this absence of practice-improvement effects, he might have noted that of the sixty-seven subjects, fifty-four were chronic psychiatric patients "suffering from conditions labeled as anxiety states, depression, or hysteria, nine were schizophrenic, three had an obsessional neurosis, and one was epileptic." Sargant and Blackburn did not reveal how their subjects were distributed among the three groups (two amphetamine-treated groups and one control group of only nineteen), remarking only that eight of the schizophrenics received amphetamine, which suggests the possibility that the other eighteen controls may have been largely or entirely selected from the remaining forty-six psychologically disturbed patients. Perhaps because of similar suspicions, Barmack decided to give separate versions of the Otis Self-Administering Test of Mental Ability (Otis SAT) to two large groups of psychologically "normal" and physically healthy male college students after administration of either 10-mg Benzedrine or placebo pills, using a "rotation method of control" designed to insure that no subject knew the nature of the pills and also to minimize any practice bias. The average Otis test score after amphetamine was about 2 percent lower (65.8 as against 67.4 out of a maximum of 75 points) than it was after placebos; Barmack concluded that "under the conditions of the present experiment the 10 mg of benzedrine did not favorably affect the ability of the subject to score on this examination."[30]

In 1941 R. Hecht and S. S. Sargent noted that early findings of striking effects on intelligence scores had not been duplicated, although the *Benzedrine Sulfate Protocol* mimeograph release from Smith, Kline & French still claimed that amphetamine heightens learning ability. They also noted that Turner and Carl Hill had found no positive amphetamine effect on rote memory, but had concluded that "where more complex memory functions, involving analysis, deliberation, 'thought,' or intention are concerned, the situation is in doubt." Hecht and Sargent set out to reduce this doubt by devising and borrowing special tests measuring "higher mental processes, in the sense of thinking, reasoning, or problem-solving." Two "reasoning tests," constructed from models devised by Dr. L. L. Thurstone of the University of Chicago, employed the ancient, unsophisticated anagram test, which duplicates, in a very simple format, everyday problem-solving experiences. The ninety-one subjects were "normal," healthy students at the Central YMCA College in Chicago; two thirds to three-quarters of each of the three groups (control, placebo, and amphetamine) were males. The twenty-one placebo recipients believed that they too were receiving Benzedrine, a methodological procedure tending to give a placebo-effect in the direction of improved performance. However, all subjects took similar but not identical tests under standarized, true control (nondrug, nonplacebo) conditions two days before thirty-eight of them were given 10 mg of Benzedrine, and the third subgroup (32 controls) received no medication or pills on either occasion. On the "reasoning" tests, the twenty-one placebo-administered students showed the least drop in scores. (The authors pointed out that "the second form of both the reasoning and disarranged word test . . . [was] more difficult than the first," which helped to counterbalance any practice bias.) The thirty-eight members of the Benzedrine group showed a relative drop in scores, although their performances were not quite as poor as the thirty-two controls. On the anagrams the amphetamine group did the worst. None of these shifts were judged statistically significant. It was "clear that, judging from these two types of test material, . . . benzedrine sulfate has no reliable or consistent facilitative or inhibitory effects upon higher mental functions."[31]

In 1943 Charles D. Flory, who had been investigating amphetamines in the general psychology laboratory at Lawrence College since 1938, quoted an excerpt from a long, handwritten, anecdotal account by a student. He and his coauthor, Jane Gilbert, considered it to have a direct bearing on the problem of evaluating the comparative effects of racemic amphetamine sulfate and caffeine citrate with regard to "speed of action, reading rate, reading comprehension, and thinking ability":

> I have been drinking a lot of coffee for the last six days in an effort to stay awake late at night. At first it worked quite satisfactorily but now it no longer has the desired effect . . . Last night I stayed awake with the aid of coffee and determination until four A. M. I slept two hours until six A. M. . . . at . . . eight-forty-five . . . I took one benzedrine sulphate pill prior to writing my exam. [He does not specify the dosage; it was possibly only 10 mg.] I felt no noticeable effects until about nine-thirty. I began to get an anxious feeling in the upper part of my stomach. My mind worked very rapidly and seemed to be able to consider one idea after another with great speed. My hands were sweating. I felt impatient at the slowness of my writing, but I was writing at top speed. I wasn't confused. I felt "hot" intellectually, as though I were at my very keenest. My mind was racing, yet I felt that I had complete control of the sequence of thought and was capable of ordinary thinking. It seemed that my memory was clearer and working better than ever. About ten-thirty I reached the climax of stimulation. I felt happy, powerful, quick—every faculty sharpened. I took a deep breath and resisted an impulse to laugh and tell my neighbor how good I felt . . . Gradually, but not noticeably, I began to lose my excited feeling. By twelve noon, I could feel the contrast.[32]

Flory and Gilbert's knowledge of the student's poor performance on this exam convinced them that his feeling of well-being was more apparent than real, since it was obvious that his "achievement did not agree with the reported efficiency." This anecdotal report encouraged Flory and Gilbert to undertake a more carefully controlled experiment. Accordingly, they evaluated the amphetamine-test reactions of ninety-four Lawrence college students under rigorously controlled, double-blind conditions. Table 5 summarizes their findings. From these data it was impossible to attribute any consistent performance enhancement to amphetamine; the statistically insignificant increase in reading speed and analogies scores was balanced by the superiority of the control group in multiplication speed—as well as by its higher overall accuracy on the analogies test (not mentioned by the authors).

Flory and Gilbert also obtained verbal reports, which they did not analyze but presented as long, open-end first-person accounts. Parts read as follows:

1. "I was expecting a period of clear thinking, but found a great deal of confusion.

2. "The subject's belly began to ache like hell. The next morning the ache was removed from the belly to my head. The ache was dull and throbbing. It felt as if the subject had been on a three-day drunk. A decided letdown was experienced and the subject felt like a wreck for the past two days."

3. "After leaving the lab I felt nauseated. I became quite talkative and talked continuously. I acted very silly and gay. During the evening . . . I never studied so well or accomplished more in my life. I translated 45 pages of French in 45 minutes. I could not go to sleep all night long . . . about 8 A.M. and against my will I began to cry."

Table 5. The effect of benzedrine sulphate on reading, multiplying, and analogies scores.

	Benzedrine group means	Sugar group means
Words read per minute	458.0	453.0
Seconds required to multiply six problems of four-place digits	368.0	318.0
Number of analogies attempted	24.4	22.9
Number of analogies correct	19.2	18.3
Percentage of accuracy for analogies	79.0	82.0

Source: Charles D. Flory and Jane Gilbert, "The effects of benzedrine sulphate and caffeine citrate on the efficiency of college students," *J. Appl. Psychol.*, 27 (1943), 122.

4. "I seemed to think faster than I could keep up with myself. I felt foggy and became dizzy after smoking. I made mistakes, for I was unusually far ahead of myself."

5. "I felt light-headed and numb . .·. There was a queer prickling feeling in my skin and a feeling of restlessness. When I retired my body felt as if it were asleep, but my brain would not stop working. I finally got to sleep about 4:30 A.M. Two days later I experienced a tremendous letdown."

6. "I experienced an increase in speed but little increase in accuracy and efficiency. I was dopey and slap-happy. I felt dizzy and had a kind of buzzing in my head."

7. "At 4:30 my mind became a sort of a blank and I stumbled over everything that I wanted to say. About 5:30 I grew nervous and jumpy. Everyone seemed far away from me. The following day I was very foggy."[33]

They noted that the incidence of adverse effects was higher among female students, but did not present any further data or theories regarding sex-linked differential responses.

In another major experiment, Flory and Gilbert tested 129 college students, divided into three groups "equated as to intelligence and sex." Group I received 15 mg of Benzedrine; Group II received five grains of caffeine citrate (approximately 325 mg or about the equivalent of two cups of strong black coffee); Group III received inert (sugar) pills. Reading speed and comprehension were measured with the I. A. Booker Reading Test (Forms 1 and 4). None of the groups differed significantly in reading speed either at the start (no-pill conditions) or during (drug or placebo conditions) the testings. Although all groups showed some improved understanding, in every case the slowest readers improved the most, regardless of whether or not they recieved amphetamine. The reading comprehension test was used to check on the suggestion that "speed of reaction increases with drugs [specifically, with amphetamine, and only secondarily with caffeine] but the accuracy of work decreases." Benzedrine-treated subjects did worst on this test, although the differences were slight. The results failed to support the student opinion "that either benzedrine or caffeine are beneficial to speed of thinking as measured by vocabulary or analogies tests." Three points stand out: (1) when subjects "are aware of the contents . . . and . . . told that each pill should be stimulating, the non-drugged . . . improve practically as much as the benzedrine and caffeine groups;"

(2) no evidence can be found "to indicate that students in general can improve their efficiency by the use of either benzedrine or caffeine citrate. There are probably individual differences, but the non-drugged groups showed as much variability as the drugged"; (3) "the euphoria reported by many students who have used benzedrine . . . has little relation to the level of their efficiency. Reported clearness of thinking and rapidity of work are not substantiated by the group results."[34]

A 1963 study at the Harvard Anaethesia Laboratory at Massachusetts General Hospital confirmed these results. They gave 14 mg per 70 kg body weight of amphetamine sulfate (Benzedrine) to seventy-eight male college students of superior mathematical abilities, and found that the drug had slight (though statistically insignificant) detrimental effects on high-level performance as measured by a series of calculus tests. They concluded that the evidence "concerning the effect of amphetamine on performance on relatively high level intellectual tests is mostly negative." After each calculus test, a digit-letter coding test was given; on this amphetamine produced a highly significant improvement in performance. This apparent enhancement of simple thought processes did not contradict the "null hypothesis" with respect to advanced intellectual functions. The weight of available evidence strongly suggested that amphetamines, at least in low to low-moderate doses, could improve noncomplex mental functioning slightly in fatigued or bored subjects; also since the four-minute coding test followed a sixty-minute calculus test, it is possible that the sensitivity of the coding test to amphetamine was enhanced by fatigue produced by the calculus test.[35] Subjective data were also collected from an eighty-one-item "mood and feeling" adjective checklist. The results were consistent with an earlier report "of increased physical and mental activation, elation, boldness, and friendliness." Of the items, 37 yielded significant effects. It was therefore apparent that the failure of amphetamine to improve calculus scores could not be attributed to any lack of perceived amphetamine "lift."

W. O. Evans and R. P. Smith subsequently incorporated a similar self-descriptive checklist into what they called a " 'structure of intellect' model," for determining the effects of drugs on intelligence.[36] It is easy to criticize such attempts to break down intellectual functioning into naive categories subsumed by these artificial constructs; and there are further limitations in the factor-analysis technique, which assumes that there is one correct or fully adequate composite picture of a person based on a limited number of distinct traits or psychological and mental clusters. They believed, however, that this approach would be more fruitful in studying drug effects than methods based upon the concept of a simple over-all "intelligence." Eventually they used fourteen tests: eight measured cognitive powers; three, aspects of judgment; and one each for memory or learning, "need to achieve excellence," and "mood activation." The only "mental operations" improved by 10 mg of dextroamphetamine in their sixty male and female undergraduate student volunteers were "consequences" and "spatial orientation"; "logical reasoning" and "perceptual speed" were ($p<0.05$) impaired. Smith and Evans found that amphetamines had done nothing to improve general intellectual performance. They attributed all its observed beneficial effects on general intelligence to its "usual action of preventing a decrement in performance due to fatigue since performance declined in the placebo group with repeated testing," and to a distinct enhancement of the subjects' "need to achieve," as measured by the adjective checklist. They concluded that the effect of amphetamine on decisionmaking (and intellectual or mental functioning in general) resulted from its ability to cause changes in a person's "utility scale," and, furthermore, that these changes were probably related to greater felt need to achieve and higher level of aspiration rather than to improved ability to estimate probabilities. [37]

Physical Endurance

The question as to whether amphetamines increase physical endurance and capacity has been given less attention. In 1959 G. M. Smith and H. K. Beecher conducted six experiments on athletic performance. The first, involving swimming, was the most rigidly controlled. Each of fifteen college swimmers swam his preferred event twice a day for a period of twelve days; for the first four days he received amphetamine sulfate (14 mg/70 kg body weight); for the next four days he received a control medication; for the final four days he received secobarbital (100 mg/70 kg). The interval between medication and exercise was two to three hours for amphetamine and fifty-five minutes for secobarbital.

The time between swims was fifteen minutes. Fourteen of the fifteen subjects swam faster with amphetamine than with placebo on their first swims of the day. On the second swims, amphetamine improved times only in the shorter distances. It is also interesting that the improvement was less when the subjects were swimming in competition rather than alone. Needless to say, secobarbital was found to impair performance. Experiments two, three, and four concerned running. In a study of nine trackmen, three ran six hundred yards, three ran one thousand yards, and three ran one mile. Eight of the nine ran faster with amphetamine sulfate (same dose as above) than with placebo. The outcome with other track events and a marathon run was similar, and combining these three studies resulted in a statistically significant difference in favor of amphetamine.[38]

Not all studies along these lines have shown significant improvements in physical endurance and capacity. In experiments with treadmill running, swimming, and various track events, P. V. Karpovich found that amphetamine given one hour before testing (10 mg), or thirty minutes before testing (20 mg), produced no improvement. Weiss and Laties suggest that his results might have been similar to those of Smith and Beecher had he allowed more time to elapse between administration of the drug and testing. Haldi and Wynn also failed to detect improvements in athletic performance. Swimmers given 5 mg of Benzedrine ninety minutes before swimming one hundred yards swam no faster than those given placebo, 250 mg of caffeine, or 100 mg of Metrazol.[39] (This was a rather small dose; amounts similar to those used by Smith and Beecher might have produced different results.)

It is not clear from the literature whether an athlete's physical endurance and capacity are favorably affected by amphetamines. It may be a matter of psychological set; if an athlete expects to have greater endurance, he may experience it. The anticipated effects of a pill can spur an athlete on to greater heights of performance, like the psychological impact of an inspiring pep-talk, or of competition itself. Some athletes may perform better for longer periods of time under the influence of amphetamine because it masks fatigue and allows them to push their bodies beyond normal limits. Laties and Weiss cite a number of studies which indicate that amphetamines prolong the amount of time during

which an individual can perform physically exhausting work. The
dangers in this situation are obvious. Fatigue is the natural protective device the body uses to indicate that an activity cannot
safely be continued. By masking fatigue, amphetamine jeopardizes the athlete's—or the student's, soldier's, or truckdriver's—
health. As early as 1941 a paper by F. A. Hellebrandt and P. V.
Karpovich opposed the use of amphetamines by athletes. These
authors cite a statement by O. Bøje in the Bulletin of the Health
Organization of the League of Nations: "In the field of sport it is
essential . . . 'to avoid the use of any artificial stimulants whose
action is associated directly with risks of intoxication or indirectly
with the danger of whipping up the organism to extreme exertion.' " Bøje, whose work was done at the Laboratory of Theoretical Studies on Physical Training of the University of
Copenhagen, reviewed methods used to raise levels of
performance in athletics and concluded: "It seems likely that any
substance capable of stimulating the body to exertion beyond the
normal limits of fatigue set by the body will prove injurious."[40]

The sense of well-being produced by the drug may lead an
athlete to believe he is performing in a superior fashion when he is
not. Recently basketball player Bill Russell revealed that he had
twice used Dexedrine before a game. He considered it bad for
both his health and his game. The aftereffects were unpleasant;
he was unable to sleep, he had "dysentery," and he felt as though
he was on "a roller coaster ride." Where his game was concerned,
Russell recalled, "I was so bad that I was performing like an ordinary player . . . I didn't jump any higher . . . I just felt like I did."
After the first dose, he was so fatigued from sleeplessness that he
had to take another Dexedrine to stay awake for the next night's
game.[41]

Between 1962 and 1965 there was a rash of amphetamine use
by athletes. Adverse publicity compelled school and professional
management to investigate and at least reduce the use of drugs by
coaches and team physicians in preparing teams for competition.
Nonetheless, amphetamine abuse by athletes continues. The
team physician of the New York Jets, James A. Nicholas, has
pointed out a secondary, exclusively modern, danger of drug use ;
"Should an athlete require surgery, such drugs [as alcohol, barbiturates, and amphetamines] can complicate his anesthesia
severely, sometimes causing death." Dr. Nicholas relates the

story of a football player who took amphetamine, reportedly for the first time, before a game in which he suffered a concussion. It led to severely increased blood pressure; and he later went into coma for several hours. Without the amphetamine this crisis might not have developed.[42]

It appears that amphetamine can improve performance, mainly on simple and tedious tasks, by masking fatigue and increasing interest and confidence. It may increase the endurance of the athlete and enhance his performance in the short run, at the possible cost of overstraining his physical capacities. It does not help with more complicated intellectual work and may even make it more difficult by inducing anxiety, restlessness, or overestimation of one's capacities.

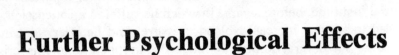

4

Further Psychological Effects

*"The first time I rushed I thought I
was in nirvana. I was tired and suddenly
my head was light. All the heaviness
and dust in my brains cleared out.
Everything was empty. Anything
that was to happen was fine, because
it was so easy to do anything."*

Sexuality

The relation between amphetamines and sexuality occupies a
small place in the literature. This is an especially difficult area,
because the connections between sexual impulses and behavior
and the central nervous system are obscure and complex. Amphetamine's sexual effects seem as varied as those of alcohol, and
depend as much on dosage, personality, and setting. Connell's
findings are illustrative: of the seventeen of his patients who reported on sexual effects, seven felt an increase in sexual tension,
five a decrease, and five no change.[1]

On one side are findings like that of S. P. Waud, who states
that "benzedrine in toxic doses reduces libido moderately after
sympathetic stimulation subsides." P. Schilder, in observations
on two patients who took amphetamine while in psychoanalysis,
found that sexual desire was diminished for both, despite an in-
tensification of diffuse object relations, or a general feeling of
being loved. Elsewhere it has been noted that "amphetamine in
the usually recommended dose will cause inability to have an e-
rection in some patients while not preventing an orgasm." One of
seven cases in Knapp's study of amphetamine addiction spoke of
a decrease in sexual feeling, and another of an increase in desire
but a decrease in satisfaction. E. Guttmann mentions "certain effects which are *not* produced by benzedrine. There is no measurable improvement in sensory perception, no evidence of sexual
excitation nor impairment of moral inhibitions."[2] One nine-

teen-year-old abuser has given anecdotal support to such statements:

> Well, I went around with this girl, see you don't want
> to stay with girls when you're high like that see? Like I say,
> you'd rather be with somebody else—me and this—uh—this
> kid had a girl friend too, y'know and we'd made arrangements
> to pick up Friday night, and then we'd get high and we would
> never show up— you know, like say we were supposed to pick
> them up 7:30. We'd be high, y'know, we'd get some beer and
> we'd sit in this party talking, and all of a sudden I'd look at my
> watch and see its 8:00 or something and say, "Aw the hell with
> picking 'em up—I don't wanna go there and get 'em, y'know."
> We wind up sitting in the park the rest of the night just talking,
> so I'd never, like uh, after a while you can't stand up a girl like
> that and expect to stay with her. But you don't care. It takes
> away your sex urge almost 100 per cent because another thing
> —like when you have so many of these amphetamines and your
> heart is beating so fast, y'know if you was to hold on to some-
> body, y'know it's like an uncomfortable feeling, even like if you
> kiss a girl you feel like you're suffocating, y'know, that's the
> feeling it gives you, y'know? And even if she presses against you
> tight it feels like she's crushing your chest, so I figured the hell
> with girls. [3]

On the other hand, the majority of references state that amphetamines definitely increase libidinal drive. W. H. Hampton
writes that "several patients reported an increase in their sexual
desire, and several indulged in elaborate sexual fantasies during
their toxic state." J. Norman and J. T. Shea, note, in a case report
of an amphetamine addict, that "during the period of addiction
to amphetamine sulfate his sexual desires and potency were increased." Rylander reports:

> The injections cause strong sexual stimulation in most addicts.
> According to my experience, Preludin and other central stim-
> ulants taken in this way are the most powerful aphrodisiacs
> known. The shot goes straight from the head to the scrotum, as
> one of my rather experienced addicts said, and another one sta-
> ted that sex stimulation is up to 50% the cause of abuse. The
> addict's term is a "fucking pump.""After a fucking pump I al-

ways need a couple of girls at the same time," two criminals confessed to me. Sometimes sex crimes follow the sharp arouse [sic] of sexual mechanism. One rape and one attempted rape were committed in 1966 on such grounds without the offenders taking any notice of the impending risk of being caught immediately.[4]

In their study of fourteen cases of amphetamine addiction, D. S. Bell and W. H. Trethowan suggest an interesting hypothesis as to why sexuality is observed to increase in some cases and decrease in others. It is based on the premise that amphetamines increase libidinal drive.

All patients in the present series demonstrated a psychosexual immaturity in keeping with their disturbed personalities. The increase in libidinal drive resulted in a disturbance of equilibrium with a breaking down of defenses and, in some cases, regression. In these instances, perverse trends became overt or exaggerated. Where the previous defense was in the nature of inhibition of sexuality, overt regression was either prevented by reinforcement of inhibition or denial of this by promiscuity. Thus some cases demonstrated the apparent contradiction that stimulation of sexuality resulted in overt inhibition.[5]

E. H. Ellinwood reported that increased libido "and polymorphous sexual activity most often preceded the [amphetamine] psychoses," although "the nonpsychotic group reported that amphetamine use either decreased libido or had no effect."[6] Although no basic hormonal change as the result of amphetamines has been shown, numerous reports suggest that a definite change in sexual performance can occur. C. Cox and R. G. Smart summarize this as follows: "Amphetamines have been reported to create or enhance sexual pleasure, although there is some disagreement as to the frequency of these effects. After speed use, ejaculation and female orgasm may be delayed so that sexual activity may continue for hours. When orgasm finally occurs it has been described as being far more pleasurable than without the drug."[7] This has been reported to result in "marathon" sexual relations lasting up to eighteen hours with only one or two orgasms.

If for many people amphetamines increase libidinal drive and make sex more pleasurable, it is easier to understand why the drugs are so popular. Sidney Cohen mentions their use by "ineffectual couples to enhance the sexual interval." Angrist and Gershon describe a female patient who "claimed that she had become orgasmic only after using amphetamine."[8] L. E. A. Berman, in a well-documented psychoanalytic case study of a woman in her early twenties, discusses the importance of amphetamines in her sexual life. She had started using amphetamines at age thirteen to relieve menstrual cramps, continued to use them as diet pills, and found that over the years she was using steadily increasing amounts: "In her social life it was the pill that made her vivacious, sparkling, and sexually active. It served to defend her against the intolerable feeling of weakness and femininity. She often took an extra pill before dates to prevent herself from feeling tired, uninteresting, and like a 'lousy lay.' She had to adjust her dosage carefully to avoid feeling too sexually overpowering."[9] One wonders how many people have tried amphetamines because of their supposed aphrodisiac powers, and how many more, who started to take amphetamines for other reasons, find that they provide relief from feelings of sexual inadequacy or boredom. The obligation often felt in our culture to be a sexual powerhouse and the high value placed on novel experiences could be leading many to experiment with amphetamines.

The controversy concerning the effects of amphetamines on sexuality has been confused by the fact that many high-dose abusers who administer these drugs to themselves by intravenous injection (mainlining) describe the intensely pleasurable "rush" or "flash" that they almost immediately experience in specifically sexual terms. Users have described it as a "full (or total) body orgasm," or an "orgasm all over your body." A twenty-year-old woman is quoted as saying: "When it is done right, when the needle goes into your arm, it hurts but it's like a sexual excitement—when the speed goes into your veins, you flash out—that's sort of like a shock—like an electrical shock or any kind of shock. It jars you but it's a speed shock. Then you get the rush which is accompanied by a feeling of euphoria."[10] Cohen says users who absorb amphetamines via the genital mucosa refer to this method as "balling speed." Such descriptions suggest that high doses of amphetamines may be perceived as so intensely pleasurable that the abuser is at a loss to convey the intensity of his enjoyment except through the use of sexual metaphors. An interesting point is that the "rush" is often described as superior to sexual orgasm,

which suggests that amphetamines may sometimes provide a substitute for sex. This hypothesis is consistent with the findings of
J. M. Henslin—although his sample (forty-two college students,
five of them amphetamine users) was much too small to confirm
it—that amphetamines do "not appear to be too conducive to
sexual relations." Three of the males were negative about the effects of amphetamine on sex. The fourth considered it, in and of
itself, a sexual experience, and the sex act miserably inferior by
contrast; for him, "speed *is* sex." "It's a sex drug. You get so
fucking—feels like you've got bubbles starting to feed and going
up and coming up the top of your head. Running underneath
your skin, you know—and you can, you just touch some chick,
you just run your hand down her arm or vice versa, and just
whew! It just tears you up! And it's all, you know, all a sex
thing."[11]

In a paper on amphetamines and sexuality, Bell and
Trethowan studied fourteen addicts. None had used other
psychotropic drugs and all had had psychotic episodes during
their period of addiction. In five cases amphetamines were reported to have no effect upon sexuality; an increase in sexuality
(marked by greater interest and activity) was noted in another
five, a decrease in three, and insufficient data in one. However,
the sexual adjustment of all but one of these patients was abnormal before use of the drug. Seven were frigid or sexually inhibited
(in two of whom, promiscuity appeared to be an attempt at denial
of frigidity). In another, a "heterosexually frigid woman, autoe-
roticism was enhanced" by amphetamines: "when given an intravenous injection of methyl-amphetamine this immediately promoted sexual fantasies and produced erotic sensations similar to
those experienced during masturbation." Two patients experienced intense conflict concerning homosexual urges. A third, already actively homosexual, became highly promiscuous under the
influence of amphetamine. "Although married she embarked on
prostitution, preferring cunnilingus with men she liked and coitus
with strangers. Despite her homosexuality she claimed she enjoyed her heterosexual relationships except with her husband
whom she could not tolerate after marriage. Like some of the
male patients . . . amphetamine markedly increased her sexual
desire but delayed orgasm sometimes for as long as 9 hours."[12]
Where deviant sexuality was inhibited before addiction, use of the

drug resulted in no change or else regression to a more infantile level, which caused the perverse trends to become overt or exaggerated. One user demanded intercourse up to twelve times a day, in addition to masturbating extensively. He became so annoyed at his difficulty in achieving ejaculation that he cut his penis with a razor blade and forced curling pins into his urethra. Another man, who had previously had an incestuous relationship with his thirteen-year-old daughter, bribed young neighborhood girls to allow cunnilingus. A third, who had been a nonpracticing homosexual since adolescence, after beginning to take amphetamines made a model of a boy's anus and external genitalia which he used for sexual activity. A fourth became an exhibitionist while addicted to amphetamines.

Obviously the abuse of amphetamine by individuals with poor or abnormal sexual adjustment presents a serious problem. This leads to the problem of its use by the young person who is passing through a crucial stage of psychosexual development when he comes into contact with the drug. In a study of 612 adolescents admitted to Remand Homes in London P. D. Scott and D. R. C. Willcox reported that: "in three cases parents complained that their sons had, on returning home in amphetamine intoxication, openly masturbated. 'He sat down in front of the television, opened his trousers and started playing with himself . . . his sister was in the room; he didn't seem to know we were there.' Another lad was observed to masturbate in the hospital waiting hall. This when it occurs is very suggestive of amphetamine intoxication."[13]

It is unlikely that such temporary lessening of inhibition does any great harm. But what of those youths who use the drug for long periods of time? Unfortunately, little has been written on this subject, and the reports that do exist are often anecdotal and much too general. Griffith found

> the attitudes of this class of people toward sexual intimacy to be very similar to middle-class attitudes toward food. They freely indulge in such behavior according to impulse. There is little courting ritual and such acts, although pleasurable to both partners, are rarely a concomitant of an implied lasting personal relationship. They cluster together when in groups—exchanging conversation, food, money, and drugs—and close physical contact is inevitable.

Such behavior gives a false impression of genuine intimacy. Behavior indicating affection, kindness, or love is quite rare and, if expressed at all, is very clumsily done.[14]

Fiddle paints a chilling picture of youths who view each other as "hostile or tempting sexual objects," the women treating their bodies as "dispensible objects."

From Haight-Ashbury observations Smith and Luce conclude that amphetamines isolate young people from one another. Many abusers substitute amphetamines for all interpersonal relationships after they have alienated their acquaintances by selfishness, paranoia, and psychotic behavior:

They sometimes had sex, but their lives were ego trips dominated by speed. A twenty-two-year-old needle freak named Terry later described this state to Roger Smith.

"It's a very personal thing to me. I always used to refer to myself as we, in the third person [sic] and when I did that, someone would say, 'What do you mean, we?' I said I'm so great that I can consider myself more than one person. The 'we' was essentially the needle, like, we're going to go home and enjoy ourselves, aren't we?

"It's a real party. You find with speed that you're your own best entertainer. To me it was a love affair. I was in love with shooting up; I was in love with myself. At times I would think of these sexual acts, like, female, come in here and let me do all those weird things to you, but when the final orgasm takes place I don't want you here—I want it all for myself. I want you to help anoint me in oil and prepare me for this, except that you rarely find a chick that will prepare you for this thing and then let you kick her out. I reached orgasms by myself at times under meth, but I didn't realize it until I took my pants to the coin-op laundry."[15]

It is difficult to know how to evaluate such reports. When Griffith describes sexual exchanges among these young people as "performed with the enthusiastic warmth of empty Pullman cars coupling or uncoupling in some dingy switchyard,"[16] one wonders to what extent his objectivity has been impaired by personal revulsion at their life style. Nonetheless, if the basic substance of the reports is considered true, there is cause for concern. Amphetamines, when abused by adolescents or young adults, may stunt their psychosexual development, possibly by impairing their capacities for meaningful intimate relationships.

Thus, a consideration of amphetamines and sexuality leads to several conclusions. First, many persons experience sexual effects from ingesting the drugs, whether these be increases or decreases in libidinal drive. Second, the fact that people experience (or believe they experience) an increase in libidinal energy, improved sexual performance, and greater sexual pleasure may be an important reason for the spreading use of amphetamines. Third, amphetamines are particularly dangerous in the hands of persons whose sexuality is abnormal or overtly perverse. And, finally, the question of whether the use of amphetamines retards or distorts normal psychosexual development deserves more attention.

Stereotyped Behavior

Amphetamine use may cause absorption in activities that strike observers as boring, repetitive, or meaningless. This is so common that a world-renowned Swedish forensic psychiatrist, G. Rylander, has suggested that the word *punding* (or *to pund*), invented by him, be officially recognized as a psychiatric descriptive category for a "new type of disease."[17] Punding is behavior induced by massive doses of amphetamines after the abuser has lost the capacity to perform complex sequential acts in a rational manner determined by the gestalt of the object or process at hand. Instead, he persists in repetitive and compulsive, but subjectively rewarding, manipulative tasks for hours or even days.

Many investigators have observed this behavior. E. H. Ellinwood has given some interesting examples of the strange collecting, analyzing, sorting, polishing, taking apart, and (sometimes) reassembling of objects—especially mechanical devices—to which amphetamine abusers become overcathected:

Watches, doorknobs, television sets, radios and phonographs, tape recorders, typewriters, and children's toys were among the common items of curiosity and analysis. Some were valueless, such as old television sets from the junk yard. Many were quite expensive, one man dismantled a $1200 hi-fi set. Another sorted, filed and put on display repainted electronic parts, both new and worthless ones. This same man polished and painted everything around. He tiled his apartment, including the walls, in Armstrong vinyl pebble tiling, then painted the individual pebbles red, yellow, gold, and black. Besides this concrete expression of curiosity, analysis and obsession with detail, more abstract visual constructive trends were noted. One patient loved to read blueprints; others analyzed materials for their weave, make-up, pattern, color and space. Two patients analyzed "in 3-D."[18]

Other descriptions of punding vary in minor details, although many place greater emphasis on its pleasurable nature. One speed abuser took apart dozens of radios, intending to build a new perfect composite. Although he failed to assemble his invention, "he cheerfully kept himself busy and nothing could divert him from this foolish task." Many "happy days and nights" were spent by another man "rebuilding" his car "by attempting to interchange even the most unrelated parts available in the repair shop."[19] Rylander goes so far as to state that punding is so intrinsically rewarding for the speed freak that, when they wish to persevere, "the majority do not have any feeling of compulsion, unless they are disturbed." But he emphasizes that, even when the amphetamine abuser finds punding unrewarding or unpleasant, he continues, describing how a thief began to pund in the middle of a burglary and persisted, although he felt "an increasing fear that someone would discover him."[20]

Recent medical and scientific articles on the amphetamines use the phrase "stereotyped behavior" when discussing the effects of amphetamines on experimental animals. Rylander stated in 1968 that the Danish neurophysiologist A. Randrup had "recently observed . . . behaviour in animals after large doses of amphetamine . . . which he thinks corresponds to my description of punding."[21] Indeed, as early as 1963 Randrup had contributed a paper on the mechanisms of amphetamine-induced abnormal behavior in mice, and since then has published numerous excellent reports on this effect. Working with I. Munkvad, he first demonstrated that subcutaneous injections of 5 mg/kg of dextroamphetamine in mice and rats resulted in clear-cut, definite, easily identified, and highly reproducible behavior patterns. (In one series, this sterotyped behavior was detected in all two hundred rats injected.) All amphetamine-treated rodents sniffed continuously, licked or bit at their wire cages, their own forepaws, or at times even their bodies,* and also "groomed" themselves incessantly, beginning about twenty minutes after the injection and continuing for the next two to three hours.[22] Increasing the dose to 10 mg/kg (that is, by a factor of two) intensified this stereotypy so that it appeared qualitatively different: during a period beginning almost immediately after injection and lasting about two hours, the rats not only displayed even more intense continuous sniffing, licking, and biting behavior but also crouched down and attempted to squeeze themselves against their cage walls or into corners; even exaggerated "normal" behavior like grooming ceased. Randrup and Munkvad conducted similar experiments on cats. Twenty minutes to two hours after injections of 13 mg/kg of amphetamine, eight male and female cats all began steretoped head movements which persisted and became increasingly intense for the next four hours. They did not move their bodies like the rats but merely turned their heads persistently and repetitively from side to side in apparent attempts to look at everything in the environment at once. But perhaps the most noticeable feature of their behavior was the hissing and spitting. Even a cat who had previously been the laboratory pet and was described as "otherwise very tame and friendly," began to hiss and spit violently about forty minutes after receiving medication.[23]

Ellinwood and O. D. Escalante have extended and refined Randrup's experiments recently, using much larger doses (10 to 50 mg/kg) of methamphetamine, and have differentiated two "stereotyped" patterns. First, after single injections of 10 to 30 mg/kg, all their cats developed the same stereotypy described by Randrup and Munkvad. However, the animals' sniffing was even more peculiar:

> The . . . pattern of behavior was that of compulsive sniffing movements usually consisting of repetitively sniffing the same

---

*In a letter to the editors of the *British Medical Journal* three physicians suggested a "simple physical sign" of amphetamine abuse which they claimed was "already widely recognized amongst the 'amphetamine fraternity' ": a characteristic "continuous chewing or teeth-grinding movements, with rubbing of the tongue along the inside of the lower lip, often leading to trauma to the tongue and lip, with ulcers visible to inspection at both sites." (G. Ashcroft, D. Eccleston, and J. Waddell, "Correspondence: Recognition of amphetamine addicts," *Brit. Med. J.,* (1965), 57.

2-5 square-inch area continuously for three to four hours after the injection . . . Often . . . a repetitive but abortive grooming response was interspersed with the chronic sniffing. For instance, one cat had a repetitive sniffing sequence . . . then suddenly looking [sic] to his right which then was followed by an abortive grooming response of his right hind leg. This sequence was observed to occur over 600 times during a 2½-hour period.[24]

Second, after chronic (daily) injections of as much as 50 mg/kg methamphetamine the cats were separable into two groups, depending on whether their *first dose* of amphetamine had elicited primarily sniffing or "side-to-side looking and fear responses." In other words, the cats no longer alternated from sniffing or "glancing" to hissing and spitting, but became "locked" into either chronic sniffing or "aggressive and fearful" behavior, depending on which type of activity had been primary during their first methamphetamine treatment.

In summary, it would appear that amphetamines, especially in large doses, can cause repetitive grooming or stereotyped behavior in many species of animals, and that tongue-licking, teeth-grinding, and "punding" may all be forms of a general, probably central, cross-species effect.

Perceptual Effects

Perhaps the most basic psychopharmacological property of the amphetamines is their ability to produce a hypervigilant state, characterized by a general heightened awareness of visual, auditory, olfactory, and tactile sensory input. Peripheral vision is greatly enhanced, especially for very slight movements at the edges of normal vision, and this increased visual awareness can become, during later stages of abuse, the stimulus from which paranoid delusions evolve. Colors may seem brighter and hues more distinct, and objects frequently stand out sharply delineated from their backgrounds. Intensified olfactory perceptions may evolve into systematized delusional mentation: one man believed that he could not only tell who had been in his room by lingering odors, but even "ferret out the smell of women, their sex and powder; he identified men by their body odor and could also 'sniff out evil like a bloodhound.' "[25] The "auditory threshold" is lowered considerably—the user hears sounds he normally could not hear—and this "hyperacousia" often causes discomfort. Although amphetamine users are notoriously loquacious and, unlike LSD users, rarely sit still, they are intolerant of sounds produced by others. Although most of the vivid and unusual sensory experiences caused by LSD have amphetamine analogues, one important difference is that while LSD and mescaline "slow down," "stop," or even "reverse," the passage of time, amphetamines usually speed it up, so that two or three hours may in extreme cases seem like ten or fifteen minutes.[26] Synesthesia is also less frequently reported with amphetamines than with LSD.

Tactile perceptions are considerably augmented by amphetamines. Even at subhallucinatory doses this may cause discomfort, and at higher doses it often leads to delusions of "parasitosis"—intense sensations of tingling, creeping, or itching of the skin. Many amphetamine abusers develop excoriative dermatitis or *acne vulgaris* because they unconsciously and compulsively rub, pick, and dig at their hands and faces. After chronic high-dose abuse, they may come to believe that they are infested with parasites. Ellinwood has observed that some of them gouge out pieces of skin and flesh with knives and surgical instruments, in order to kill these imaginary bugs under the skin, called "crank bugs." ("Crank" is one of the older Midwestern or Western slang expressions for amphetamine.) R. C. Smith, who has observed that one of the first adverse reactions to the drug is often the appearance of "crank bugs," includes the following description by a twenty-four-year-old speed freak: "It's just that when you're shooting speed constantly you start to feel like there's bugs going around under your skin and you know they're not there, but you pick at them anyway. You go through all these changes scratching. Once in a while you'll see a little black spot and you'll watch it for 10 minutes to see if it moves. If it doesn't move it isn't alive. You can feel them on your skin. I'm always trying to pick them out of my eyebrows."[27] Some amphetamine abusers not only feel them on their bodies, but see them everywhere in the environment. But, despite these distressing sensations, the amphetamines' extraordinary capacity to make people feel that they are supremely in control of almost any situation is in sharp contrast to the feeling generated by LSD, that something inexplicable, wonderful, or terrifying, is happening *to* one.

Volubility

Associated with this sense of control is another phenomenon, volubility, often so intense and compulsive that the user is too preoccupied with what he is saying to consider ordinary conversation as anything but inconvenient and frustrating—unless he adopts an attitude of superiority and condescension. Even when he seems to be listening, he may not be thinking about what is being said. Smith quoted one user's analysis of his own perception of these speech transactions: "Like, when you're talking constantly, you always think people will be glad to listen and you're sure that you know everything. If you listen, it's out of a sort of deference, it's because you're humble too." Carey and Mandel quote a "self-characterized Meth-head, age 20": "I take it especially because it creates within me this need to talk for hours. In fact, that's the quality of it. Lord help you if you ever have a friend who likes Methedrine and gets on it and comes over and talks to you the entire night." [28]

Insightfulness and Religiosity

Like LSD, amphetamine can produce a great expansion of the realm of "meaningful" or "significant." Ellinwood has observed a dose-related "sense of portentousness and significance," even in extreme amphetamine abusers who have not developed full-blown paranoid episodes. Many people in his sample intensively examined trivial or incidental aspects of their environments (especially stray words or phrases) and became deeply involved in elaborating what Ellinwood considered unsophisticated philosophical ideas about "beginnings, meanings, and essences." They reported profound and emotionally charged "Eureka!" insights into the "meaning of life." One exclaimed exuberantly, if somewhat incoherently, that "everything became relative to some truth; a light ray would prove unity; a light ray breaking up would prove why men break up . . . I suddenly discovered how the world began." "Future orientation" was common: one intravenous abuser remarked, "I began to put details together from the past and present. Now I think I know what is going to happen to this world." There was a strong emphasis on religion, particularly small or arcane cults, and astrology; many abusers have adapted traditional studies of the zodiac to fit private, complex, and incessantly discussed "systems." [29]

Seymour Fiddle believes this search for significance represents a pathology which is becoming more and more prevalent in our mechanized, specialized society, and which is related to the problem of expanding "leisure" time. He sees the speed freak as a caricature of the frenetic urban or suburban "time stuffer." Somewhat condescendingly, he describes how drug abusers "hunt around for mystical meanings and objects, play Japanese musical instruments to Buddhists' tunes, search in Chinese texts for occult meanings, and weave the whole into an elaborate time-stuffing mumbo-jumbo that keeps everyone on the precipice of meaning." But an amphetamine-induced increase in suggestibility rarely leads to hypnotic or slavish adherence to the precepts of a "leader" or "code," because the impatience and self-confidence engendered by the drug prevent the formation of any long-term, hierarchical, subgroup stratifications. As Fiddle points out, conventional or systematically rigorous religion holds very little appeal for amphetamine abusers, because these stimulants so easily "give one aspect of the religious experience to the abuser, namely, intensity of feeling toward the sacred."[30] This amphetamine-induced religiosity is characterized by a *focus* much more compelling, though more transient, than any "centering device" offered by most institutionalized sects or religious organizations. Furthermore, these philosophical, religious, and magical involvements or manias often degenerate—sometimes with amazing rapidity—into paranoid delusions, and eventually full-blown amphetamine psychoses, so stable group relationships are impossible to maintain. A reporter for *The Village Voice* noted that most drug cognoscenti recognize the vast difference between the religious value of amphetamine and that of LSD, mescaline, and other hallucinogens: "the Underground takes amphetamines seriously. Amphetamine heads are a distinct group, semi-quarantined and often regarded with apprehension by fellow hippies. Amphetamine is not a psychedelic drug like marihuana and LSD. The drugs seem to occupy opposite poles in the underground, in almost a Blakeian perspective of heaven and hell . . . An amphetamine comedown is not compatible with the love-joy-ecstasy trip."[31]

When amphetamines are used intravenously it is often difficult to determine the exact nature of the experience from the user's description. Carey and Mandel quote one speed freak's account of his initial injection: "The first time I rushed I thought I was in nirvana. I was tired and suddenly my head was light. All the heaviness and dust in my brains cleared out. Everything was empty. Anything that was to happen was fine, because it was so easy to do anything."[32] One could infer with equal justification that this person had undergone a genuine spiritual experience or that he had merely felt intense euphoria after a period of depression. Indeed, one of the major problems in evaluating the psychedelic experience is that for many—Huxley, Watts, Baba Ram Dass, Burroughs, and Ginsberg, for example—the experience was significant mainly because of what they themselves brought to it. Their exceptional literary styles have, in a sense, compounded the difficulty of assessing actual drug effects. On the other hand, perhaps no clinical report will ever say more than books like Huxley's *Doors of Perception* or Watts's *The Joyous Cosmology*, when it comes to conveying a full sense of what it is like to take drugs such as LSD and amphetamines.

Amphetamines, especially at high doses, further resemble LSD in their ability to break down our boundaries between the self and the environment. The amphetamine abuser, and sometimes even the "therapeutic" user, may experience distortions and gross alterations in his body image which are often (probably more often than with LSD) frightening. These changes vary from slight alterations in the perception of size, consistency, weight, or color of body parts to the conviction that one is transparent or invisible. Some amphetamine abusers have reported that the right and left or lower and upper halves of their bodies seemed separate or even antagonistic in action or capabilities. A few become convinced that they are totally ethereal and can transport themselves to distant places at will; others believe they can control distant objects and persons by thought, or are themselves being controlled. Ellinwood has observed that this "manipulation-countermanipulation takes more bizarre forms with some self-appointed shamanistic speed freaks informing others—especially initiates to the 'speed market-place'—that ' . . . you're a power generator. We can transmit through you.' Patients feel that they are not only being monitored, but are also being manipulated by hypnosis, radio, television, transmitters, and unknown power sources, with which they, in turn, manipulate others." One hundred percent of his sample reported "marked distortions of facial percepts";

these sound much like the more unpleasant LSD effects: "Faces melted, faded, appeared with stockings or masks on them; blood and bones appeared; eyes changed their slant or shone; faces became hairy, developed deep crevices and lines; they glowed and were transformed into those of witches or monsters."[33]

Another psychedelic amphetamine symptom is false recognition. Amphetamine abusers often mistake strangers for friends or even family members, accost them on the street, and initiate intimate conversations. Eventually almost everyone may come to look like an intimate acquaintance—or a powerful and treacherous personal enemy.

When amphetamines are taken at doses high enough to mimic some of the "hallucinogenic" effects of LSD, they invariably cause equal or greater impairment of body coordination, performance on even very simple intelligence, psychological, and psychomotor tests, memory, ability to change by comprehending past experience and applying general principles to new cases, willingness to persevere in practice, and other modes of acquiring and using information. Even at doses only slightly above the manufacturers' recommended "therapeutic" levels, they can interfere with ability to perform complex sequential activities, to coordinate related body movements, or to shift from one task to another as the situation requires. After hallucinatory doses or chronic abuse the short-term alerting or steadying effects of amphetamines are lost, and the typical speed freak or intermittent high-dose abuser is almost completely incapacitated, although he may believe that he is more than equipped to deal with any problem or to overcome any difficulty. In this respect he is completely different from the psychedelic user, who is generally aware that normal activities are impossible and prefers to remain in a contemplative, passive, and (physically) inactive state.

Effects of Short- and Long-Term Use

"Within five years the patient
was obtaining prescriptions
from several doctors (who were unaware
of his addiction) and had increased
his dosage to 250 mg . . . he became
very restless and suspicious,
complaining that searchlights
were being thrown into his bedroom."

Amphetamine Psychosis

Psychosis is often considered a possible effect of amphetamine use. Many medical papers contain detailed case histories of observed psychoses which the authors believe to be the direct result of such abuse. In addition to the 42 cases he himself observed, P. H. Connell, in his classic monograph, reported 36 authenticated cases in the French and English literature up to 1956. O. J. Kalant, reviewing the literature, found 71 authenticated cases, up to 1958, and 118 cases between 1958 and 1963.[1] Such cases are reported increasingly.

The earliest report of a relation between amphetamine and psychosis appeared in 1938, three years after the drug's introduction for the treatment of narcolepsy, when David Young and W. B. Scoville concluded that a latent paranoid tendency in two of three narcoleptic patients had been turned into a paranoid psychosis by Benzedrine. One, a thirty-four-year-old man, had suffered from narcolepsy more than ten years. About five years before the onset of his psychosis he began taking ephedrine; two years prior to hospitalization he became noticeably suspicious and began imagining plots against his life. Two months before hospitalization, Benzedrine at 20 to 30 mg per day was prescribed, and within a few weeks he had doubled the dose on his own. He began to fear that his family was in danger, that his house was wired, and that he was being poisoned. Medication was stopped upon admission; he improved rapidly, and five weeks later was discharged. In the other case, a twenty-five-year-old man had been suffering from narcolepsy for three years. He feared that he had developed a brain tumor or epilepsy and that the doctors were withholding the truth from him. Six weeks before hospitalization he began taking large doses of Benzedrine, again in place of ephedrine. He had hallucinations of voices calling him "homo." His hospital course was described as follows:

> Mentally he was alternately affable and irritable, depressed and appreciative. At times, he was demanding, suspicious, threatening and trying to escape. He often appeared preoccupied and bewildered. He was overactive and occasionally reacted to hallucinations. His talk was fragmentary and circumstantial. He told of his hallucinations, that people were accusing him of sexual crimes and of his delusional ideas that the doctor would torture him and emasculate him. His trend was homosexual and paranoid but not systematized. During his three weeks' hospitalization he became more at ease, although he impulsively smashed a pane of glass. He was convinced that the "voices" were real, arguing that otherwise he must be crazy; that was the extent of his insight. His hallucinations continued during his hospitalization and have persisted for over a year after discharge.[2]

The authors concluded that it might be better for such patients to endure the narcolepsy rather than be treated with a drug which makes manifest their latent paranoia.

In the late 1940s a few cases of psychosis occurred among prison inmates ingesting the contents of Benzedrine inhalers. J. M. Schneck encountered one case in an inmate population of 1,200 at the United States Disciplinary Barracks. Monroe and Drell, studying a similar population, found 25 percent of the men using the inhalers, four of whom were paranoid and had hallucinations. They emphasized the difficulty in differentiating toxic amphetamine reactions from the homosexual panics, transitory paranoid reactions, and acute anxiety reactions common in a prison population even in the absence of drug use. Nevertheless, the authors of both reports believed they had encountered genuine cases of amphetamine psychosis. Monroe and Drell detailed two case histories: in one, the patient admitted to ingesting 250 mg two or three hours before the onset of his overt paranoid psychosis; in the second, the patient ingested 93 mg in thirty-six hours and became confused, heard threatening voices, and refused to eat or drink, fearing he might be poisoned. They categorized fifteen of the amphetamine abusers in terms of personality defects. "All showed some pathologic trends in the personality structure. Nine were of the inadequate personality type. Six were considered immature personalities, with reactions manifested by aggressiveness (2), passive aggressiveness (2), emotional instability (1), and passive dependency (1)."[3] However, such data are unreliable because the authors did not control for psychiatric problems in nonamphetamine users or consider the influence of the prison itself on "personality."

Schneck's case was a twenty-six-year-old inmate with a premorbid history of a personality disorder involving aggressive and antisocial features. His activities ranged from juvenile delinquency as an adolescent to charges of theft and burglary as an adult, and he was said to have consumed alcohol to excess on occasion. His psychotic state, relatively acute and transient, developed after he had swallowed the contents of one and a half Benzedrine inhalers within thirty-six hours. He experienced paranoid delusions as well as visual and auditory hallucinations for two days. Schneck concluded, as had Monroe and Drell, that Benzedrine taken in excessive amounts by "psychologically predisposed individuals" could precipitate an acute transient psychosis.[4]

Norman and Shea reported the case of a forty-nine-year-old man who had been a heavy smoker and drinker for many years. When he was forty-four, a physician prescribed amphetamine sulfate, 40 mg per day, to relieve his fatigue and "all-gone feeling." The patient increased the dosage without his physician's approval, and within five years was obtaining prescriptions from several doctors (who were unaware of his addiction) and had increased his dosage to 250 mg per day. Four months before being admitted to a mental hospital he became very restless and suspicious, complaining that searchlights were being thrown into his bedroom, that his home was being watched, and that cars were following him to and from work. He became so fearful he quit his job. A month before admission he began to experience visual and auditory hallucinations. He heard the voice of his son (in the Armed Forces, stationed in Europe) and believed the boy was flying overhead in an invisible helicopter and that the stars were signals from him. He also decided that he was being tested by the government for a secret service position. He remained in the hospital for thirty days before his symptoms cleared sufficiently for discharge. The authors noted the similarity between this patient's symptoms and those of acute alcoholic psychosis; the visual hallucinations were the most prominent.[5]

In 1945 H. J. Shorvon wrote about the "Use of Benzedrine Sulphate by Psychopaths." Although he refers to the patient as a "psychopath," the data Shorvon presents suggest schizoid personality as the correct premorbid diagnosis. The patient was described as a reserved man with few friends, an anxious nail-biter, high-strung, sensitive, and easily depressed. From 1939 until his hospitalization he was a firefighter and went through the London blitzes expecting each raid to be his last. His general condition deteriorated until he finally reported sick. He had bad dreams, felt people were talking about him, and was confused and agitated. He admitted that he had been taking 125 to 150 mg of Benzedrine a day since the 1940 air raids. He reported that "it stimulated my sense of perception, imagination, and formulation of ideas" and provided the energy and sense of well-being needed to perform his job. Shorvon implies that the man could not have endured his war experiences without Benzedrine, comparing his need for it to a diabetic's need for insulin.[6] The article's primary purpose was to describe the drug's *usefulness* to a patient Shorvon considered a "psychopath," but Connell and others cite it as evidence of amphetamine-induced psychosis.

P. M. O'Flanagan and R. B. Taylor presented a case of a thirty-two-year-old man, who began taking 10-15 mg of amphetamine sulfate daily under a doctor's supervision. After nine months he was admitted to a hospital, and during the next six years he was admitted sixteen times to various mental hospitals, each time with the features of excitement, confusion, distractibility, and marked paranoid delusions; hallucinations were never recorded. Each admission was preceded by ingestion of a large dose of amphetamine sulfate occasioned by some stress in his life.[7]

A 1954 paper by R. B. Carr details the first reported case of amphetamine psychosis attributed solely to the inhalation of methamphetamine. A forty-one-year-old man was admitted to the hospital, acutely hallucinating and anxious, after using five Methedrine inhalers to relieve nasal congestion. After seven days of hospitalization he was asymptomatic, but agreed to remain and undergo a diagnostic test. He was given thirty mg of methamphetamine intravenously and once again experienced hallucinations for several days. After discharge he used inhalers again and had a third hallucinatory episode. In Carr's opinion this man's premorbid personality "predisposed" him to a psychotic breakdown, but no data are presented to support this statement.[8]

A.H. Chapman, also writing in 1954, emphasized that:

> it is often difficult to say whether the misuse of amphetamine is symptomatic of an incipient psychosis or precipitated the psychosis in an emotionally unstable person.
>
> It has been suggested . . . that amphetamine compounds, by inducing a state of distractible alertness, facilitate feelings of personal reference from the environment, and thus precipitate paranoid episodes in emotionally predisposed persons; whether the episode is transitory or becomes chronic would depend on the severity of the prepsychotic tendency toward paranoid, projective processes.[9]

A significant report by M. Herman and S. H. Nagler presented the largest series of cases of "psychosis due to amphetamine" published up to 1954. The authors observed seven instances of amphetamine psychosis and noted that many such reactions go unrecorded or are improperly diagnosed. Like many before them, they concluded that the typical clinical picture was a "paranoid psychotic reaction with a minimal disturbance in the intellectual and cognitive functions," and that the prepsychotic personality of these patients showed many abnormalities usually associated with psychopathology. Although five of the cases had used alcohol excessively, the authors considered this a minor factor in the development of the psychotic state.[10]

After in-depth interviews with twenty-five amphetamine patients at least two weeks after their complete withdrawal from all drugs, Ellinwood summarized their recollections of psychotic experiences:

Visual hallucinations started with fleeting glimpses of just rec-
ognizable images in the peripheral vision. The hallucinations
later became more individualistic: some saw God, people involved in sexual activity, tormentors, buildings crumble, animals, Martians, angels, and cities in the sky. Auditory hallucinations began with the patient's perception of simple noises
or voices which whispered or called his name . . . Often psychotic patients perceived voices as either friendly or evil, and
they devised elaborate methods to distinguish between them. In
the more advanced psychoses, the patient conversed with them.
. . . patients reported infestations of microanimals and the presence of vermiform and encysted skin lesions which they felt as
well as saw . . . The hallucinations became integrated into delusional material as the patient became more psychotic.[11]

He reported that the patients with stable personalities tended to
have more reality-oriented persecutory ideas: "they were in keeping with the objective circumstances of an addict group persecuted by federal narcotic agents. Among the more schizophrenic individuals, delusions were more bizarre."[12]

Most early case histories (1938-1954) stress the importance of
premorbid personality. One exception is F. A. Freyhan's report of
a forty-year-old man who ingested the contents of three inhalers
in three days and then developed feelings of persecution and fears
that he was about to be killed. Although this man had a history of
alcoholism and had been imprisoned for three and a half years
(during which time he had occasionally used inhalers), the author
noted that he was *not* premorbidly paranoid and that therefore
his fears and persecutory delusions might have been effects of the
drug alone. But E. H. Ellinwood states that, except for Connell,
few authors describe patients with normal personalities prior to
the toxic state and these are usually cases which developed after a
single very large dose.[13]

Beyond question cases of amphetamine psychosis do exist
where, in view of the patient's premorbid personality, the drug
can be considered only a precipitant. The ambulatory schizophrenic or preschizophrenic is likely to find amphetamine an attractive drug that seems to combat the progressive failure in
adaptation, loss of energy, and inability to cope with work that
are symptoms of incipient schizophrenia. In such cases the drug
may either bring about psychosis or end the remission of a chronic ambulatory schizophrenic. J. M. was eighteen, in her first se-

mester at college, and overweight when a physician prescribed
Dexedrine for her, 5 mg three times a day. Before that time she
had made a fairly satisfactory adjustment to college, although
there was some suggestion that she might have been susceptible to
a schizophrenic break (she daydreamed to the point where it inter-
fered with her school performance; also she had never been able to
make friends). She considers the Dexedrine a major cause of the
decompensation she underwent and writes of her first weeks on
amphetamine as follows:

> I felt special, destined, set apart. For the first couple of weeks
> I had super concentration on my homework, particularly an-
> thropology and literature. I felt I really got *inside* what I read
> and had amazing insight. It seemed as though a genius in me
> was awakening.
>
> I also got *into* music, classical music. It seemed fragmented
> and I could see sinister aspects of it.
>
> Nature—grass, water—made me depressed to look at it.
> Thoughts of suicide came simultaneously with feelings of ela-
> tion (after three or four weeks). I tried to commit suicide by
> taking aspirin and bufferin (twenty-three pills), but forgot to
> tell the psychiatrist whom I saw a couple of days later.
>
> When my ability to concentrate on my studies disappeared, I
> often found myself staring at the walls, as though I were in a
> trance, for maybe an hour at a time.
>
> I suddenly became a good dancer, and felt real sexual urges
> for the first time in my life. I had fantasies about a man in New
> York whom I had fallen in love with, but with whom I had only
> a passing platonic relationship. I would come out of these rev-
> eries feeling all warm and erotic. The fantasies became uncon-
> trollable and I began to leave behind a real-life burgeoning sex-
> life for a deeper imaginary one.
>
> I had shown promise in creative writing (winning local high
> school's literary prize), but I decided to give it up permanently
> because I felt that the nature of writing kept one a spectator of
> living, rather than a participant.
>
> The main problem (as it had always been, only now more in-
> tensified) was that I felt separate from myself. I felt as though I
> were both involved in the action and observing it neutrally, like
> a camera. I existed on different planes. My thoughts, moods

and emotions seemed to swim by with nothing to direct them, or restrain them. I had amazing thoughts. I felt completely divided into different personalities, each one being observed by me. Sometimes the other personalities disappeared and I was totally the observer.

I often felt buoyed up to a high spiritual level by some intense mystical force.

When I tried to commit suicide the personality that was most in evidence was the one that was ridiculous, pathetic. I had often felt kind of fragmented in the past, but now, whole personalities seemed to switch on and off; I really felt like many different people. I was by turns a kind of neuter, someone who appeared to have no life of her own and no feelings, or someone completely at the mercy of romantic fantasies, etc.

It is not clear whether her ideas of reference and paranoid delusions began while she was still taking Dexedrine or after she stopped. In psychotherapy with one of us (L.G.) for several years, she had been doing quite well: she returned to college and graduated with honors; she developed an active social life; her affect (the feeling-tone accompaniment of an idea or mental representation) became appropriate and there was no evidence of thought disorder. Then, at a friend's suggestion, she took 150 mg of diethylpropion hydrochloride (Tenuate Dospan), an amphetamine congener normally used for appetite suppression but recommended to her for its amphetaminelike "high." Three hours later she experienced a return of the disintegration she had experienced with Dexedrine several years before. Sitting in a coffee shop, she began to think that two women were staring at her and described the experience as follows:

When abused and want to fight back, or stare back: sour stomach, straw feeling, head full of cotton, can't breathe very well, all stiff around ribs. Feel like a mannequin—joints don't move easily; stiff, jerky movements. Move: go onto different plane. Stopped from participating in life (people, newspaper-reading, studying anthropology) by dizzying feeling, emotional dizzyness, of "too much." My head becomes light—change from drab to vital is too much—punishment will follow. Open up dark, secret corners of life (against Mom)—too much (unwholesome) intensity of emotion, like some kind of psyched-up violin playing—not words (I'm not human after all) leads to screwed-up emotions, as a punishment—like Faust opening Pandora's little box. (Afraid, head spins) Terrible doom as a result of expanding imagination. Proof: Edgar A. Poe, V. Van Gogh.

Fortunately, this relapse was temporary; all traces of it disappeared within four days.[14]

Types of Mental Disturbance

John Johnson and George Milner provide an excellent overview of the types of mental disturbance related to amphetamine abuse. Using the methyl orange test, they screened the urines of 370 admissions to the psychiatric ward of a general hospital and found 127 in whom the test was positive. Since this test is not specific for amphetamine, the investigators consulted the patients' doctors and confirmed that seventeen (4.6 percent) of the patients with positive urine tests had ingested amphetamines immediately before hospitalization. Of these, only two were clear cases of amphetamine psychosis. A fifty-one-year-old woman, admitted as an emergency patient in an aggressive and excited state, was disoriented in time and place and had visual hallucinations. All investigations of her physical state, including X-rays of the skull and lumbar puncture, yielded normal results. Within five days of withdrawal she spontaneously recovered. Were it not for the urine test, this patient probably would have been diagnosed as an acute paranoid schizophrenic. She had, in fact, been taking Dexedrine for obesity for three months, and two days before admission she had increased the dosage to eight 5-mg tablets per day.

In addition to the cases of obvious amphetamine psychosis four more of the seventeen patients exhibited symptoms of schizophrenia. Three had previously been admitted to hospitals with diagnoses of process schizophrenia; they had taken amphetamines to relieve depression or aid in dieting. The authors classified them as ambulatory schizophrenics, functioning adequately outside the hospital, in whom the use of amphetamine had precipitated an overt psychosis. Dependence on amphetamines led to admission in four cases; two were admitted for depressive symptoms on withdrawal; the others had committed criminal offenses to obtain the drug. Of the remaining cases, four had personality disorders and had been admitted because of acute behavior disturbances;

for example, one woman tried to stab the man she was living with. In the other three cases, amphetamine consumption was considered incidental to the psychiatric disorder.[15]

The Role of the Premorbid Personality

The premorbid personality and the drug's inherent psychopharmacological properties both must be kept in mind when considering amphetamine psychosis. Although thirty of the forty-two patients in Connell's study manifested abnormal personality and psychopathology,

> to say that amphetamine psychosis occurs only in people with abnormal personalities means little, prophylactically . . . the concept of latent paranoid traits, used by many to explain the development of paranoid reactions in patients who would not have been expected to develop them, is specious and dangerous: it is often forgotten that it is merely an unverified hypothesis, and its acceptance promotes a complacency which stifles further enquiry and shifts attention from the possible disrupting influence of the drug.[16]

Ellinwood believes "sociopathic personalities and schizophrenics have a predilection to the use of amphetamines and that schizophrenics and schizoid individuals are more prone to develop psychosis." In studying addicts at Lexington Narcotics Hospital, he found that antisocial or schizoid personalities and schizophrenic reactions constituted 60 percent of the diagnoses of the patients addicted to amphetamines, a much higher percentage than in the general addict population. They were more often sociopathic and exhibited more eccentric and bizarre behavior, and he suggested that "psychopaths" might prefer amphetamine to other drugs because of an initial "paradoxical" calming effect they described, an effect produced by amphetamine "stimulating internal arousal mechanisms and, thereby, reducing the psychopath's known need for novel environmental stimuli." However, according to Ellinwood, when these arousal mechanisms become grossly hyperactive, an overt psychosis is likely to develop.[17]

Ellinwood's conclusions, based on psychological evaluations and the Minnesota Multiphasic Personality Inventory (MMPI), obtained after rather than before psychosis, measured the post-amphetamine abuse personality, which may not have been the same as the personality before abuse. In other words, amphetamine abusers may be diagnosed as having been "pre-schizophrenics" or "latent schizophrenics" on the basis of symptoms that actually result from their abuse of the drug. Also, when the diagnosing psychiatrist knows that a patient has already experienced a drug-induced psychotic episode, or even only that he has abused drugs, he is more inclined to interpret any variation or eccentricity in behavior as proof of a fundamentally premorbid, schizoid, or paranoid personality. Accordingly, when discussing "addiction-proneness," the psychiatrist may be making a disguised moral judgment. In any case, one must be cautious about using the concept of premorbid personality, and not assume that most amphetamine abusers were schizoid, sociopathic, or neurotic before their use of the drug.

In opposition to the premorbid personality view, Kalant believes that in 109 of the 201 cases of psychotic reactions associated with amphetamine, the drug alone was responsible.

In 1955 E. Martimore, et.al. reported the case of a 38-year-old doctor who was admitted to hospital with hallucinations and ideas of persecution, but aware that he was intoxicated with d-amphetamine tartrate. He had begun taking 20 mg of d-amphetamine tartrate some months earlier because of personal problems. He took the drug intravenously. At first, with doses of 50 mg daily there was hyperactivity, marked but not unpleasant insomnia interrupted by periods of deep, almost comatose sleep, disturbances of the personality, anorexia, loss of weight, and mydriasis. A few attempts to give up the drug at this time failed. "I needed my injections to regain my calm." Progressive increase in dosage to 500 mg per day was accompanied by the development of delusions of persecution and he became isolated, seclusive, and morbidly jealous. Despite a decrease in dosage to 200 mg per day his delusions persisted, and in addition visual hallucinations appeared. Voluntary abstinence for 48 hours abolished the symptoms but a single injection brought them back and this led to his hospitalization. After 4 days of drug withdrawal in hospital the hallucinations and delusions disappeared completely. The authors note that the absence of pre-existing paranoidal traits and the complete disappearance of symptoms on withdrawal indicate a primary toxic psychosis, and in cases like this they considered the prognosis good unless the patient resorts to the drug again.[18]

Multiple drug use is another important factor. Forty-eight percent of Connell's cases had drunk alcohol excessively. Therefore, "as the paranoid picture in amphetamine psychosis and that in alcoholic hallucinosis are so similar, one wonders whether alcohol may not have been the main agent in, or at any rate contributed to, the production of some cases of amphetamine psychosis."[19] Often such patients also use barbiturates, marihuana, hallucinogens, and/or heroin. It is possible that while amphetamines are too frequently exonerated on the ground of previous psychopathology, they are also too frequently indicted as the exclusive agent in cases where other drugs are implicated.

The amount of amphetamine necessary to precipitate a psychotic state varies widely. In 1957 Wallis, McHarg, and Scott reported a case in which a mere 55 mg of dextroamphetamine appeared to precipitate a psychotic state in a twenty-nine-year-old man whose doctor had prescribed the drug for the treatment of headaches and depression. He experienced auditory and visual hallucinations and became so disturbed that he required hospitalization. Kalant, Connell, Carratala and Calzetta, and Ruiz Ogara support this with findings of their own.[20] At the other end of the spectrum, H. Isbell found that subjects could tolerate up to 2000 mg of amphetamine (type not specified) a day subcutaneously, though they developed acute confusional reactions, resembling cocaine intoxication. (We suspect these patients built up to this dosage over a period of time.) Hekimian and Gershon were able to determine specific dosage in thirteen of the twenty-two cases of hospitalized psychotic amphetamine users they studied. The mean daily dose was 780 mg per day, but the range was from 30 mg to 5000 mg, taken either orally or intravenously.[21]

Regarding onset, Kalant reports that more than half of the 201 cases she considered developed a psychosis within a period of abuse of two years or less; others went ten years or more before their first psychotic episode. Still other individuals have no adverse psychiatric effects after prolonged use: J. H. Bakst reports a man who took 15 to 30 mg of amphetamine sulfate daily for approximately nine years with no remarkable effects or any perceptible changes when the drug was discontinued; and W. Bloomberg found similar results with two narcoleptic patients who took 70 mg of amphetamine sulfate for thirty-two months.[22] In most cases the onset of psychosis is immediately preceded by the taking of a larger amount than usual in a short period of time.

This seems far more significant than prolonged use of even large amounts. Even in the histories of habitual abusers, it will often be discovered that just prior to the onset of the psychosis they had increased the dosage enough to exceed their own established tolerance level. In any event, it appears that the amount necessary to produce psychoses is usually many times the ordinary "therapeutic" dose.

The worldwide frequency of reported cases of amphetamine psychosis is increasing. From 1938 to 1958 there were only 71 cited cases, as opposed to 118 (160 if Connell's are included) in the next five years. F. Askevold reported that 0.2 percent of all patients admitted to a Swedish mental institution between 1947 and 1957 were there because of amphetamine abuse. In a survey of hospitalized psychiatric patients in Dublin in 1962, W. B. McConnell noted that amphetamines played an important part in the causation of presenting symptoms in 2.1 percent of referrals. And J. Johnson and G. Milner found that 3.5 percent of all admissions under sixty years of age to a rural psychiatric hospital in England in 1964 suffered from a "psychiatric state directly related to amphetamine consumption." They believed that this percentage would be even higher in urban centers. In their work at the San Francisco General Hospital, Rockwell and Ostwald did in fact find startling percentages of amphetamine use among psychiatric patients.[23]

In 1970, A. G. Blumberg, working with Drs. Cohen, Klein, and Heaton, found that a minimum of 60 percent of 332 young (aged fifteen to twenty-five) consecutive admissions to a psychiatric hospital had abused drugs immediately before entering the institution. (The authors define detectable drug abuse as the "self-initiated administration of psychoactive drugs such as amphetamines, barbiturates, tranquilizers, and narcotics.") This was a substantial increase over the 39 percent reported by Cohen and Klein in the same hospital only two years earlier. The most fascinating aspect of their report was that treatment in an open-ward psychiatric hospital did not reduce the patients' consumption of psychoactive drugs. The investigators collected urine samples without revealing their real purpose; both staff and patients were told that levels of urinary creatine were being measured. The study continued for 72 weeks, with an average of 27 separate urinalyses performed on each patient. Urine from 60 percent of the patients showed unmistakable evidence of drug abuse at least once while in the hospital. Although urinalysis revealed that 176 patients (53 percent) had taken barbiturates at least once, compared to 80 (24 percent) for amphetamine, the authors emphasized that whereas their thin-layer chromatography enabled them to detect even a single dose of 100 mg of barbiturates for at least five days after the drug had been taken, amphetamines could not be found after forty-eight hours, no matter how large the dose: "Thus the accuracy of barbiturate determination is almost three times as great as for other drugs, and, accordingly, our comparative findings do not necessarily reflect the actual comparative incidence of drug abuse."[24] It was especially alarming that over half of those patients whose urines were "clean" upon admission, abused drugs at least once while in the open-ward hospital.

Diagnosis

We believe that for each reported case of psychosis resulting from amphetamine use, a number go unreported or misdiagnosed. Many doctors are not aware of the existence of amphetamine psychosis; in fact, it is often mistakenly diagnosed as schizophrenia or toxic psychosis from other drugs. In reviewing patient charts, Rockwell and Ostwald noticed that when a patient volunteered the information that he had been using amphetamines, he was almost invariably given an amphetamine-related diagnosis. But when use of amphetamines was discovered only through urine analysis, and the diagnosing physician was unaware of the test results, he almost invariably diagnosed the patient as schizophrenic. Amphetamine psychosis greatly resembles paranoid schizophrenia. The condition is often preceded by restlessness, irritability, and increased perceptual sensitivity. In both conditions there are delusions of persecution, ideas of reference, and visual and auditory hallucinations, frequently of a bizarre nature. Reviewing 87 cases of amphetamine psychosis, Kalant found that 83 percent had delusions of persecution, 19 percent had ideas of reference, 63 percent had some kind of hallucination, 54 percent had visual hallucinations, and 40 percent auditory hallucinations.[25] Proper diagnosis, therefore, is difficult. The most reliable technique is the methyl orange test, paper chromatographic tests, or some other means of detecting amphetamine in the urine, all of which require a great deal of time, equipment, and expertise. Also, the paper chromatographic method is not always reliable, and is entirely ineffective if more than forty-eight hours have passed since the patient took his last dose. Histories given by addicts are notoriously unreliable, and even thorough physical examinations seldom reveal amphetamine use. The cardiovascular system can adapt to very large doses of amphetamines, so the heart rate and blood pressure may not be significantly increased in the chronic abuser. Similarly, the abuser's pupils may no longer show the dilation described in most pharmacology texts as one of amphetamine's physiological effects. (Combining amphetamines with sedative-hypnotics that cause "pinpoint" pupils can result in normal pupil size.)

Without information obtained from history, urinalysis, or obvious physical signs to confirm the presence of amphetamine, amphetamine psychosis often can be distinguished from paranoid schizophrenia only by the short time it takes the symptoms to disappear—rarely more than a few days or, at most, weeks, once the drug has been withdrawn. Visual hallucinations also predominate to an extent unusual in schizophrenia; and this and the relatively appropriate affect make amphetamine psychosis distinguishable. Also, the amphetamine-induced hallucinations usually occur in a setting of clear consciousness and correct orientation; the thought disorder characteristic of schizophrenia, in which affective and conative mental functions operate independently of any conscious regard for reality, is not present.

Carl Breitner not only questions the resemblance between paranoia and amphetamine psychosis, but also suggests that the latter should be considered a separate form of schizophrenia:

> the most outstanding feature of amphetamine schizophrenia . . . is not paranoid ideation but the disorganization of the emotional life. Depression alternates with euphoria and hyperactivity, the depressive episodes prevail, and there are numerous suicidal attempts. In fact, the syndrome resembles schizophrenic reaction so much that it can rightfully be called a schizophrenic reaction even though the origin may be different from naturally occurring schizophrenia.[26]

This statement is consistent with the finding of Hekimian and Gershon that the amphetamine psychotic's affect is more fluid and shifting than the paranoid's. Both seem opposed to Ellin-wood's view that affect is "relatively appropriate." Breitner of course is also disputing Ellinwood's assertion that amphetamine psychosis is distinguishable from schizophrenia. Such disa-greement suggests strongly that misdiagnosis may be blamed not just on the physician's unawareness of the possibility of amphet-amine psychosis but on the great difficulty in differentiating be-tween it and schizophrenia.

Were it not for a tolerant milieu many amphetamine addicts might be considered paranoid enough to be hospitalized as psychotic. On the basis of interviews with addict inmates in a California Rehabilitation Center, the Kramer group concluded that no prolonged psychotic reactions had occurred in this group and that none had required hospitalization for psychoses. However, these abusers were mostly members of a drug subculture which tolerated their paranoid behavior and created a medium in which they could function in spite of their symptoms. If they had tried to live in a more conventional setting, they might more readily have been considered candidates for psychiatric hos-pitalization. Kramer writes:

> Although the addicts felt that strangers were watching them, that best friends had turned informers, that apartments were "bugged" by the police department, that shadows and trees in the streets were disguised detectives, and that parked cars were police cruisers, their references, persecutory fantasies, and il-lusions were always realistically focused on their own law vio-lations. Auditory and visual pseudoperceptions were common, particularly at night, but some realization of the delusional character of these experiences was persistently retained. Para-noid feelings, thoughts, and behavior continued but simulta-neously our subjects knew that they were paranoid and did not take it too seriously . . .
>
> Paranoid reactions appeared to be accepted by this group as a natural consequence of their use of drugs and this awareness and anticipation seemed to have modified the extent of this ef-fect of the drug.[27]

Laboratory Psychoses

It is possible to induce amphetamine psychoses experimentally in human subjects. Such an experiment was first reported by

J. D. Griffith and his associates in 1970. Concerned about the ethical aspects of administering amphetamines, they selected as subjects people who had previously taken large oral doses of dextroamphetamine. Of the six males in the study, two had experienced psychoses while using amphetamines and the others were aware of the possibility. Of normal intelligence with no history of other psychoses, none of the subjects had personality disorders of the schizoid or paranoid types. Each was hospitalized in a psychiatric ward for six weeks prior to the study to insure a drug-free interval, then given an initial intravenous injection of 10 mg of d-amphetamine, followed by 5-10 mg of d-amphetamine orally each hour. The subjects were carefully monitored physiologically and psychiatrically and were required to consume adequate amounts of food, fluids, and salt. Five of the six experienced clearcut paranoid psychosis after receiving d-amphetamine for one to five days, the total cumulative dose ranging from 120 to 700 mg.

After a prepsychotic phase of several hours' duration, during which the subjects became taciturn and reclusive, refused to answer questions, and took an abnormal interest in detail, the psychotic phase began quite abruptly:

> Subjects who had previously refused to discuss their thoughts acted as if they had gained some sudden insight and began to discuss paranoid ideas openly and without reservation. Only one subject seemed agitated, and this condition lasted only so long as he was out of his room. The rest exhibited a cold, blunted affect and attempts to reason, comfort, or distract these paranoid subjects led only to increased negativism. The delusions expressed by the subjects were fairly well organized. One patient, for example, felt that he was about to be assassinated by a friend of his wife's and asked the attending doctor to guard the door. In less than an hour, this idea dissipated and was described, in retrospect by the patient, as an unreal perception. Another patient felt that he was receiving rays from a "giant oscillator" which was controlling his thoughts and making his skin tingle. He felt that this oscillator was also controlling people in the hall.
>
> Ideas of reference were also common. For example, one patient felt that a nurse may have been an old friend "in disguise"; another subject felt that a mirror was actually a front

for a hidden camera. This feeling that he was being photographed persisted despite his freedom to examine the back of the mirror. Still another subject felt that the name of one of the psychologists, "Kar," was a subterfuge to remind him of an auto accident.[28]

All the subjects denied visual and auditory hallucinations, and all were completely oriented throughout the experience. On discontinuance of the drug, the subjects became depressed. They slept for short periods during the first day and then for eight to twelve hours at a time on the second day. Paranoid ideation in one subject continued for three days.

The investigators noted that, although substances such as alcohol also can elicit paranoid symptoms, unlike amphetamines they impair intellectual capacities. This led to the suggestion that study of the amphetamine psychosis may shed light on the etiology of the functional psychoses. Again, the importance of predrug personality is challenged, since none of these subjects were considered borderline psychotics or schizoid personalities before the experiment. All were kept properly hydrated, which makes it unlikely that dehydration and loss of fluid balance are necessary preconditions for amphetamine psychosis.

In a more recent study, D. S. Bell found that he could produce a psychosis with intravenous methamphetamine in twelve of fourteen patients who had been dependent on amphetamine; the two in whom no psychosis appeared were the only ones who had not regularly used amphetamine above the "therapeutic dose range." The amount of amphetamine necessary to produce the psychosis varied greatly from patient to patient, and the psychosis lasted from one to two days in nine cases; for six days in two others—and was intermittently present for twenty-six days in one patient later discovered to have been taking the drug secretly. Bell agreed that the amphetamine psychosis is characterized by a clear consciousness and no evidence of schizophrenic thought disorder.[29]

Sleeplessness is a common reaction to amphetamine. There has long been controversy about whether sleep deprivation can cause psychosis. A study conducted in 1968 in which four healthy young men were deprived of sleep for 205 hours found no evidence of sleep deprivation psychosis. Pasnua and his colleagues concluded that "sleep deprivation per se is unable to produce psychopathological reactions which extend beyond the period of sleep deprivation."[30] It therefore seems unlikely that any cases of apparent amphetamine psychosis have been caused by sleep deprivation. (The work of Griffith makes it even less likely, since two of their subjects became psychotic after only one night without sleep.)

Amphetamine psychosis usually occurs while the abuser is actually taking the drug; depression is more commonly associated with abstinence after long usage. But there are also occasional reports of paranoid psychoses related to the withdrawal syndrome. F. Askevold described four cases of an abstinence delirium. Three occurred from two and a half to ten days after withdrawal of the drug; in the fourth, delirium began sixty-four days after withdrawal of the drug, but the patient was strongly suspected of receiving smuggled drugs for at least the first month of his hospitalization. These patients suffered psychotic confusional states of a delirium type lasting from four to eighteen days. Three of them had a history of barbiturate abuse, and in two the serum level of barbiturate upon admission to the hospital was 3.3 and 11.4 mg percent. Their symptoms were those of the typical amphetamine psychosis—acute delirious confusion, motor hyperactivity, suspiciousness, and visual and auditory hallucinations, without the vegetative symptoms like anorexia, nausea, vomiting, loss of weight, muscle weakness, and convulsions that predominate in barbiturate withdrawal. Askevold acknowledges that the possibility that chronic abuse of amphetamine and barbiturates may have "played a modifying role in the symptomatology of a possible barbiturate delirium" cannot be ignored but concludes that an abstinence delirium peculiar to amphetamine may occur.[31]

An especially interesting case was reported by Young, Simson, and Frohman. It involved a boy given d-amphetamine sulfate (20 mg daily) for hyperkinesis for three years beginning at age nine. When the boy was twelve, his parents terminated the treatment in response to his complaints of insomnia. Ten days later he began to have difficulty concentrating on his homework, and a day later exhibited paranoid delusions, visual hallucinations, and looseness of thought associations. By the next day his behavior had become grossly unmanageable and, apparently in response to a somatic delusion, he had tried to mutilate himself. He was hyperactive and could not sleep normally. Fourteen days after termination of the amphetamine, he was admitted to the hospital in an acutely disturbed state. He was suspicious, suffering from both paranoid and somatic delusions; he was disoriented with respect to time; he was unable to do simple calculations; and his apperceptive capacities were grossly impaired. The next day he became withdrawn and mute and began to assume bizarre postures; he later became incontinent. By the eighth day of hospitalization the psychosis had ostensibly disappeared, and two weeks after admission he was discharged. He returned to school immediately and demonstrated a fair to good adjustment, even though amphetamine treatment was not reinstituted. This patient's withdrawal syndrome is particularly interesting because children do not usually have psychoses which so closely resemble adult schizophrenia. One investigator (who supports the position that psychoses result only from the presence, not from the withdrawal, of amphetamines) refers to it as the only case in the literature describing an abstinence psychosis, and suggests that it may only be an apparent case, because the onset of psychotic symptoms preceded withdrawal of the drug.[32] Presumably he is referring to the appearance of insomnia; but even if the insomnia was an early symptom, the onset of the full-blown psychosis occurred well after the excretion of amphetamines from the body was completed.

Whether amphetamine can cause a chronic or long-term psychosis remains an open question. S. Tatetsu, studying 131 hospitalized Japanese methamphetamine addicts, found that 14 percent developed a chronic (as long as fifteen years) psychosis, with clinical and histopathological (lobotomy and postmortem) evidence of permanent organic brain damage. However, these may have been ambulatory schizophrenics or preschizophrenics whose psychoses were precipitated by amphetamine.[33] Ellinwood comments as follows on long-term effects:

[Five out of six] amphetamine psychotics, after withdrawal, still felt that many of their bizarre experiences were real. The question can be raised as to the long-term effects of delusional thought that became relatively fixed during the period of amphetamine psychosis. Certainly this is a difficult question to answer because of the interaction with different predisposing personalities; however, the writer has examined at least three individuals that still have firm beliefs in their delusional systems and still believe that their bizarre experiences were real, over two years after the last amphetamine intake.[34]

The question is whether the schizophrenic patterns noted after withdrawal of amphetamines are strictly a matter of predisposing personality or, in part, represent residue from amphetamine use, either in the form of a chronic functional or an organic disturbance.

In a study of fourteen cases of "psychotic states that developed during the course of amphetamine addiction," D. S. Bell found that all had "seriously disturbed personalities, but there was no common demonstrable pattern or single abnormality to their disorders." He believes that:

> a more plausible explanation than the activation of a latent abnormal process would seem to be that continued addiction to amphetamines produces a gradual reversible change in the activity of the brain, possibly of the reticular activating system. The continued and prolonged stimulation results in a disturbance that is so stereotyped that it may be regarded as a physiological [or neurochemical] reaction rather than as unmasking psychological "latent traits." A theoretical implication similar physiological "latent traits." A theoretical implication is that a similar physiological [neurochemical] mechanism may be involved in schizophrenia, giving rise to the symptoms that are common to it and amphetamine psychosis. Chronic prolonged and excessive arousal may be a pathogenetic mechanism common to both entities.[35]

A good reason for rejecting the argument that amphetamines only "trigger" a psychosis in persons who are already predisposed is the alternative hypothesis which more fully explains why some people develop amphetamine psychoses much more readily than others. This hypothesis also supports the view that the psychosis results from the actual presence of the drug in the body and not from withdrawal. Even before Connell's observation that apparently normal people may develop psychotic reactions, a group of amphetamine experts (including Gordon Alles) had speculated in 1957 that the development of an amphetamine psychosis was determined by some as yet unelucidated "threshold phenomenon."[36] They supposed that the development of amphetamine-induced psychotic symptomatology reflected a normal capacity of the human brain. It might be true that some of the details of any particular amphetamine psychosis were determined by personality structure, and that individual personality could determine the "threshold level" at which psychotic or schizophreniclike symptoms would appear. There should be no implication that a person was "prepsychotic," simply because he showed a low threshold for amphetamine-induced psychosis. But the underlying bioneurological character of this "threshold phenomenon" remained a mystery until quite recently, when researchers compared the psychosis-producing capabilities of the dextro- and levo-isomers with those of dextro-levo-(or racemic) amphetamine in animals and humans.

The transmission of messages between brain cells appears to be accomplished by the release of neurohormones like dopamine and norepinephrine, which are normally pooled or stored in brain cells (neurons) near the synapses, the points at which the branches of one of these neurons come very close to (but do not quite touch) the receptor sites of adjacent cells. When a nerve impulse in a neuron reaches a synapse, it triggers the release of dopamine or norepinephrine, which crosses the intercell cleft and causes the adjacent neuron to fire further signals to other brain cells in a similar manner. But once the neurohormone (whether dopamine, norepinephrine, or some other chemical) has crossed the gap and caused the receptor cell to become in turn a transmitter cell, it is rendered inactive; otherwise it would cause the second (receptor turned reactor) cell to continue firing in a random or sporadic manner. In the case of norepinephrine and dopamine, this inactivation is largely accomplished by a mechanism described as a "reuptake," whereby the neurohormone is transported back to the neuron from which it originated.

Amphetamines seem to act in part by inhibiting this reuptake mechanism, so that excesses of dopamine and norepinephrine accumulate in the synaptic clefts, causing the receptors to continue firing long after they would normally have stopped. The different types of amphetamines apparently cause differing degrees of neurohormonal reuptake inhibition. Dextroamphetamine is about ten times as powerful as levoamphetamine in inhibiting the reuptake of norepinephrine but has about the same effect as the levo-isomer on dopamine reuptake. S. H. Snyder and his colleagues demonstrated that dextroamphetamine is about ten times as potent as levoamphetamine in producing behavioral stimulation in experimental animals, and their findings have been duplicated by other investigators. Accordingly, it has been suggested that the CNS stimulation and increased activity typically caused by amphetamine is caused by inhibition of the reuptake of *norepinephrine*. At the same time, dextroamphetamine is only slightly more powerful than its levo-isomer in eliciting "stereotyped" or repetitive and "purposeless" grooming, licking, and gnawing behavior in rats, which suggests that the *dopamine* brain tracts mediate the behavior considered to be the animal analogue of psychotic symptomatology in human amphetamine abusers. This hypothesis has gained some support from recent experiments conducted by B. M. Angrist and S. Gershon on a human volunteer. They found that dextro- and levo- amphetamine were almost exactly equipotent in eliciting psychotic symptoms, while the dextro- isomer caused considerably greater central stimulation before the abrupt onset of psychosis. After administration of dextroamphetamine, the subject experienced an initial euphoria lasting about four hours, followed by deterioration of his logical thought processes. Levoamphetamine caused a more slowly developing but sustained euphoria with hallucinations.[37]

It seems possible that amphetamine-induced psychoses are basically the result of accumulated excesses of dopamine in synapses; the specifically paranoid element may be due to the accumulation of norepinephrine. If this hypothesis proves to be valid, it may be that the "threshold" at which amphetamine psychosis develops depends on relative excess or deficiency of available dopamine, or, alternatively, on the ability of the neurohormonal system to withstand the dopamine reuptake inhibiting effect. Similarly, the occurrence and intensity of the paranoid elements may depend on some relative excess or insufficiency of norepinephrine or neurologically determined susceptibility in connection with norepinephrine brain tracts. The point is that there appears to be no correlation between these factors and any "personality predisposition" toward "natural" (reactive or endogenous) psychosis.[38]

Depression

The depression caused by withdrawal from amphetamines has been insufficiently emphasized, possibly because it does not resemble the heroin abstinence syndrome. This common symptom has been noted by Kalant, Bell and Trethowan, and Breitner. Often there is a vicious cycle of amphetamine use and depression. As B. W. Durrant has observed, a patient suffering from chronic depression takes amphetamine for relief, becomes dependent, tries to discontinue its use, suffers depression as a withdrawal symptom, and renews his use. Depression is an important aspect of five of the fourteen cases Durrant cites, although it should be noted that most of these patients were taking Drinamyl, a proprietary preparation which also contains amobarbital. One fifty-year-old woman had been taking a half-tablet of Drinamyl daily for nine years; after withdrawal she became depressed and attempted suicide. A thirty-two-year-old woman became acutely agitated and depressed following withdrawal of her illicit supply of Drinamyl; the exact quantities she had consumed were unknown; on one occasion she attempted suicide.[39]

Watson, Hartmann, and Schildkraut investigated some neurophysiological aspects of depression in amphetamine withdrawal and found that depression following withdrawal was associated with a decrease in excretion of MHPG (3-methoxy-4-hydroxyphenylglycol, a metabolite of norepinephrine) and an increase in REM sleep. This finding regarding MHPG is compatible with the hypothesis that "some, if not all, depressions may be associated with an absolute or relative deficiency of norepinephrine or other catecholamines at critical receptor sites in the brain." Watson and his colleagues refer to the hypothesis that REM sleep, discussed earlier, may have a role in regulating catecholaminergic neuronal systems in the brain, and the increase may be associated with an adaptive physiological response. They point out, however, the possibility that affective state, sleep patterns, and MHPG excretion could all be altered by amphetamines and their subsequent withdrawal, even if not themselves causally interrelated.

All four of Watson's subjects became depressed after withdrawal of amphetamine. The one who suffered the most severely said, "I was too depressed to cry . . . If I had been home I would have killed myself." A second patient, though she denied feeling depressed, continually made comments such as "I'm getting uglier every day." All four showed considerable lethargy. The peak of their depressions came two to three days after their last dose of amphetamine. After four days the worst was over, but all patients continued to exhibit some depression and fatigue.[40]

Physical Disease

A number of adverse physical effects are discussed in the medical literature on amphetamines, and they have been implicated in some deaths. But since the evidence is anecdotal, haphazard, and complicated by the use of other drugs and the possibility of undetected pre-existing pathology, such reports must be considered with a good deal of circumspection. From the year 1932, when amphetamine (Benzedrine) was introduced as a therapeutic agent, to 1945 only three reported fatalities were attributed to it. The first, published in 1939, concerned a twenty-five-year-old college student, who collapsed and died while taking an examination. This young man was a good athlete and only a year earlier had been granted a preferred risk rating after a complete medical examination. His habit had been to take 5 mg of Benzedrine before examinations, and he had probably ingested 30 mg during the few days before his collapse, 10 of which were taken that particular day. Noting that it is highly unusual for such a small dose to be lethal, Smith mentions other factors that may have enhanced the toxic effects of the medication; the subject was tired and nervous about the examination, and had had a large meal just before it. As we shall see, fatigue increases the toxicity of amphetamine, as does increase in body temperature, which may also have been present. The death was described on autopsy as due to dilatation of the right auricle of the heart and gastric and splanchnic dilatation.[41]

In a 1943 report, a year-old child died after she accidentally ingested a minimum of 40 mg of Benzedrine and an unknown amount of ferrous sulfate. On hospital admission she was cyanotic and semicomatose. Respiration was difficult and ceased temporarily but was re-established by artificial respiration. Erythematous blotches appeared on her skin, and extreme dilatation of her pupils was noted. Nineteen and a half hours after admission she died. An autopsy revealed recent hemorrhage in the gastric wall and adrenals and edema of the lungs; examination of the brain was not permitted. Since ferrous sulfate can be toxic in children, it is impossible to say with certainty that amphetamine was the sole cause of death. The third report, which appeared in 1945, concerned a thirty-six-year-old soldier with a long history of alcoholism, who, with suicidal intent, ingested about 120 mg of Benzedrine. An autopsy found subdural and subarachnoid hemorrhage, petechial hemorrhages of the cerebrum, hemorrhage of the pons, congestion of the lungs, spleen, and kidneys, and pulmonary edema. The immediate cause of death was given as subdural and subarachnoid hemorrhages. Since we do not know the details of this man's alcoholism, it is unsound to assume that at the time he ingested the Benzedrine he was in perfect health.[42]

There are more recent reports of fatalities caused by amphetamine. In 1965 the *British Medical Journal* contained a brief account about a thirty-year-old woman, already taking phenelzine three times daily (15-mg tablets) and trifluoperazine, 2 mg at night for treatment of depression, who ingested 20 mg of dextroamphetamine. Within fifteen minutes she complained of a severe headache, called her doctor and told him her head was "bursting." She became comatose and her blood pressure rose to 170/100 mm Hg before her death. Autopsy showed a hemorrhage in the left cerebral hemisphere disrupting the internal capsule and adjacent areas of the left corpus striatum. A case reported in 1969 further indicates the difficulty of causal determination when multiple drug use is involved. R. W. Jelliffe reported the death of a nineteen-year-old boy on a weight-reduction regimen of thyroid preparations, digitalis, amphetamines, and diuretics. Death was attributed to hypokalemia with myocardial irritability and cardiac arrhythmias. "It is quite possible, however, that each medication, if taken by itself in similar doses, probably would not have caused death."[43]

E. G. Zalis and L. F. Parmley in 1963 added a tenth account of death by amphetamine poisoning to the nine already reported in the medical literature. It concerned a twenty-two-year-old man who, in order to "avoid military service," had ingested twenty-eight 5-mg tablets of methamphetamine five hours before his hospital admission. Intense efforts had to be made to maintain his blood pressure; he developed fever as high as 108° F; there was acute renal failure, and, when jaundice developed, peritoneal dialysis became imperative. However, ventricular fibrillation developed, and cardiac massage and electric countershock were required to restore normal sinus rhythm. The dialysis was performed, but the patient again developed fibrillation and this time resuscitative measures failed. Zalis and Parmley found that autopsies of the previously reported cases shared some significant details: "Diffuse petechial hemorrhages, cerebral edema, acute internal hydrocephalus with dilated ventricles, alcoholic fatty liver with central and midzonal necrosis, subdural and subarachnoid hemorrhage, acute gastric and splanchnic dilatation, hemorrhagic gastritis, and tubular degeneratation."[44] In Zalis' patient the striking pathologic features included diffuse petechial hemorrhages, cerebral edema, tubular degeneration, and centrolobular hepatic necrosis. Zalis and Parmley discuss what should properly be considered the lethal dose of amphetamine. At the time of their writing it was considered to be 20 mg/kg, but they point out that in the reported fatalities the dose was never that high, and in fact may be as low as 5 mg/kg for individuals who are particularly sensitive to the drug. Obviously, the factor of tolerance as well as individual differences must be considered.

In addition to the reported fatalities there have been a great many reports of nonfatal amphetamine poisoning. From 1939 to 1952 at least fifty-four cases of *acute* physical poisoning were reported in American and British journals, and there were many additional reports from Japan and Sweden. B. H. Ong noted that in 1958 alone thirty-eight cases of acute amphetamine poisoning in children under five years of age had been reported to the Boston Poison Information Center. Fifty-two cases of very young children suffering from acute physical reactions to amphetamine were admitted to one Toronto hospital from 1960 to 1963. P. H. Connell has drawn up a list of physical signs and symptoms of amphetamine poisoning which includes: flushing, pallor, tachycardia, serious cardiac problems, gastrointestinal disturbances, tremor, ataxia, anorexia, dryness of the mouth, insomnia, headache, dizziness, vasomotor disturbances, excessive sweating, muscular pain, rapid or slurred speech, irritability, dilation of pupils, fever, and profound collapse.[45] The 225 or so reported British and American cases of acute amphetamine poisoning probably represent only a small fraction of the actual number. Almost half of the cases reported in Great Britain are from the period 1956-1958 alone, and all the case histories from the United States were published before 1954. At least three factors have contributed to this erratic pattern of reporting. First, the

AMA has been loath to impugn the value of the drug. Second, a-cute amphetamine poisoning has become so common that hospital personnel regard the cases as routine and hardly worth writing up. Third, many of these cases also exhibit psychotic symptomatology which is hard to distinguish from acute paranoid schizophrenia; these are generally admitted to psychiatric hospitals and often misdiagnosed. The same considerations apply to the mere 252 reported cases of physical toxicity resulting from long-term or chronic use of amphetamine, the symptoms of which are similar to those of acute poisoning but more severe.

The amphetamines have also been incriminated as the cause of a number of blood dyscrasias; however, the evidence is not compelling. Myerson, Loman, and Dameshek mention a mysterious and astonishing polycythaemia—ten million red cells per cmm—produced by a daily dose of 40 mg of Benzedrine for ten days. This phenomenon may be related to the observations of S. L. Simpson, who, in some 1937 experiments on the effects of ephedrine on guinea pigs, found that the drug "probably causes extrusion into the circulation of erthrocytes, leucocytes, and platelets from the storage and haemopoietic centres, including the bone marrow." More recently, J. N. Berry has linked amphetamine to a number of blood disorders. He presents the case of a twenty-four-year-old man suffering from acute myeloblastic leukemia, and speculates that the condition might be related to his use of eight to sixteen Benzedrine tablets (strength uncertain) daily for two and one half years. There was no past or family history of hematologic disorder. We could find no other reports supporting Berry's speculation, but he includes substantiating evidence from the medical literature.[46]

The first report of severe muscular fibrillation and fasciculation linked to ingestion of amphetamine sulphate appeared in an Australian journal in 1959. The young man in question took up to 600 mg per day for two and one half weeks, in an effort to maximize his study time. When examined upon admission to a hospital he had severe fibrillation, and with percussion of any muscle there was a tremendous and sustained spasm and fasciculation of the segment percussed. The authors believed that this syndrome was very similar to that of motor neuron disease, and noted that before this case the central action of Benzedrine had "never been known to stimulate both the motor area of the cortex and possibly the anterior horn cells of the spinal cord, to produce severe muscular spasm and fasciculation."[47]

Nine years later four cases of a movement disorder associated with use of dextroamphetamine (5 to 20 mg per day) were reported. The movements were dystonic, grimacing, ticlike, or choreo-athetoid. Although muscle tremors are frequently reported in cases of amphetamine use, these dyskinesias, which are a fairly common side effect of the phenothiazines, to the authors' knowledge had never before been reported in connection with amphetamines. Three of the patients had evidence of prior (perinatal) organic brain disease, which suggests that dextroamphetamine may have unmasked a subclinical extrapyramidal movement disorder.[48]

Hyperpyrexia or high fever has also been observed in amphetamine poisoning. In a case reported in the *British Medical Journal*, a young woman of twenty-five was admitted to the hospital with a temperature, taken in the axilla, of 109° F (42.8° C). Her friends described her as "full of life and energy" for a number of days preceding her admission. Two hours before arrival at the hospital she had complained of headache and taken two aspirin. On admission she was comatose, her skin was hot and moist, and there was intense shivering with some neck retraction. Her pulse was rapid (132), and her systolic blood-pressure was low (80 mm Hg). The pupils were dilated and nonreactive, and respiration was stertorous and rapid. After tepid sponging and intravenous administration of 100 mg of chlorpromazine, her temperature fell to 102° F (38.9° C), but she died an hour later. Autopsy revealed 310 mg of amphetamine in her stomach. Since there seemed to be no other reason for the hyperpyrexia, the authors suggest that it was a manifestation of amphetamine poisoning. They cite seven other cases in which hyperpyrexia was associated with amphetamine poisoning; we found additional references.[49]

Some experimental work along these lines has been done. Although several investigators have demonstrated that some animals die of amphetamine poisoning without any significant rise in body temperature, studies by B. M. Askew have shown a relation between the degree of elevation of body temperature and the death rate of mice treated with amphetamine; death usually resulted when the animal's body temperature rose to 108.3° F (42.4° C). Environment has been shown to play an important role here: mice placed in an aggregate situation or isolated mice forced to exercise require relatively low doses of amphetamine to produce hyperpyrexia and resulting death; it takes larger amounts to kill animals placed in cold or isolative environments in which they are less active. As muscle temperatures rise, the spontaneous yield of lactic acid is increased. In experiments with muscle tissue from rats, D. I. Peterson and his colleagues found that increased concentration of lactic acid due to muscle fatigue or increased muscle temperature enhances the ability of amphetamine to produce neuromuscular block *in vivo* and suggested that this may be a cause of death from amphetamine poisoning.[50]

As early as 1935 reports began to suggest that Benzedrine might cause serious cardiovascular disturbances. The first concrete evidence was published a year later by E. W. Anderson and W. C. M. Scott. Immediately after ingestion of either Benzedrine (10-30 mg) or a control substance, the pulse and blood pressure (both standing and lying) of twenty physically healthy subjects were recorded. These readings were repeated throughout the day. Some of the changes noted in the individuals receiving Benzedrine were pallor, flushing, palpitation, and both increases and decreases in the pulse-rate and blood pressure. In six cases the effects were more severe and included collapse, multiple extrasystoles, heart-block, and pain in the chest radiating into the left arm. An illustrative case is that of a male, thirty-five, who after 20 mg of Benzedrine had a blood pressure change of 125/85 to 153/94 and a change in pulse from 85 to 115 in four hours while lying down. He experienced pain in the left chest after one and one half hours and in the left axillary region after ten hours.[51]

The 1936 Myerson studies firmly established that Benzedrine causes a rise in blood pressure (especially systolic), a rise in spinal fluid pressure, a decrease in pulse-rate, and a variable increase in the white (chiefly polymorphonuclear) and red blood counts without a corresponding change in cell volume or hemoglobin content. And J. H. Fisher, investigating the effect of 30 or 40 mg of Benzedrine, taken orally, on healthy persons observed a moderate rise in blood pressure which returned to normal after four hours in all of the subjects. (The majority also experienced a slight increase in pulse rate after one half hour, but after one to two hours the pulse rate was slowed in all individuals and was in fact at its slowest when the blood pressure was highest.)[52]

More severe effects of amphetamines on heart action were examined in detail in eight experiments by S. P. Waud. A healthy young man was given Benzedrine by means of inhalers at intervals of seven to ten days. The amount absorbed each time was estimated at 4-5 mg per kg. The toxic signs included: many extra-systoles for four to five days; paroxysmal tachycardia on two occasions after cessation of inhalation; rhythm of heart unstable and sinus arrhythmia present; slight exertion producing marked tachycardia and moderate tachycardia at rest for two days; and orthostatic hypotension for twenty-four hours after cessation of stimulation. A case report by G. A. Curry confirms these observations. A twenty-three-year-old man complained of numbness within three hours after swallowing the contents of a Benzedrine inhaler. After several days tachycardia with extra systoles developed, and he found it hard to get his breath. He experienced a severe anxiety depression and slowly improved when given large doses of barbiturates.[53]

An interesting case report of pulmonary hypertension, possibly induced by amphetamines, concerned a Swedish woman who, over a ten-year period, used a number of drugs including dextro-amphetamine, phenmetrazine, diethylpropion, kloforex, and phentermine to suppress her appetite. She first became aware of marked lassitude and breathlessness about three years before her death. Autopsy revealed very prominent atherosclerosis in the pulmonary artery and its larger and medium-sized branches which was clearly lumen-narrowing. Microscopy of lung sections showed pronounced hyperplasia of the intima of the smallest artery ramifications. The authors write, "the consumption of appetite suppressing drugs is large enough to be striking per se and since the disease she contracted is rare, we felt that a certain suspicion of a causal relationship should be entertained." Accounts of cardiovascular effects are corroborated by studies of laboratory animals, for example, the Rumbaugh team's study of five Rhesus monkeys, published in 1971.[54]

Some of the deleterious organic effects of intravenous injection of dissolved amphetamine tablets are produced by the talc or cornstarch filler rather than by the drug itself, and in a 1969 study two patients who had been injecting dissolved methylphenidate hydrochloride (Ritalin) tablets showed granulomas of talc in the lungs and heartvalves on autopsy. Another study demonstrated this phenomenon, in which aggregates of granulomas form larger lesions composed of histiocytes and foreign-body giant cells. There have also been reports of deposits of talc in the liver, spleen, and kidneys. In a very recent study W. E. Atlee found ocular involvement in seventeen patients using intravenous methylphenidate hydrochloride. Although only one of them had complained of any visual difficulties, upon examination characteristic embolic particles concentrated in the macular regions could readily be seen ophthalmoscopically in all seventeen. The number of particles was roughly correlated with the amount of the drug taken and the duration of its use. In addition, macular edema, venous engorgement, and several blotch hemorrhages were seen. An autopsy on one of the patients confirmed histologically the presence of these talc particles in both the retina and the choroid.[55]

Perhaps the most startling data concern the brain. We have already referred to the possibility of permanent organic brain damage in connection with psychosis in chronic amphetamine abuse. Although the reported amphetamine users often had been using other drugs as well or had pre-existing organic conditions, there is compelling evidence that amphetamines can cause severe brain damage. B. P. Citron, who noted deterioration of the small blood vessels of the brain in fourteen hospitalized drug abusers, demonstrated that this pathology was necrotizing angiitis, and could also be found in the renal and other visceral arteries. Necrotizing angiitis is a sometimes fatal vascular disease characterized by inflammation and fibrinoid necrosis. Four of Citron's subjects died of this disease, and postmortem findings on them (all of whom had used large amounts of amphetamine) are detailed. Dr. Citron cautiously concludes: "An inescapable inference from this report is that drug abuse may be a factor in necrotizing angiitis."[56] (Though concerned mainly with amphetamine, he realizes it is not possible to establish a single cause when a number of drugs are being used.)

Alarmed by soaring stroke rates among fifteen- to twenty-five-year-olds in southern California, R. C. Rumbaugh and his associates at the University of Southern California Medical Center, have done considerable work in the area of drug-induced brain damage. They have found that stroke frequently occurs in young people who have a history of drug use, in particular the intravenous injection of methamphetamine. Amphetamines cause a constriction of small blood vessels which, if massive, can block or deform the vessels of the brain. **Rumbaugh** points out that, although this may be partly responsible for the stroke pattern, in his nineteen case histories many other factors were involved. Often these abusers were using other drugs such as heroin. The role of impurities was uncertain. When the drugs are diluted with urine or tap water, foreign protein sensitivity with antigen-antibody reactions may arise. Sepsis is another frequent complication with intravenous drug abusers, and home remedies for drug overdose can cause brain damage. Patients have arrived at hospitals comatose from injections of milk and even mayonnaise. The authors summarized their findings:

> Cerebral arteriography demonstrated a beaded, irregular appearance of many of the cerebral arteries, with irregular segmental changes of caliber and contour of the vessel walls. The most common finding in these patients, however, was small artery occlusive disease. One could observe numerous small caliber cerebral arteries (1 mm and less in diameter) with short segments of slow flow and/or complete block. At these sites, a faint smudge or stain could frequently be identified. This smudge or stain may represent slow flow in surrounding capillary beds or actual extravasation of contrast medium through the endothelial lining of the arterioles, capillaries, or venules at these sites of vascular injury.
>
> Whether these changes actually are residua of embolic phenomena with resulting vascular endothelial damage and ischemia, whether they represent a primary vasculitis, which in turn results in small vessel occlusions, or whether both mechanisms of vascular injury are occurring is not yet established.

Three illustrative case histories follow:

A thirty-seven-year-old man was admitted to the hospital in coma, with a laceration of the skin over the left eye. He had a history of drug abuse with intravenous heroin and intravenous Methedrine. Cerebral arteriography demonstrated extensive small artery occlusive changes. A repeat cerebral arteriogram one week later showed no change.

A thirty-two-year-old woman was admitted in coma. The drug abuse history consisted of intravenous amphetamines and barbiturates in addition to alcohol abuse. Cerebral arteriographic findings consisted of a moderate number of small artery occlusive changes.

A twenty-four-year-old man presented with a right hemiparesis. There was a drug abuse history with barbiturates and amphetamines. Cerebral arteriographic findings consisted of a minimal number of beaded irregular arterial changes and an extensive number of small arterial occlusive changes.[57]

In their work with Rhesus monkeys, the Rumbaugh team noted that in some of them, within ten minutes of amphetamine injection, many of the very small arterial branches of the anterior and middle cerebral arteries and of the lenticulostriate arteries decreased in caliber as shown by carotid arteriography. After injections of 1.5 mg/kg body weight of methamphetamine (tablets dissolved in normal saline) or of pure normal saline (for the controls) every other day for two weeks, the monkeys were killed and autopsied. The two controls showed no evidence whatsoever of brain damage, whereas the others had irreversible brain damage in the areas around the small blood vessels including focal areas of ischemia and infarction and generalized areas of cerebral edema and ischemic nerve cell changes. This is similar to the damage found in human stroke victims. The authors were amazed that animals suffering from such extensive brain damage were able to function as well as they did by the end of the two weeks.[58] The amount of amphetamine was about the same per unit body weight as that of a fairly low dose (50 to 100 mg intravenously) taken by a typical speed freak.

S. J. Goodman and D. P. Becker presented two cases of intracranial hemorrhage after ingestion of amphetamine. In one, an eighteen-year-old boy was admitted to a hospital suffering from a severe bifrontal headache after a single seizure. For several months he had been taking two to three 10-mg dextroamphetamine sulfate tablets a day. Two days before admission he had taken 50 mg orally in less than an hour. A lumbar puncture was performed, and the findings of an opening pressure of 470 mm and grossly bloody cerebral spinal fluid with supernatant xanthochromia established the diagnosis as intracranial hemorrhage. In the second case a twenty-six-year-old man, who in the past had taken up to fifteen tablets ("bennies") a day (strength unknown), was admitted to a hospital complaining of progressive lethargy and left-sided weakness. One month earlier he had begun taking speed intravenously (dosages again unknown), noticing severe right frontal headaches after each injection: "A carotid angiogram showed a large avascular right frontoparietal mass with a 10 mm anterior and posterior midline shift. At right frontal craniotomy, a 75 to 100 cc partially clotted intracerebral hematoma was evacuated from a deep basal frontal location . . . Also noted were multifocal areas of pia-arachnoid adhesions that suggested some preexisting inflammatory disease." In these cases, as well as in three similar cases of subdural and subarachnoid hemorrhage which occurred within hours of the ingestion of amphetamine, the authors believe that two factors are involved: the hypertensive effect of the drug and a pre-existing vascular lesion. "Either an intracranial aneurysm or an arteriovenous malformation could serve as a locus minoris resistentiae in an individual suddenly become hypertensive." They suggest that the first patient may have had a small aneurysm that ruptured, and the second patient a pre-existing vascular lesion. S. R. Weiss and his colleagues reported two additional instances of intracerebral hematoma which they concluded were caused by metamphetamine (in one case taken intravenously, in the other orally).[59]

Teratogenic Properties

The effects of d-amphetamine sulfate on the fetus have been explored in a number of animal studies. R. W. Bell and his colleagues injected a number of pregnant female Long-Evans Hooded rats with 3.0 mg/kg body weight of a 0.9 mg/1.0 cc solution of d-amphetamine sulfate. The injections were administered either between six and nine days postconception (when the fetal stomach and intestine are developing), or between twelve and fifteen days postconception. The offspring were characterized by modified emotionality as measured by activity level in open field trials and a greater tendency to develop gastrointestinal ulcers. Other rats injected with 1.5 cc/kg body weight of distilled water did not produce offspring with these characteristics.[60]

In 1962 a warning was issued by the manufacturer of Preludin (phenmetrazine hydrochloride) that the drug should not be used in early pregnancy until a possible causal link with congenital malformation had been investigated. Shortly thereafter the *British Medical Journal* published the case history of a mother who had taken phenmetrazine for approximately the first six weeks of her pregnancy; her child was born with deformities of the lower limbs and one hand. Another case history cited in the same journal presented convincing evidence of teratogenic properties. During two of six pregnancies, a woman took Preludin, three 25-mg tablets per day, from the fourth to the twelfth weeks. Her first, second, third, and fifth pregnancies, during which she took no medication, resulted in normal children; the fourth and sixth pregnancies, during which Preludin was ingested, produced infants with almost identical abnormalities.[61] As a result of this report, the sale of phenmetrazine was temporarily banned by the Italian government, and a letter was sent by the manufacturer to all physicians in West Germany and France warning against the use of the drug by pregnant women.

In a more recent study two hundred forty women were studied during their pregnancies following initial prenatal visits to a hospital. Thirty-one of them (13 percent) took an appetite suppressant, most often dextroamphetamine sulfate, during the first trimester; and 65 sometime during pregnancy. Eight delivered babies with major malformations. Three of these eight took an appetite suppressant in the first trimester, and a fourth took one in the second trimester. However, the authors relied on the women's memories, which may have been unreliable; also there was a high incidence of multiple drug use.[62] Data like these, although they may not establish a causal link, do cause suspicion, and the fact that almost all these women had taken the amphetamines on prescription suggests a lack of knowledge or good judgment on the part of many physicians.

In summary, there is substantial evidence for the psychological and physiological damage that can be caused by the use of amphetamines. Numerous studies suggest that there is an amphetamine psychosis, although multiple drug use and premorbid pathology complicate the investigations. Regarding physiological reactions studies with humans implicate amphetamine misuse in cases of blood dyscrasia, movement disorder, and hyperpyrexia. Animal studies corroborate instances of damage to the fetus, the brain, and the cardiovascular system. Although evidence is not sound and is clouded by the possibilities of pre-existing pathology and the use of other drugs, fatalities have been attributed to amphetamine abuse. Despite all the qualifications, research to date points unquestionably to the harmful effects of short- and long-term amphetamine misuse.

Habituation, Dependence, and Addiction

"The symptoms of withdrawal were so severe that at times I couldn't think who I was and other times where I lived; the floor was coming up at me and the walls seemed to move. At night people would break in or just come into the room and terrify me, while to an onlooker I slept peacefully next to my husband."

Scientific debate about "drug addiction" has been plagued by a confusion of terminology reflecting the confusion in underlying concepts. Drugs have been described as "addictive" rather than "only habituating" or "dependence-producing" on the most varied grounds and for the most diverse reasons. Understandably, where physiological, psychological, and social issues are so inextricably entangled, conceptual clarity is hard to achieve. And in this case the confusion has been compounded by two factors. One is the tendency to regard opiates as the pardigm or model for *all* drug dependence. The other is that moral attitudes toward the use of psychoactive drugs have hardened into legal misclassification and culturally approved definitions of "addictiveness" that have little relevance to either the pharmacological nature of the drugs or the needs of society.

Terminology

As there is no medically recognized criterion of addictiveness there is no disease, with clearly defined symptoms, called drug addiction. The classification is basically a social and moral one. Because of this and because of the term's misleading connotations, the World Health Organization (WHO) has recommended substituting "dependence" for it. The very vagueness and neutrality of this word is a virtue. Questions about psychoactive drugs and their abuse focus on the most complex and least easily definable issues in the relation between mind and body or individual psychology and social setting, and a term like dependence is helpful because it makes few premature ideological or pseudoscientific commitments but leaves the field open for exploration. We will use it wherever possible. Nevertheless, we will continue to use "addiction" because of its currency in popular speech, and because its association with the opiates helps to emphasize the similarities between opiate and amphetamine dependence. Recalling Aristotle's comment that it is the mark of an educated mind to demand no more precision than the subject warrants, we choose to give not a precise definition but a general working characterization of "addiction": drug dependence that does some harm to the user and society and is associated with a fairly severe physiological abstinence syndrome or "withdrawal reaction," usually connected with the development of tolerance to the drug's effects and therefore a tendency to increase the dose.

In 1931 A. L. Tatum and M. H. Seevers, noting that much confusion existed concerning the significance of terms employed in discussing drug addiction, differentiated addiction from habituation in nontechnical terms: "Habituation is a condition in which the habitué desires a drug but suffers no ill effects on its discontinuance. Addiction is a condition developed through the effects of repeated actions of a drug such that its use becomes necessary and cessation of its action causes mental or physical disturbances." Thirty-one years later Seevers admitted that neither he nor Tatum had ever been satisfied with these simple definitions.[1] The difficulty in distinguishing between addiction and habituation continued to plague commentators. In 1937 C. K. Himmelsbach and L. F. Small suggested new definitions, using several technical terms that appear in most subsequent versions:

> By habituation is meant the psychical phenomenon of adaptation and mental conditioning to the repetition of an effect. Habituation to opiates is probably more intense than habituation to other substances. In a sense habituation represents psychical dependence.
>
> Addiction to opiates embraces three intimately related but distinct phenomena, namely tolerance, habituation, and dependence. These phenomena make up the psychosomatic complex known as addiction and are intricately interwoven and interdependent.[2]

Since this attempt to distinguish drug addiction from drug habituation, numerous and increasingly complex definitions have been advanced. The one most often referred to is that of the WHO's Expert Committee on Addiction-Producing Drugs, first stated in 1950, reformulated in 1952, and given final form in 1957:

> Drug addiction is a state of periodic or chronic intoxication produced by the repeated consumption of a drug (natural or synthetic). Its characteristics include: (1) an overwhelming desire or need (compulsion) to continue taking the drug and to obtain it by any means; (2) a tendency to increase the dose; (3) a psychic (psychological) and generally a physical dependence on the effects of the drug; (4) detrimental effect on the individual and on society.
>
> Drug habituation (habit) is a condition resulting from the repeated consumption of a drug. Its characteristics include: (1) a desire (but not a compulsion) to continue taking the drug for the sense of improved well-being which it engenders; (2) little or no tendency to increase the dose; (3) some degree of psychic dependence on the effect of the drug, but absence of physical dependence and hence of an abstinence syndrome; (4) detrimental effects, if any, primarily on the individual. [3]

These definitions did not *require* physical dependence—it is said to occur "generally"—for a diagnosis of addiction, but most writers have ignored this point, partly because the definition of habituation explicitly excluded physical dependence; it was therefore natural, though incorrect, to assume that the Expert Committee was implying that in addiction it must always be present.

This interpretation was reinforced by the British Interdepartmental Committee (sometimes known as the Brain Committee, after its chairman, Sir Russell Brain). In 1961 this group formulated definitions of addiction and habituation very much like those proposed by the WHO in 1957, except that both "physical dependence" and "the appearance of a characteristic abstinence syndrome" were specified as necessary criteria of addiction. [4]

Actually, there is no clear way to identify physical dependence and distinguish it from psychological dependence apart from the abstinence syndrome. Besides, by "abstinence syndrome" these official bodies meant chiefly the *opiate* withdrawal reaction; the very different amphetamine abstinence syndrome simply was not classified as one. The shortcomings of these official definitions became obvious when cases of abuse of the drugs called merely "habituating," especially the amphetamines, proved to be as chronic and difficult to treat as the classic addictions; the relapse rate was often as high and the prognosis as discouraging. Abuse of amphetamines and other "habituating" drugs could damage society as much as heroin abuse. In addition, the proliferation of new drugs with varying modes and durations of action made it difficult to determine whether any particular case should be regarded as habituation or addiction. The official terminology also led to such clinical and logical confusions as "habituation to addiction-producing drugs" (for instance, heroin and morphine) or "addiction to habit-forming drugs" (for instance, barbiturates, some of the "minor" tranquilizers, and amphetamines).

So the definitions were changed again. In 1963 the AMA's Council on Drugs recommended replacing the terms "addiction" and "habituation" with "descriptions of the characteristics reported, or considered likely, to occur."[5] One of its purposes was to emphasize the dangers of amphetamines without using the word "addiction," which was too closely associated with the abstinence syndrome peculiar to opiates. In 1964 the WHO substituted for its 1957 definitions a new term, "drug dependence," described as: "a state arising from repeated administration of a drug on a periodic or continuous basis. Its characteristics will vary with the agent involved and this must be made clear by designating the particular type of drug dependence in each specific case—for example, drug dependence of morphine type, of cocaine type, of cannabis type, of barbiturate type, of amphetamine type, etc."

The Expert Committee characterized "drug dependence of amphetamine type" as a state arising from repeated administration of amphetamine or an agent with amphetaminelike effects on a periodic or continuous basis. Its characteristics were said to include:

(1) a desire or need to continue taking the drug; (2) consumption of increasing amounts to obtain greater excitatory and euphoric effects or to combat more effectively depression and

fatigue, accompanied in some measure by the development of tolerance; (3) a psychic dependence on the effects of the drug related to a subjective and initial appreciation of the drug's effects; and (4) general absence of physical dependence so that there is no characteristic abstinence syndrome when the drug is discontinued.[6]

There were several virtues in this change. It recognized that a continuum of degrees of dependence had to be substituted for the old concepts of habituation and addiction. The differences between drugs were more clearly spelled out, so that the misconception of "drug addiction" as a disease could be more easily combated. Unfortunately, the definition of "drug dependence of amphetamine type" was confusing. It still assumed that amphetamine did not produce "physical dependence" because it did not lead to an opiatelike withdrawal reaction. The ambiguity in (4) of the definition evades the question of whether "physical dependence" means anything apart from an abstinence syndrome, much less what qualifies as an abstinence syndrome.

This matter of the abstinence syndrome is important less for its own sake than because it is a major component of the public's idea of "addiction." Most of us see the drama of the withdrawal reaction to opiates as a condemnation of the drugs as well as the users: since many of the symptoms are strong involuntary reactions, we feel that something is being done to the user or imposed on him by the drug. When withdrawal symptoms are less obvious or less obviously "physical," many consider the user "weak-willed" or "intemperate." So "addictiveness" comes to incorporate a premature fixing of blame. By using "addiction" in something like its traditional sense, we lay ourselves open to this kind of misinterpretation, so we want to emphasize that a withdrawal reaction is no more than a fairly well-defined set of physiological symptoms, different for different drugs. It is neither the major cause nor the most important medical or social consequence of drug abuse, and its presence or absence should not be a criterion for moral judgments.

Tolerance and Withdrawal Symptoms

Withdrawal symptoms are usually preceded by another physiological reaction: acquired tolerance. This is a kind of adaptation of the body to the drug, so that to achieve the same effects it becomes necessary to increase the dose. Tolerance almost always arises with prolonged use of opiates, barbiturates, alcohol, and amphetamine. Its development is usually a sign that physical symptoms will appear on withdrawal; so, if the drug is considered harmful, it is a criterion of "addictiveness." (It is not a universal one: LSD, for example, produces tolerance very quickly but has no withdrawal reaction.)

Tolerance seems to have several physiological sources. One that operates in the case of opiates, barbiturates, and alcohol is an a-daptive increase in the rate at which the drug is metabolized to inactive products ("drug disposition" or "metabolic" tolerance). Amphetamines are largely excreted unchanged in the urine, so metabolic tolerance does not develop. A more important form, common to most psychoactive drugs, is an adaptation at the cel-lular level in the central nervous system that makes the user less sensitive to the drug's effects ("pharmacodynamic," "tissue," or "cellular" tolerance). For depressant drugs like narcotics and sedatives this means an increase in the nerve cells' excitability; for amphetamines, a decrease. In the case of amphetamines there may be another mechanism of tolerance. High doses can inhibit ap-petite to the point where the body is near starvation, and in star-vation the urine is strongly acidic. Since excretion of amphet-amine apparently occurs much faster when the urine is acidic, the heavy user who does not force himself to eat more than he wants must keep increasing the dose.

When the amphetamines were first introduced it was some-times said, with characteristic overoptimism about new drugs, that they produced little or no tolerance. But as early as 1938 P. Bahnsen discovered tolerance to the euphoric as well as the minor unpleasant "organic" effects after one to three weeks. Although the euphoric and anorectic (appetite-reducing) effects often dis-appear quickly, amphetamine's effectiveness in the long-term treatment of narcolepsy (as well as the insomnia usually exper-ienced by steady users) indicates that the awakening action is less easily inhibited. There is wide variation in the development of tolerance to the toxic effects of the amphetamines. The upper limit beyond which tolerance will not develop also varies, but there are some indications that, at least for certain people, there is practically none. For example, although the average daily "therapeutic" dose of methamphetamine is 15 mg, at least one substantiated case of self-administration of 15,000 mg in twenty-four hours has been reported.[7]

Acquired tolerance and physiological withdrawal symptoms are usually (though not always) linked, yet the false belief that amphetamines produce no abstinence syndrome has had much wider and longer circulation than the view that they produce no tolerance effect. Even writers attempting to warn against the dangers of amphetamines have found themselves admitting that they are not "technically addictive." The reasoning goes as follows: there is no opiatelike withdrawal reaction; therefore there is no withdrawal reaction; therefore "technically" there is no addiction. The beginning of wisdom was recognition that "drug addiction" is not a useful term. But an inchoate sense of some basic difference between opiates and other drugs remained, until it was accepted that several kinds of abstinence syndrome exist.

Medical research and literary reporting that concentrated excessively on opiates helped prevent the recognition of alcoholic delirium tremens and barbiturate hallucinosis as true withdrawal reactions. The problem has been even greater with amphetamine, because the abstinence syndrome of a stimulant drug is, as one might expect, almost the opposite of that produced by a depressant like heroin. Instead of agitation, nonfocal hyperactivity, and insomnia, the abuser experiences lethargy, sleepiness, and depression. This has resulted in claims, like that of E. Stungo, that the 1957 WHO definitions did not "sufficiently emphasize the occurrence of abstinence symptoms on withdrawal of an addictive drug," which he thought distinguished "between addiction and habituation." According to Stungo, addiction to the amphetamines rarely occurs, since even prolonged use results in no "characteristic" abstinence symptoms. He admitted that depression and sleepiness had been seen "occasionally" after the discontinuance of amphetamine therapy, but attributed this to a natural exhaustion that would follow any period of prolonged overstimulation and claimed that they "do not necessarily constitute evidence of physical dependence." He concluded that it could be "categorically stated that addiction or habituation to amphetamine alone is extremely rare and that when it does occur the patient is suffering from a condition which is not specific to the amphetamines," and that someone can ordinarily be said to be addicted to amphetamine only in the sense that he may be described as "addicted" to tea, coffee, or tobacco. [8]

Another example of this peculiar blindness is the report on a fifty-two-year-old woman who had been abusing amphetamine sulfate for about five years. She had rapidly developed tolerance to its effects and after only a few months had increased her daily dosage from 5 to 50 mg—but even then complained that the drug was much less effective than it had been. By the end of her first year she was taking 700 mg each day in single doses of 50 mg and had begun to experience visual and tactile hallucinations of worms crawling over her body and small animals everywhere. She tried to stop using the drug but found that even a reduction of her usual 700-mg daily dose caused extreme fatigue, almost total lack of energy or motivation, and inability to concentrate. Physical examination revealed fine and gross tremors, dry mouth, vasomotor instability, difficulty in breathing, excessively rapid heartbeat, and high blood pressure. She managed to reduce her intake of amphetamine to some degree, but could not completely discontinue its use. The authors decided that this was not an instance of true addiction on the grounds that the woman did not display the "classic" symptoms of habituation: craving, "characteristic" abstinence symptoms, and "perversion." [9] This conclusion is astounding. Although the evidence presented is somewhat scanty, it is nevertheless clear that the woman experienced a strong craving, suffered a depression and other symptoms of a "characteristic" abstinence syndrome, and, most important, could not stop taking the drug. The inclusion of "perversion" as a criterion of addiction is unique, to say the least. The only conceivable justification for the authors' conclusion is that in France in 1947 nobody was called an addict unless his or her behavior was in some obvious way grossly reprehensible. The unstated assumption seems to have been that only excessive use of opiates leads to "true addiction."

In a study of amphetamine abuse in Newcastle-upon-Tyne, England, L. G. Kiloh and S. Brandon quoted some statements about the drug's "non-addictiveness," then continued: "It is the purpose of this paper to demonstrate that these statements are dangerously inaccurate and that a considerable abuse of the amphetamines and phenmetrazine exists, habituation and addiction occurring very frequently in our society." Repeating the 1957 WHO definition of addiction, they commented: "It must be conceded that a number of patients taking excessive quantities of amphetamine fulfil this definition. They certainly suffer an overpowering desire to continue taking the drug, they take it in amounts far exceeding the usual therapeutic dose, they may be prepared to break the law to obtain supplies, they are dependent upon it, and they sometimes become psychotic. Furthermore, withdrawal symptoms may occur, notably states of depression in which suicide may occur."[10]

Although discomfort intense enough to cause resumption of use can arise even when amphetamine has been taken only for a short time and the dosage has not been increased, the withdrawal symptoms are most distressing when the user has been taking high doses intravenously. Unlike the hyperstimulated withdrawing heroin addict, the "crashing" amphetamine abuser lacks the energy to complain and may seem to be merely exhausted and in need of sleep. Recently investigators have looked more closely, and the emerging picture is unpleasant and painful. Extreme lethargy and fatigue are almost invariably reported. Although the "crasher" may sleep for several days, he never sleeps well, and often wakes screaming from nightmares. On awakening, he may experience anxiety attacks and suicidally severe depression. His psychic disruption and loss of self-control may lead to violent acting out of sexual conflicts and aggressive impulses. He often experiences acute fear and terror and is as likely to turn homicidal as suicidal. He is apt to be extremely irritable and demanding, driving people away just when he most needs their help. His head aches; he may have trouble breathing; he sweats profusely; his body is racked by alternating sensations of extreme heat and cold and distressing muscle cramps. He may feel so exhausted that he is unable even to stand. He is chacteristically constipated, and suffers painful gastrointestinal cramps. Very often he develops severe secondary reactions: hepatitis (with intravenous abuse), influenza, pneumonia, and various vitamin deficiency states are common. If he is alone, despite sometimes incredible hunger, he may lack the strength to eat. If he has been taking other drugs (including alcohol) to excess, his agony is compounded, and he may die a most unpleasant death.[11]

One woman described her amphetamine problem thus:

> At the age of twenty, amphetamine was first prescribed for me for weight reduction. At the time, I was a vocational nurse at a private hospital. I became almost immediately addicted.
>
> Now I am forty years old and have been off the drug for less than one year, but I now understand how to stay off.
>
> In the years between, I have gone through all the symptoms you describe in withdrawal, including hallucinations.
>
> Mostly what I want to tell you is of my lonely battle against amphetamines. I was convinced from remarks he had made about other doctors' wives who were drug abusers that my husband (a doctor) would leave me if he knew, so I knew I'd have to secretly get help.
>
> . . . I went to two psychiatrists and flatly insisted I was addicted and begged for help in getting off. All of them (one at a time of course) pressed new prescriptions for the drug on me, saying I was not addicted. This after I told them I knew I was because I had forged a prescription with my husband's name and even I realized that was the clearest indication of addiction.
>
> At last, after numerous attempts and indescribable suffering (over this period of eighteen years), I went to a psychiatrist for marital counseling with my husband. Privately, I saw the doctor and again expressed my desperate situation. He also denied I could be addicted but said a friend of ours could be trusted with the knowledge of my "thinking I was addicted."
>
> I went to him and he simply demanded that I stop the abuse at once and prescribed antidepressants instead. I wasn't able to stop quickly like he said, but gradually I got so I could go longer and longer and suffer more and more without taking the amphetamine.
>
> The symptoms of withdrawal were so severe that at times I couldn't think who I was and other times where I lived; the floor was coming up at me and the walls seemed to move. At night people would break in or just come into the room and terrify me, while to an onlooker I slept peacefully next to my husband.

All this and more, much, much more I went through without my husband knowing or being able to give understanding or support. I've hurt him and god only knows what I've done to my children or to my own brain. Do you suppose I have permanent brain damage?[12]

After discontinuing her use of amphetamine, the woman gained fifteen pounds. Although this upset her husband, she felt that being off the drug was more important than being slim. "If he knew what I've been through," she wrote, "he'd know it is a small price to pay to be free."

We believe amphetamines do cause physical dependence, unless "physical dependence" is regarded as synonymous with "dependence produced by opiates." It is true that the amphetamine abstinence syndrome is not always so obviously painful or apparently life-threatening as the opiate or barbiturate abstinence syndrome. This difference appears to be related to the rate at which different drugs are eliminated from the body. For drugs like heroin and morphine, which are quickly degraded and excreted, there is a very short time between the cessation of drug use and the onset of abstinence symptoms. But when the rate of excretion is low, as with amphetamines, the interval between suspension of intake and disappearance of the drug from the system is prolonged. During this time (for amphetamines, a matter of days or weeks) the individual experiences gradual rather than abrupt development of withdrawal symptoms. His situation is like that of the opiate addict who is slowly withdrawn from his quickly eliminated drug in an institution by medically supervised step-by-step reduction of the dosage. Even among opiates, the severity of the abstinence syndrome depends on the rate at which the particular drug is eliminated. Methadone is excreted much more slowly than heroin or morphine, and its abstinence syndrome is correspondingly milder.[13]

The unpleasantness of the heroin abstinence syndrome has been vastly overestimated. Until recently the strongest heroin available to most addicts in this country was only about 3 percent pure, and physical dependence produced by such dilute preparations is quite weak. According to D. P. Ausubel and G. Gay, the typical heroin abstinence syndrome is "seldom more severe than a bad case of gastrointestinal influenza."[14] (Reportedly the heroin used by American servicemen in Vietnam was

much stronger—up to 96 percent pure—and the resulting abstinence syndrome correspondingly more severe.) The suffering
has been exaggerated by the addict himself, because the ordeal is
considered a peculiar badge of courage indicating membership in
a group of dangerous and daring people. Thus:

> Many addicts discuss their own and others' withdrawal ex-
> periences with heavy humor and boastful exaggeration, not
> unlike children who compete in describing the rigors of their
> measles or draftees who boast about the meanness of their non-
> commissioned officers in basic training. We are not suggesting
> that they regard the withdrawal experience as pleasurable, but
> rather that its occurrence and severity become integrated in
> their self-images as a valid, interesting, and necessary aspect of
> themselves. Though the nonaddict may regard the withdrawal
> experience as a terrible deterrent to addiction, the addict de-
> velops the same attitude toward dependence on opiates as the
> organization man does toward the "rat race" of business life in
> large corporations.[15]

Furthermore, almost all observed opiate abstinence symptoms
occur in a hospital setting, where the addict suspects that if he
puts on a good enough act he will receive a narcotizing dose of
tranquilizers or barbiturates—or even opiates.

Sleep

A major breakthrough in the clarification of the physiological
correlates of withdrawal reaction in drugs usually considered
"addictive" occurred with the publication in 1963 by Ian Oswald
and V. R. Thacore of "Amphetamine and Phenmetrazine Addiction: Physiological Abnormalities in the Abstinence Syndrome." After noting that "amphetamine addiction is common, though the readiness with which such addiction develops is
not as widely recognized as one could wish," they state: "Addiction to these drugs ('drinamyl' and 'preludin') is common in Edinburgh, and it is our purpose to demonstrate that *physical dependence* and characteristic, persisting, and easily measurable
'physical' or physiological abnormalities form part of the *abstinence syndrome.*"[16] They noted that research had revealed the
existence of two separate phases of normal human sleep, easily
distinguishable on EEG recordings, and referred to as REM

(Rapid Eye Movement) sleep and non-REM sleep. Non-REM sleep, characterized by tense muscles, motionless eyes, and increasing voltage and synchronization and decreasing frequency relative to the waking EEG, occurs first in each night of sleep, and lasts about seventy minutes; then there is an abrupt shift to REM sleep, which is characterized by a low-voltage, mixed-frequency EEG pattern somewhat resembling that of drowsiness, inhibited muscles, and jerky rapid eye movements. REM sleep recurs from four to six times throughout the night and occupies about ten minutes of the first two hours and about 22 percent of the whole night's sleep. When people are awakened from REM sleep they usually report that they have been dreaming. Some sleep-deprivation experiments suggest that we need a certain minimum of REM sleep to maintain normal psychological functioning; the need for non-REM sleep seems more elastic and more directly related to physical performance.[17]

Oswald and Thacore studied the sleep patterns of six women who were chronic abusers of amphetamines. Admitted to a hospital for drug withdrawal and treatment, they were told beforehand that they would be allowed to continue their drug use for a short time. This was done "in order to allow a doctor-patient bond to develop, strong enough to sustain them on drug withdrawal." The early nocturnal EEG, eye-movement, and muscle tonus recordings showed that all of the women had been taking the drugs for so long that their bodies had compensated for the usual effects of amphetamines on sleep (a decrease in both REM and total sleep), and they were all sleeping normally. But after they were withdrawn, their sleep patterns became markedly abnormal. They not only slept much longer, but their REM sleep began as soon as four minutes after the beginning of sleep, and occupied up to seventy minutes of the first two hours and up to 48 percent—237 out of a total of 494 minutes—of the night's sleep. The return to normal sleep patterns took from three to eight weeks. If the amphetamines were again given to the patients during withdrawal, their sleep patterns immediately returned to normal, becoming markedly irregular once more when the drugs were removed. The authors concluded that the women were physically dependent upon amphetamines:

To establish the existence of "physical" dependence on a drug it is necessary to demonstrate some physiological function which is within normal limits in the fully addicted patient but which becomes abnormal upon drug withdrawal, and which returns to normal if the drug is again given. The physiological function we have chosen to measure concerns a basic brain process—sleep. . . . The central nervous systems of our patients had evidently become so accustomed to drugs that a normal pattern of sleep was present. In each case . . . upon withdrawal a huge increase in R.E.M.-time occurred, reversible by reinstituting the drug. . . . Alternatively, the passage of time brought about a decline to fairly steady individual normal values. The addicts were therefore dependent on their drugs for normal function. . . .

We do not understand the basis of the abnormalities we have observed; for, notwithstanding its fundamental role in our economy, the significance of our need for sleep remains a mystery. We believe this to be the first demonstration of an abnormality both easily measurable and long-persisting (one to two months) in any kind of human abstinence syndrome.[18]

These findings provide the first evidence of an abnormality of function causally related to the ability of a drug to produce addiction. Oswald noted that all addictive drugs seem to "suppress REM sleep with an increase following withdrawal." The same pattern has been observed after use of some of the newer "diet" drugs such as phenmetrazine (Preludin), diethylproprion (Tenuate), and chlorphenteramine (Pre-Sate), as well as the antidepressant amphetamine derivative tranylcypromine (Parnate). Suppression of REM sleep has also been reported for the amphetamine-related stimulant methylphenidate (Ritalin); although most of these drugs have been available for a relatively short period of time, instances of abuse, psychotic reactions, and addiction already have been reported for each. The same suppression and subsequent rebound of REM sleep has been observed for drugs long known to have a high addictive potential: heroin, morphine, alcohol, barbiturates, the sedative-hypnotic glutethimide (Doriden), and one of the oldest of the "minor" tranquilizers, meprobamate (Miltown). Delerium tremens may be a state of acute "over-rebound" from a chemically induced deprivation of REM sleep: that is, the alcohol has suppressed REM sleep, and the extremely vivid hallucinatory state the alcoholic suffers on withdrawal is a kind of "over-effort" to catch up on lost REM sleep (and hence perhaps lost dreaming as well). Since dreaming is the state par excellence of escape from reality and wish-fulfillment, it is at least possible that the use of addictive drugs—all of which offer at least an alteration in the sense of, if not a direct escape from, the tensions of waking reality—should somehow lead to a change in the amount and frequency of dreaming, or even act as some kind of substitute for it. Thus, the delirium tremens of alcoholism, the hallucinations and delusions of extreme barbituratism, and the amphetamine abstinence syndrome may all be examples of a rebound-overcompensation of suppressed REM sleep. (Heroin addicts seem to be let off quite easily.)[19]

A. F. Mirsky has noted that addictive drugs produce a low-voltage, fast-activity EEG reading, while nonaddictive drugs with a strong effect on the brain and nervous system (for example, chlorpromazine) produce a high-voltage, slow activity reading. Amphetamines produce the pattern typical of addictive drugs, which is close to the EEG of normal individuals during REM sleep—when they are dreaming. Mirsky suggests that a study of EEG recordings taken from subjects under the influence of various drugs may provide a key for determining these drugs' addictive potentials.[20]

Sleep research on nonaddicting drugs with a strong effect on the central nervous system has shown that, although many of them suppress REM sleep to some extent, they do not cause a REM sleep rebound following cessation of medication. Sleep and EEG research appears to be one of the most promising fields of inquiry in the search for a truly safe anorectic drug. Only one amphetamine derivative or amphetaminelike drug—fenfluramine (Ponderax)—can be classified as even potentially safe; significantly, it has no effect on REM sleep. Oswald and his associates recently discovered that two antidepressant drugs, phenelzine and imipramine,[21] which so far appear to be nonaddictive, cause some REM sleep rebound. However, it is yet to be shown that there is any drug that produces a withdrawal reaction but not both REM sleep suppression and a later rebound overcompensation.

The mechanisms and adaptations behind the phenomena of REM suppression and rebound have been at least tentatively explicated. Japanese researchers have found a decrease in anaerobic and aerobic *in vitro* glycolytic activity in the brain tissue of rats and guinea pigs for over forty-five days after methamphetamine withdrawal. Oswald speculated that in REM sleep the brain is synthesizing protein. He noted that a fifteen-day half-life for human brain protein was suggested by the findings of studies on radioactively labeled amino acids. Thus, damaged enzyme systems would make a 94 percent recovery in two months—about the maximum time that it had taken for the REM sleep of withdrawing amphetamine addicts to return to a normal level. Accordingly, he suggested that "the REM sleep rebound after drug-withdrawal indicates a reshaping of neuronal machinery through protein synthesis, a process of repair within brain cells." The three-or-four-day troubled sleep of the withdrawing amphetamine addict may therefore be a manifestation of brain cell damage.[22]

Craving

The "craving" associated with withdrawal is sometimes considered to be the main defining characteristic of addiction. It is an ambiguous term connoting both physiological symptoms and psychological dependence. A. R. Lindesmith, who suggests that we "think of the tendency to relapse and other commonly emphasized features as corollary aspects or consequences of it," believes this craving results from the addict's "experience of relief of withdrawal distress which follows within a matter of five to ten minutes after an injection . . . the craving develops in this situation only when the individual understands the withdrawal symptoms and attributes them to the proper cause. A person who remains ignorant of the source of withdrawal symptoms and interprets them in some other way will not become addicted." According to him, "instead of saying that the addict craves drugs because he likes their effects, it may be nearer the truth to say that he likes the effects because he craves the drug"—and he craves it because he has learned that it will stave off an abstinence syndrome.[23]

Because Lindesmith's discussion dealt only with opiates, he could be interpreted as saying that they alone produce a genuine drug craving, and therefore addiction. Animal experiments conducted by M. H. Seevers and reported by N. Bejerot supply evidence not only that the desire for amphetamines may be as strong—or last twice as long—as the desire for heroin, but ___ that it cannot be explained adequately by Lindesmith's theory. In Seevers' experiments, Rhesus monkeys were attached to devices enabling them to self-administer drugs intravenously; half received heroin and the other half amphetamine, by means of systems of flexible tubes and injection devices. The monkey received his injection by pushing a button inside his cage; each was left to discover this by accident. All soon were exhibiting chronic drug-induced behavior; they acted addicted. The monkeys provided with amphetamine would push their buttons to receive doses of amphetamine continuously, day and night, going entirely without sleep and eating or drinking very little for from six to eight days. After a week-long amphetamine "run" they would collapse into exhausted sleep that lasted, on the average, two days. When they awoke they would immediately show interest in food and drink, and then resume another week-long period of intensive amphetamine self-administration.

Seevers then took both sets of monkeys out of their experimental cages, provided rest and high-nutrient diets for a few weeks, and returned them to the cages. This time he did not connect the drug-administration apparatus to the buttons. The monkeys who had received heroin pushed the buttons an average of two thousand times before they gave up; but those who had received amphetamines persisted an average of four thousand times. None of the monkeys had been given the opportunity to "learn" that readministration of either heroin or amphetamine would alleviate their drug withdrawal distress. Therefore, according to Lindesmith's theory, none should have experienced a drug craving. Their continuing to push the buttons thus suggests that drug craving does not entirely depend on learning that readministration of the drug will alleviate an unpleasant psychological or physical state. Here the attainment of euphoria was the primary factor. Evaluating these experiments, Bejerot writes: "In this way Seevers has shown that the psychological dependence is stronger in amphetamine than in heroin addiction, and it is the strength and duration of the psychological dependence which is the central problem in addiction."[24]

A physiological aspect of craving also exists, especially when associated with an abstinence syndrome. Oswald and Thacore state:

> Unfortunately we cannot measure another neurophysiological abnormality—namely, that which directly underlies the most significant feature of the syndrome, the *craving*.
>
> After withdrawal of amphetamine, patients describe listlessness, depression, and sleepiness, but cannot easily formulate their craving: "I feel terrible, I miss them so" (Case 4); "I can't get them out of my mind, I think about them all the time" (Case 6). It is this craving that drives them to antisocial acts; to obtain their drugs without prescription from small-time traffickers and unscrupulous pharmacists; to alter, steal, and forge prescriptions; and to call in rotation on different doctors from whom they conceal their addiction. . . . Persons taking these drugs certainly experience an intense craving to continue so to take them, and to obtain them by almost any means.[25]

As early as 1949 F. A. Freyhan raised the question whether the craving for amphetamines might not reflect an acquired physiological need rather than a purely psychological desire, and suggested that psychiatry alone could not explain its mechanism. Craving is probably best defined as an aspect of psychological dependence rather than identified with an abstinence syndrome—which too often means the opiate abstinence syndrome. Such a craving for amphetamines has been reported too many times to be ignored or denied. Almost every report on amphetamine abuse mentions it; it seems to be no less compulsive than the craving experienced by heroin addicts. Descriptions run like this: "subjects want to continue" their use of amphetamines; they "would like to continue taking the drug"; they experience a "compulsion to continue"; terminating use "appears to be very difficult"; they experience an "overpowering need"; they "are impelled toward return to use of their drug with a force comparable to that of heroin users"; they "can't do without them every morning"; they make importunate demands for prescriptions because of an "overpowering desire"; they insist that they need the drug; they feel "unable to maintain any contact without it," or are "no longer able to face life without [its] help."[26]

Lindesmith's emphasis is misplaced, even for opiates. If the craving can be entirely accounted for by the addict's having

learned that administration of more opiates will forestall or eliminate the unpleasantness of the abstinence syndrome, why do
heroin addicts notoriously take much more of the drug than they
need to prevent or end withdrawal distress? As Ausubel notes:
"the amount of morphine required to prevent withdrawal symptoms is characteristically no more than one-half to one-tenth the
actual dosage used by most addicts. How, therefore, can one account for this surplus dosage if the drug is merely taken, as addicts claim, just to stay normal?"[27] The only sensible answer is
that the craving is multidetermined; although the addict may
claim he takes the drug merely to avoid withdrawal symptoms, he
also wishes, consciously or not, to recapture his first euphoric experience. Many addicts take two separate injections of the same
opiate, the first to forestall withdrawal symptoms and the second
for the kick or "rush". Although the addict wants to limit tolerance and avoid withdrawal pains, he wants even more to "get
high":

> It is the tightrope walk between these three positions that in-
> volves so much of the junkie's waking moments. In this con-
> text, a little withdrawal reduces tolerance and produces a
> better "high"; a complete withdrawal may eliminate tolerance
> if it has not become fixed, and again make possible the earliest
> virgin "bang." The latter is a state much to be desired, but to
> respond to the siren's song of euphoria leads to its loss through
> tolerance and its reawakening through withdrawal only. The so
> called "cure," then, is a vital stage in the reinforcement of ad-
> diction, since cure is too frequently only a euphemism for the
> reduction of tolerance and the recovery of euphoric potential,
> also euphemistically called "relapse," for which the addict
> periodically strives.[28]

Physiological dependence, once established, may strengthen a
drug craving, but "craving, as clinically observed, unquestionably
develops in persons who liked and wanted opiates prior to any
indications of pharmacological dependence on these drugs;
craving much more typically leads to the pattern of use which
establishes dependence than vice versa."[29]

Lindesmith is the victim of his own wish to formulate an absolutely inclusive theory of addiction; his theory becomes so general
that it is finally merely tautologous:

Lindesmith's theory is based on the research method of analytic induction. This procedure is aimed at the discovery of generalizations which apply to every single case of the behavior studied, rather than generalizations which state relationships in terms of frequency or probability. An inherent danger in the method is that, to avoid exceptions, the definition of the problem being investigated is gradually narrowed to exclude those of its aspects which originally aroused interest in the problem, and which are most in need of being explained.

As one example, Lindesmith holds that a general theory of addiction must apply equally to the Oriental opium-smoker and the English opium-eater of a century ago, the physician addict of today, and the young minority-group heroin addicts in metropolitan slums. This is a legitimate goal and a useful one, but a completely satisfactory theory should also explain the differences among these types. Further, as Turner points out, "Lindesmith provides us with a causal complex which is empirically verifiable *in retrospect*, but which does not in itself permit prediction that a specific person will become an addict nor that a specific situation will produce addiction."[30]

Lindesmith's theory is untenable for another reason.

If physiological dependence were the primary etiological factor in perpetuating the drug habit, how could one explain the fact that at least 75 percent of the drug addicts discharged from federal hospitals start using the drug again almost immediately after release? By this time it is usually at least a year since their physical dependence was broken. If they really find withdrawal symptoms tolerable only by surrendering to chronic addiction, why should they start all over again when they obviously do not have to? We can only assume that various positive and pleasurable gratifications are associated with the practice, among which is the satisfying experience of alleviating the distress of withdrawal symptoms.[31]

Some investigators attribute this high relapse rate to the difference between the environment in which the addict undergoes withdrawal and the one he returns to. T. Thompson and W. Ostlund, after experiments with albino rats, concluded: "readdiction is more probable if the opportunity for readdiction is presented in a home environment rather than in a new environment, and read-

diction is also more likely if withdrawal has taken p.
miliar surroundings with respect to the readdictic
ment."[32] Other aspects of addiction that seem indepenc
vironment also contradict Lindesmith's hypothesis. A
clinical evidence indicates that even after an addict has co...pletely
lost all craving for a drug, and even if a long time—say fifteen
years—has elapsed since he abused it, if he should take even a
small amount, he will resume the addiction at the advanced point
at which he left it. In other words, even when conscious craving is
completely extinguished, the addiction persists latently by some
mechanism not yet understood. This latent drug hunger has been
observed in the case of opiates, alcohol, and cigarettes (presumably nicotine), and there is some indication that it may also occur
with amphetamines. The basic mechanism may be an irreversible
physiological or biochemical (physical) change or set of changes
resulting in the development of "permanent tolerance."[33]

Another argument is that many addicts, without any treatment, simply stop using heroin. The exact nature of the changes
enabling an addict to "mature out" of his heroin (or other opiate)
addiction is not well understood, although the phenomenon has
been reported many times.[34] However, if craving were entirely
determined by the addict's learning that readministration of
heroin brings relief from abstinence symptoms, there would be no
self-terminating addiction, because the steady increase of dosage
necessitated by the development of tolerance would make the
abstinence syndrome progressively worse, and the craving would
become unbreakable.

In sum, Lindesmith's attempt to reformulate the theory of addiction fails because it overemphasizes the opiate abstinence syndrome, cannot account for the craving experienced by those addicted to drugs other than opiates, and generally oversimplifies
the constellation of subjective feelings, tendencies, and urges
that constitute craving. His theory relies too heavily on an exaggerated and inaccurate conception of physical dependence:

> But even apart from the fact that the abstinence syndrome is
> neither catastrophically severe nor long lasting, there are many
> reasons for believing that physiological dependence does not
> play a central etiological role in drug addiction. The popular
> misconceptions that addicted individuals deprived of the drug
> suffer the tortures of the damned, and that once caught in the

iron grip of physiological dependence the average person is powerless to help himself, are beliefs that have been foisted on a credulous public by misinformed journalists and by addicts themselves.

In the first place, unless other subjective satisfactions were derived from the habit, it is difficult to believe that any individual would be willing to pay the fantastic price of the drug and risk imprisonment, social disgrace, and ostracism merely to avoid a moderately severe ten-day illness. Second, it is well-known to most practicing physicians that every year thousands of patients suffering from protractedly painful illness receive opiates regularly over sufficiently prolonged periods of time to develop marked physical dependence on the drug. Nevertheless, despite frequent awareness of this state of affairs, the vast majority are able to sever their dependence quite easily following gradual reduction of the dosage. Unlike addicts, they do not claim that they are compelled to continue using the drug because of the intolerability of the abstinence symptoms. . . . To explain the fact that most persons who develop physiological dependence after receiving opiates for therapeutic purposes do not become addicted, he [Lindesmith] speculates that some individuals are differentially sensitive to withdrawal symptoms. However, as long as the differential sensitivity is not explained, this explanation merely begs the question, for on what basis are some persons more sensitive than others? Furthermore, the fact that all addicts appreciate the connection between injection of opiates and relief of withdrawal symptoms does not prove that this is the only or central causal factor in addiction.[35]

It is extremely difficult to determine the relative strengths of different users' "desire" or "need" to continue taking the same drug, or of a single user's "desire" or "need" for two different drugs. Unless the researcher excludes all evidence not expressed in overt, quantifiable action, he is left with verbal reports like "nothing could be worse than this monkey on *my* back." Craving cannot be explained purely in terms of pharmacology; it occurs even after the relief of physiological dependence. Perhaps use of the drug provides a sense of personal indentity, associations based on a common purpose, a feeling of belonging to a group, a means of filling an empty life.

Psychology of Drug Dependence

The psychology and sociology of drug dependence are the real heart of the matter. Here all assertions should be tentative, because all the terms used imply moral and even political judgments; they are "loaded" words which should not be burdened excessively or with the wrong connotations. In this context the question of "addictive personality" arises. The label has been confusingly used as both complement and contrast to "addictive drug": in the case of opiates, as a complement (the inadequate personality is inclined to take the harmful drug); in the case of other drugs, especially amphetamines, as a contrast (the defective personality makes bad use of a good drug). This is the same evasion of issues and premature blame-fixing we have already mentioned. But it is not absurd to speak of personalities, as well as drugs, that tend to produce drug dependence. Some people cannot gain respite from psychological pain unless they are under the influence of a drug. They may suffer from character disorders, anxiety, depression feelings of inadequacy, or intolerable life situations. However, when considering amphetamines we must not fall victim to the fallacy of the reversed apparent equation. When Emerson wrote, "to be great is to be misunderstood," he did not mean that everyone who is misunderstood is great. It may be true most amphetamine abusers have some psychological deficiency, but we should not assume that only and all persons who are in some unique way "addiction-prone" will abuse amphetamines or other drugs.

There is no single pre-addictive personality and there is no such person as "the" addict. Any man, woman, or child will develop addiction to certain psychoactive substances upon exposure to sufficiently large doses for a sufficient length of time. It may well be that certain kinds of persons are more likely to become amphetamine addicts, but it is extraordinarily difficult to describe just what such a personality consists of, or to predict exactly who is likely to become addicted. Many people with personality structures and early family histories indistinguishable from those of addicts do not resort to drug abuse. Or, in Cohen's words, "what must be remembered is that many youngsters with a so-called addictive personality profile are not, and will not become, dependent on drugs."[36] It is almost impossible to arrange satisfactory control groups, or to devise methods to account for the differential availability of amphetamines (and other drugs) for different segments of the population. A glance at Lindesmith's characterizations of addicts proves the futility of such an attempt: "alienated," "frustrated," "passive psychopath," "aggressive psychopath," "emotionally unstable," "nomadic," "inebriate," "narcissistic," "dependent," "sociopath," "hedonistic," "childlike," "paranoid," "rebellious," "hostile," "infantile," "neurotic," "overattached to the mother," "retreatist," "cyclothymic," "constitutionally immoral," "hysterical," "neurasthenic," "hereditarily neuropathic," "weak character and will," "lack of moral sense," "self-indulgent," "introspective," "extroverted," "self-conscious," "motivational immaturity," "pseudo-psychopathic delinquent," and finally, "essentialy normal."

One label popular in reports of amphetamine abuse during the late 1940s, "psychopathic personality," is no longer in official use. This catch-all term usually was applied after someone had engaged in some specific antisocial or destructive behavior; for example, most prisoners were grouped as psychopaths. But no one had discovered a way of determining which individuals were "psychopaths" *before* they got into serious difficulty, so the label lacked diagnostic value. The concept has been convincingly attacked as meaningless.[37]

But the inclination to insist that anyone who abuses amphetamine must be "abnormal" in some clearly definable way persists. In their study of Benzedrine inhaler use, Monroe and Drell conducted interviews with fifteen of their subjects to determine the personality type which would use amphetamine. The sample was small and they gave no indication that it was random, but they concluded that "all showed some pathologic trends in the personality structure. Nine were of the inadequate personality type. Six were considered immature." According to the War Department diagnostic guide used by these investigators, persons classified as having "inadequate personalities" are "characterized by inadequate response to intellectual, emotional, social, and physical demands. They are neither physically nor mentally grossly deficient on examination, but they do show inadaptability, ineptness, poor judgment, and social incompatibility." What this really means is that nine of the fifteen were judged to respond inadequately to the demands of life in an Army jail, and may have been socially "incompatible" with fellow inmates. What of the six

with "immaturity reactions"? According to the
"this category applies to physically adult individua.
able to maintain their emotional equilibrium and
under minor or major stress."[38]

Monroe and Drell were apparently aware of a repo
by H. B. Gwynn and W. M. Yater in 1937, on their adr ____ation
of 20 mg of amphetamine sulfate per day for three days to 147 apparently "normal" medical students. Of these, 113 reported
"peppiness," 72 said the drug caused them to feel exhilarated, 61
that it greatly increased their powers of concentration, and 42
that it made them feel more verbal and talkative. Furthermore,
118 (80 percent) stated that they would like to take the drug
whenever possible to help them study for examinations.[39] If
persons who because of educational attainment and professional
prospects are rarely charged with having severely "inadequate" or
"immature" personalities would seek out amphetamines in a free
environment, it cannot be considered abnormal that military
prisoners, trapped in a frustrating and degrading environment,
should try to relieve feelings of tension, boredom, anger, or
diffuse malaise through the use of amphetamine. Clearly these
men resorted to inhalers because, unlike their fellows outside the
barracks, they did not have easy access to Benzedrine in pill form.
Military incarceration is one of the most intensely lonely, directly
stressful, and personally traumatic situations any American can
expect to encounter, and it is obvious that Monroe and Drell's
subjects should not have been labeled psychologically "inadequate" or "immature" because they resorted to amphetamine
abuse.

The essential "normality" and general reliability of the initial
euphoric effect of amphetamine is what makes the drug so likely
to produce dependence. No peculiarities of personality need be
involved. Consider Blum's characterization of amphetamine
users in his California campus studies:

> Higher prevalence occurs among students who are older, are
> upperclassmen, are arts, humanities, and biology majors,
> come from wealthier families, have one or both parents dead,
> are from unsettled families, are either without religious affili-
> ation or are Jewish, are without interest in religion, have a reli-
> gion different from their father's and their mother's, find ath-
> letics unimportant, do not participate in religion or in politics,

seek new experience, find academic-career activities unimportant, are politically left wing and actively involved in politics, are undergoing a political change to the left, differ politically from their fathers and mothers, are not in agreement with their families on issues. Amphetamine users are also more often found, in proportion, among students who perceive their parents as having been reluctant to give drugs—or in other cases quick to do so—who found childhood illness satisfying, see parents as having been little concerned over their health as children . . . Prevalence of amphetamine experience is greater among students who view as nationally dangerous the Establishment, other presently powerful cliques, or middle-of-the-roaders, and who are also among those students seeing good reasons to take illicit-exotic drugs.

Reviewing minor drugs, we find a greater prevalence of amphetamine users among those who drink coffee often, drink tea, and take stay-awakes. Regarding drug functions, there is a greater prevalence of users among those who take drugs to gain courage, to explore themselves, to have religious experiences, to satisfy strong cravings, to relieve boredom, to combat depression, to relieve nervousness, to facilitate moods, to combat anger, to facilitate friendliness, to alter appetite, to seek to feel stronger, to combat feelings of dullness, to improve sexual appetite, to reduce sexual desire, to combat panic, to attempt suicide, to enhance intelligence, to improve performance, to prepare for stress, and to exclude stimuli. [40]

Obviously no composite "profile" of the "typical" amphetamine user is possible—even among a relatively homogeneous group of college students. As many different kinds of people use amphetamines as use tobacco or alcohol, and for as many different reasons.

One reason for apparent similarities is that most drug abusers become known to the medical community only after they have been arrested or have agreed to voluntary confinement. Characterizations of their personalities often reflect this social situation rather than anything accounting for their drug dependence. When drug abusers are observed in less authoritarian settings—in private medical practice, for example, or on the street—they represent a wide variety of psychological types. The importance of the social setting is also suggested by the fact that some abusers of opiates and other drugs, especially physicians and medical workers, manage to avoid any associated personal and social disorganization.[41] This may be, Scher suggests, a clue "to the avoidance of the degenerative development of the life"—which elsewhere he calls the "core-addict" life. "If the addict functions effectively in work and family, he will probably not get into serious difficulty until he begins to develop reduced euphoria, elevated tolerance, and/or withdrawal anxiety in significant proportions. As one addict put it, 'Is it not possible that in many addicts the psychological disturbances develop after addiction or drug dependence occurs rather than before it?' " And M. Schmideberg believes that "the argument that it is only 'inadequates' who become addicts is wrong. Many become inadequate as a result of the addiction on which they embarked through curiosity, temptation or 'social' pressures, in the same way that habits of social drinking are responsible for quite a number of alcoholics."[42]

We must avoid indiscriminately assigning "personality types" to drug users. Nevertheless, even terminology that has little clinical or diagnostic value and indicates a distaste for cultural deviance rather than an understanding of drug abuse tells us something important: that the observer does not consider himself or other "normal" people as likely to become addicted to this drug. The difference between heroin and amphetamine in this respect, like the difference in initial perceived euphoric effect, is striking. C. W. M. Wilson describes heroin addicts as "self-centered and narcissistic," "interested only in satisfaction of [their] own primitive needs," "not matured in a healthy way," "not interested in giving to anyone," "interested only in receiving," unable to "accept a mature heterosexual role," and unable to initiate or maintain "meaningful relationships with loved ones." By way of contrast, he refers to a study comparing fifty adolescents admitted to a reformatory who had amphetamines in their urine (positive subjects) with one hundred who did not: "No obvious differences of personality between positives and negatives were apparent. The average intelligence quotient was a little lower in positives than negatives (97:99). Inspection did not suggest marked differences in type or severity of problems."[43] Comparing narcotic and stimulant abusers at the California Rehabilitation Center, V. S. Fischmann, although he found few differences between the two groups with regard to psychiatric diagnosis, judged the amphetamine abusers to be participating more intensely and sincerely in the treatment program and considered them more sociable, adaptable, sensitive, verbal, and intellectual. He also discovered that they were more literate, had completed more years of formal education, had higher intelligence quotients, and came from families of higher income level.[44]

In other words, amphetamine abusers seem more "normal" (or more like the observer) than opiate abusers. This judgment was made by von Felsinger, Lasagna, and Beecher, whose findings were confirmed subsequently by most investigators. Noting that four of twenty student volunteers had dysphoric reactions and consequently did not like amphetamine, they characterized these "atypical reactors" as "conspicuously lacking" in the "high degree of motivation and goal orientation" characteristic of their sixteen fellow students. Descriptions like "low motivation" and "drifter" appeared in their records; "their academic achievement was low"; they revealed "a pervading sense of failure or inadequacy in meeting life's demands." All four "felt a release of pressure from drinking alcohol, and they were suspected of having neurotic causes for their drinking." Rorschach testing confirmed "passivity and dependence" and "fear of loss of control under any type of pressure" for all four. The authors particularly noted a "striking emphasis on restrictive control," which they considered to be connected with the subjects' high anxiety-hostility scores. They stated:

> It is not unreasonable to assume that such a personality structure, already inadequate to deal with everyday stresses, fraught with impulsivity and anxiety, and fearing loss of control, may be alarmed by the surge of stimulation and energy associated with amphetamine, which would but add to the tension and further threaten precarious controls. A well-balanced personality structure, on the other hand, could conceivably integrate such stimulation into ongoing activity without disturbance and with pleasant effect.[45]

The Lasagna, von Felsinger, and Beecher studies also included thirty "postaddict" prisoners at the United States Public Health Service Hospital at Lexington, Kentucky. Most of them had been addicted to heroin or morphine, and a few to cocaine. About half found it pleasant and about a third distinctly unpleasant. The results for heroin and morphine were not much different. On the questionnaire, morphine (+ 27) was rated more euphoric than heroin (+ 16) or amphetamine (+ 19). All the drugs were judged to improve mental functioning about equally, and willingness to repeat the experience was about the same for all three drugs (about half of the prisoners in each case). Amphetamine, however, was most often chosen as the most unpleasant of the three drugs (for the "normal" volunteers, the worst was morphine).

It is interesting that even a group composed mainly of opiate addicts should enjoy amphetamine almost as much as heroin or morphine. Still, the differences between their reactions and those of the students are clear, not only in their expected greater liking for opiates but also in their lower regard for amphetamine. Certainly these prisoner-addicts can be considered socially "atypical" in an even stronger sense than the four students who had a dysphoric reaction, whatever psychological or psychiatric terms one chooses to apply. Again, although most people enjoy the effects of amphetamine, people seen by investigators as "normal" and "healthy" enjoy them more often than others.

In his monograph on amphetamine psychosis, Connell reported that thirty of the forty patients for whom there was information "showed a background of factors usually associated with the development or manifestations of abnormal personality and psychopathy." However, he emphasized that this does not mean that only persons of abnormal personality will become addicted to amphetamines. He noted that six of the forty had backgrounds and personalities that appeared normal and that "the majority of patients appeared to be extraverts, since twenty were described as friendly and good mixers and only eight were said to have no friends." He considered this important "in view of the opinions expressed in standard textbooks of psychiatry and in the literature emanating from drug houses that amphetamine addiction and psychosis occur only in persons of abnormal or psychopathic personality."[46]

The prisoners in Lasagna's study indicated that they had had to learn to perceive opiates as euphoric, in the face of nausea and other distress, with the help of encouragement and "instruction" by friends. The taste for heroin or morphine is an acquired one; to use a frivolous analogy, it is like a taste for olives or oysters. The taste for amphetamine is more like a taste for chocolate layer cake—easier to come by and possibly more dangerous. Not everyone will take the trouble to learn to like opiates. And the fact is that amphetamines are much more likely to produce damaging drug dependence than opiates.

The different kinds of drug dependence are not mutually exclusive. Barbiturates are used by amphetamine abusers who feel too "strung-out" or jittery, encouraged by the drug industry's "combination" products like Dexamyl. Amphetamines are also often used in conjunction or alternation with opiates. Both these substances can be "mainlined," dissolved and injected directly into a vein. (The self-administration of drugs by injection appears to be uniquely pleasurable for some persons, perhaps because of its sexual connotations.) Many heroin addicts mix their opiate with amphetamines or use amphetamines alone when they cannot obtain opiates. As a British physician pointed out: "the dependence potential of 'meth' is such that a heroin-and-methyl-amphetamine abuser or addict when confronted by a treatment-centre doctor with the choice of cutting down on either 'H' or 'meth' prefers to reduce 'H' rather than 'meth'; and some addicts receiving 'H' from a treatment centre exchange some of it on the illicit market for 'meth.' "[47]

In a letter to the editor of *The New England Journal of Medicine*, a young médical school student, temporarily in charge of the drug-abuse program at Cermak Memorial Hospital in Chicago (the only accredited prison hospital in the country), described a process of moving from heroin to amphetamine addiction:

Recently, I received several reports from the men on the program that there is a new thing turning on their particular micro society. Their term is "West Coast." Many have at least tried it, and an increasing number are becoming addicted to it.

I was informed by one prisoner who has a 20-year-old heroin habit that he mainlined "West Coast" just once and that he was finding himself "running" (the vernacular for trying to buy it on the street) for it. The same man told me that it is not covered by the drug-abuse laws. A second inmate, who is an addict both to heroin and to "West Coast," but mostly to "West Coast," told me today that in the two months that he was out of jail he lost 14 kg (30 pounds) and got little or no sleep (he also has the abscess problems that virtually all these men have from "shooting" quinine and using dirty needles). He is nervous and jittery and seeks only more "West Coast" to keep him going.

One of the main reasons I am writing this letter is that all the prisoners I have talked to about this increasing problem got the drug with a doctor's prescription. Many of them are getting it with their aid privileges and selling what they don't use to earn money to support themselves and their habit. This menacing drug is being released to these men by careless physicians, who, I hope, will read this letter and act on the knowledge I am trying to impart.

The more proper name for "West Coast" is methylphenidate, or perhaps doctors know it as Ritalin. Yes, it is the most highly addicting and dangerous drug that any of these men can think of, and they have had much clinical experience in the matters of intravenous addiction.[48]

To "graduate" from heroin to amphetamine abuse is to exchange a bad situation for a worse one. Heroin, with its "normalizing" rather than intoxicating effect on the body, has never been shown to produce any disease, or tissue or organ damage; and heroin-related deaths are usually caused by infections from dirty needles or other conditions not connected with heroin's pharmacological properties. But amphetamines can cause psychoses and serious depression and can debilitate the abuser enough to render him susceptible to a number of organic syndromes, sometimes leading to death.

Literature that relies on the ideas of "addictive drug," on the one hand, and "addictive personality," on the other, has created much confusion. It is less misleading to speak of social conditions and cultural settings that tend to sustain drug dependence of a particular kind and particular attitudes toward that dependence. In a culture where energetic active striving is considered more desirable than passive acceptance, people considered "normal" will prize the effect of a stimulant like amphetamine more than that of a depressant like heroin. The comparison with alcohol, a more socially acceptable depressant, is interesting. The primary effect of alcohol is to decrease ability to monitor incoming information and general alertness to environmental stimuli. In small doses this produces mild relaxation and disinhibition of thoughts and feelings, convivality, and animated conversation—a euphoriant effect not unlike amphetamine's, although the underlying mechanism is entirely different. But alcohol does not increase energy or concentration or improve work performance in any way; in fact some of its physiological effects resemble the onset of sleep. It is a drug for play, for "after hours," for forgetting one's troubles. Its use or overuse is often regarded with amused tolerance, but never as a virtue. Amphetamine, on the other hand, by its alerting effect helps people to get on with what is regarded as the *business* of society—studying for examinations, driving trucks for long distances, athletic performances—so the notions of pleasure and usefulness, of feeling good and doing something right, are fused. It is possible to deny that one uses amphetamine for mere "pleasure" at all. When combined with rampant moralizing on the subject of "addiction," such an attitude can lead to real absurdities; for example, one German investigator dismissed all the cases of methamphetamine dependence he found in the medical literature as not true instances of addiction because the users said they had begun taking the drug to increase endurance rather than to achieve euphoria.[49] Amphetamines can easily come to be approved as useful for reasons hard to distinguish from the ones that make people like them immediately, and this mixture or confusion of motives is particularly effective in producing drug dependence.

Social rules and customs may not only contribute to the causes of psychoactive drug abuse and provide opportunities for it, but also, in the most literal sense, define the consequences. That is why we have the unfortunate but unavoidable word "addiction," which has too often meant little more than "the consequences of opiate use." And of course many of the worst consequences of opiate use are produced by the punitive legislation that makes it necessary to embark on a criminal career to obtain the drugs. It is sometimes said that only very high doses of amphetamine, not medically therapeutic ones, lead to "addiction." But the same could be said, *a fortiori*, of opiates, if laws and social attitudes were different. Low-dose chronic use of amphetamines usually is not described as addiction simply because it is not as expensive as injecting weak solutions of heroin or as likely to lead to prison, and therefore not as disruptive of the user's life and society's routines. To use such a criterion for addiction is to impose a moral judgment on a social situation in the guise of a medical diagnosis.

There is a pattern in the medical community of optimism about new psychoactive drugs followed by disillusionment. A drug is introduced as "nonaddicting"; its capacity to produce dependence is not observed. When evidence of abuse gradually accumulates, legal controls and sanctions are applied, whereupon an illegal traffic arises. Meanwhile, physicians begin to debate whether or not the drug is "truly addictive." In 1898 heroin was introduced as a "nonaddictive" cure for opium and morphine addiction, its name derived from the word "hero." Twelve years later it was already considered more dangerous than the other opiates. Similar claims of panacealike powers, harmlessness, and capacity to "cure" other kinds of drug abuse were made at one time or another for morphine, cocaine, barbiturates, "Demerol" (meperidine hydrochloride), and "minor" tranquilizers like "Miltown" (meprobamate) and "Librium" (chlordiazepoxide hydrochloride).[50] It has been the same with amphetamines. We have reached the point where their dangers are obvious. They have a remarkable power to reinforce occasional or sporadic use with sensations of euphoria that can establish a pattern of abuse. Whether this dependence is defined as "drug addiction" is not important. What matters are the psychological, social, and medical consequences.

Crime and Violence

"From all evidence, amphetamines
do tend to set up conditions in
which violent behavior is more
likely to occur than would be the
case had the individual not used
it. Suspiciousness and hyperactivity
may combine to induce precipitous and
unwarranted assaultative behavior.
Under the influence of amphetamines,
lability of mood is common, the user
abruptly shifting from warmly congenial
to furiously hostile moods for the most
trivial of reasons."

The crime rate in the United States has risen steadily over the past several decades. During this period, and particularly since the early 1960s, there has been an enormous increase in drug abuse. To what extent is drug abuse a causal factor in the commission of crime? How, and in what ways, is the abuser or addict apt to be or become a criminal? Is there anything about the psychopharmacological properties of certain drugs that makes them, when abused, more criminogenic than others? More specifically, is there a relation between amphetamine abuse and criminal behavior, and, if so, how does it compare with the relation between heroin and crime?

Public Attitudes toward Drugs and Crime

In the 1930s the Federal Bureau of Narcotics' "educational campaign" described marihuana as so potent a criminogenic agent that even a single use could drive a previously law-abiding person to violent crime. Later, official anxiety concerning the criminogenic properties of drugs focused on heroin. And now social scientists, medical authorities, and law enforcement officials have begun to express concern about other drugs, especially amphetamines and barbiturates. Is this simply the latest manifestation of a general disposition to assume that the abuse of any drug will lead to crime and violence, or are these drugs uniquely criminogenic?

In surveying marihuana's reputation as a drug which leads to crime, one is struck by the tremendous and disproportionate influence of a nine-hundred-year-old myth. This myth, introduced to the Western world by Marco Polo, concerns the eleventh-century Persian "Assassins," and has served as the source for many persons seeking to connect cannabis and crime. In 1937, while Commissioner of the Federal Bureau of Narcotics, H. J. Anslinger made the following statement: "In the year 1090, there was founded in Persia the religious and military order of the Assassins, whose history is one of cruelty, barbarity, and murder, and for good reason. The members were confirmed users of hashish, or marijuana, and it is from Arabic 'hashashin' that we have the English word 'assassin.' "[1] This brief, incorrect version has had the strongest impact on nearly all who are aware of any part of the myth, or even of any connection between the words "hashish" and "assassin." It is difficult to believe there can be any rational justification for basing an important twentieth-century prohibition on misunderstood eleventh-century folklore.

There are no valid data indicating that cannabis is criminogenic, or that its use leads to acts of violence. Dr. Walter Bromberg, a psychiatrist at Bellevue Hospital, studied all convictions (over 91,000) in the Courts of General and Special Sessions from 1932 to 1937, looking for any evidence indicating a causal relationship between marihuana use and crime. He and his team also interviewed about 17,000 offenders, several hundred of whom had used marihuana. He concluded that "the earlier use of marihuana apparently did not predispose to crime, even that of using other drugs . . . The expectancy of major crimes following the use of cannabis in New York County is small, according to these experiences."[2] Two earlier studies conducted by the Army in the Panama Canal Zone in 1925 and 1931 found that "delinquencies due to mariajuana [sic] smoking which result in trial by military court are negligible in number when compared with delinquencies resulting from the use of alcoholic drinks."[3] The investigators observed that marihuana caused no tendency to combativeness or destructiveness and was no threat to military discipline.

In 1946, Bromberg and T. C. Rodgers, then serving in the United States Navy, denied any relationship between marihuana and aggressive crime in one of the best reports to date on what is described as the "controversial point" of "the influence of marihuana on the antisocial impulses of its users, and its influence on crime causation." After a well-documented study of 9,280 convicted naval offenders, they concluded:

> 1. There is no positive relationship between aggressive crime and marihuana usage in the Naval service . . . 2. . . . there is no significant causal relationship between aggressive crime in civilian life (of the naval offenders studied) and the use of marihuana . . . 3. Marihuana usage is but an aspect of some type of mental disorder or personality abnormality.[4]

R. N. and G. S. Chopra, who studied cannabis in India for years, found that:

> so far as premeditated crime is concerned, especially that of a violent nature, hemp drugs in some cases may not only not lead to it, but they may actually act as deterrents . . . one of the important actions of these drugs is to quieten and stupify the individual so that there is no tendency to violence . . . The result of continued and excessive use of these drugs in our opinion is to make the individual timid rather than lead him to commit a crime of violent nature.[5]

In the case of the opiates, there is very definitely a relation between drug abuse and the commission of crime, but it is not a simple one, since heroin and other opiates do not possess, as a psychopharmacological property, the ability to induce violent behavior. Unlike marihuana, all opiates are fairly strong central nervous system and motor depressants, so a person under the influence of heroin is probably even less capable of committing a crime than one who is using cannabis. Our present national attitudes toward heroin addiction result from the historical convergence of a number of social factors which, in themselves, have nothing at all to do with the effects or dangers of the drug. There is a curious ambivalence in our view of the heroin addict:

although we often give lip service to the notion that he is sick or psychologically disturbed, our more basic emotional response is fear and hatred. Heroin is commonly believed to cause "moral degeneration" and great deterioration in physical health, violent aggressive behavior, "strong-arm" crime, and sexual assaults. Although these views may be slowly changing as the heroin abuse problem spreads from the slums to suburbia, the public attitude is summed up in the term "dope fiend."

Somewhat ironically, the roots of contemporary attitudes toward heroin addiction can be traced to another civil war. In the early 1860s many wounded soldiers became drug addicts as a result of the newly discovered technique of hypodermic administration of morphine for pain. Morphine addiction was so common among veterans that it was called the "soldier's disease." Respect and pity conflicted with apprehension and revulsion for a while, but public judgment swung strongly to the negative side when Chinese laborers, imported to the West Coast between 1852 and 1870 to work on railroad construction, introduced opium to this continent. By the time opium use had become widespread among the loose-living pioneers along the Pacific frontier (the amount prepared for smoking and imported to the United States rose from 20,000 pounds in 1860 to 298,000 pounds in 1883), opposition to the practice was tinged with racial prejudice. Many viewed it as an indulgence of an inferior and debased people, a habit contrary to white supremacy and white morality. This view of opiate use as foreign and menacing was strengthened by racial and national prejudices against immigrants of Italian, central European, and Jewish descent, who made up most of the opiate addicts on the East Coast and especially in New York City.[6]

At the end of the nineteenth century the American public gradually became aware of the existence of a growing drug problem. Preparations containing opium and opium derivatives were available without prescription at pharmacies and grocery stores. In the days before the advent of large-scale, scientifically oriented medicine based on careful diagnosis and specific treatment, such home remedies were extraordinarily popular. A few of these patent medicines were "Dr. Fowler's Strawberry and Peppermint Mixture" (contining morphine), "Dr. Grove's Anodyne for Infants" (morphine sulfate), "Dr. Moffett's Teething Compound" (powdered opium), "Adamson's Botanic Cough Basalm" (heroin hydrochloride), "Gooch's Mexican Consumption Cure" (morphine sulfate), and "Professor Hoff's Consumption Cure" (opium).[7] The "medical addicts" (estimates vary from a low of 264,000 to a high of 2,000,000 addicts at the turn of the century) were thus provided with further remedies which "cured" by maintaining their addictions. Many of these contained the newly synthesized opium derivative heroin; others were "secret formulas" of old standbys, morphine and opium. Eventually public indignation over these proprietary medicines was aroused, and their ineffectiveness and dangers were publicized.

Another factor contributing to heroin's present reputation was the rapid growth of large-scale illicit traffic. An ideal drug for smuggling, heroin is three times as potent, weight for weight, as morphine, so can be concealed in a small space. Greater potency meant greater profit, since more doses could be obtained from the same amount of basic drug. Furthermore, the crystal structure of heroin salts made it easier to dilute ("cut") this drug with lactose or quinine. Many of the men engaged in this illegal traffic were recruits from the underworld, and the public attitudes toward them were readily transferred to the drug they smuggled.

At the Hague Conference of 1912, most of the major nations decided to limit production and trade in opiates to the amounts required for medical purposes. To fulfill United States obligations under this Convention, Congress passed the Harrison Narcotic Act in 1914. This statute, based on federal power of taxation, established a licensing system to control the importation, manufacture, distribution, and sale of opiates. Properly licensed physicians were allowed to prescribe or dispense opiates only in the course of their medical practice and only to bona-fide patients. After World War I many addicts began to patronize a small number of "script" doctors, who prescribed opiates for profit and made no attempt to treat their clients. Many of these "script" physicians were arrested and prosecuted. A number of rulings by the Supreme Court on these cases upheld the constitutionality of the Harrison Act and declared that dispensing opiates to an addict without attempting to cure his addiction constituted improper medical practice. Public authorities, forced to do something for addicts who urgently needed drugs but were being refused them by their physicians, established out-patient clinics in various cities to administer opiates (and sometimes cocaine) to addicts otherwise unable to obtain drugs legally. Most of these clinics were understaffed and had little direction or purpose and even less knowledge. Those in charge were rarely interested in trying to cure addiction and found it easier to give an addict a week's supply of his drug than to see him every day. The results were an increase in illicit traffic, a rise in the number of addicts, and a migration of many addicts to cities where clinics existed, with a consequent disruption of their lives. The medical profession was soon united in vigorous opposition to the clinics, and in 1920 and 1921 two special committees of the American Medical Association condemned them and called upon the government to act. The Treasury Department complied by closing the clinics.

One such clinic in Shreveport, Louisiana, survived almost four years. A letter written in 1920 from the Shreveport Commissioner of Public Safety to the Louisiana State Board of Health states:

> I wish to write you and express how the Police Department of Shreveport feels in regard to the Louisiana State Board Dispensary, known here as the Narcotic Clinic, same being under the direction of Dr. Willis P. Butler. The writer feels that this letter is due the State Board, as well as simply an act of justice toward Dr. Butler, for upon the institution of the clinic I had grave doubts as to its efficacy, and in fact expressed myself as being bitterly opposed to it . . .
>
> I wish to say that from a police standpoint, the City of Shreveport is greatly benefited by its being here. It has practically eliminated the bootlegger who deals in narcotics, and in this way alone has reduced the number of possible future dope users . . .
>
> Before the establishment of the Clinic a great number of criminals prosecuted through this department were those addicted with the use of opiates. Now, however, it is very seldom that we have to prosecute this class, and we are able to keep a direct line upon anyone who might sell morphine, cocaine, and such other drugs as are prohibited by law . . .
>
> Our records show that the Clinic here has cured a number of those afflicted with this habit, and some are working here and are citizens that respect themselves and are respected by this department. The authorities in charge of the Police Depart-

ment in Shreveport would regard it a calamity should this Clinic be removed from this point, and we are as earnestly for it at the present time as we were bitterly opposed to it upon its institution here. We cannot speak in too high terms of Dr. Butler and his methods used at the dispensary.[8]

It is clear that it was the medical profession, not the police, which took the initiative against the clinics. Furthermore, it was at the explicit request of the AMA that in 1921 the Attorney General brought before the Supreme Court the famous Behman case, in which the Court ruled that to supply drugs to an addict for self-medication constituted improper medical practice. This firm stand by such an influential group as the American Medical Association undoubtedly strengthened the general public impression that heroin addiction was evil. Moreover, it was on the AMA's recommendation that the federal government established two "prison hospitals" (at Lexington, Kentucky, and Fort Worth, Texas) for institutional "treatment" of arrested addicts. Although voluntary patients were admitted, the tight security and the authoritarian and custodial relationships with "patients" strengthened the public's impression that there was a direct causal link between heroin addiction and criminal behavior.[9]

At the end of World War II, there was a sharp increase in heroin traffic and addiction. Racial and social prejudices again helped solidify national attitudes. Most of the new addicts came from the slums and ghettos of a few big cities, where the majority of people were blacks or of Spanish descent. The public seemed eager to believe that heroin was a "cause" of crime and violence, without considering that addiction in the slums and ghettos might result from the same discrimination and repression that led to violent and criminal behavior. Today, use of heroin and other opiates continues to be dealt with primarily through prohibition and criminal penalties. Addicts (with the exception of a few, like physicians and pharmacists) must seek illicit sources. The more effective the obstacles to producing and distributing the opiates, the scarcer they become. The greater ingenuity and risk needed by the pusher as well as the addict are reflected in higher prices, and addicts turn to prostitution or crime (almost invariably against property, and only accidentally against person) to raise money for drugs. Thus the more successful the enforcement of prohibition, the more crime will be associated with a drug of addiction, even when the capacity to induce antisocial behavior is not one of its inherent properties.

Amphetamine and Crime

Contrary to much medical and popular opinion, the amphetamines are probably as addictive as heroin. If they were as difficult to obtain as opiates, crime (again largely against property) related to amphetamine abuse would be as frequent and as widespread as crime related to heroin is. Moreover, since the amphetamines have psychopharmacological properties which potentiate or disinhibit aggressive impulses and promote paranoid thinking and even delusions, they have much greater potential for producing violence than opiates or marihuana. Nevertheless, the Federal Bureau of Narcotics and the AMA, while devoting much energy to establishing marihuana as a "killer drug," have paid little attention to them.

Still, there is considerable literature relating amphetamines to crime. Some of the earliest reports appeared in the Japanese literature. In June 1954 it was estimated that the number of Japanese abusers of "wake-amine" was between 500,000 and 600,000, and the Japan Pharmacist Association placed the number at 1,500,000. A number of scientists have investigated the impact on Japanese society. H. Noda, after studying 136 amphetamine addicts in the city of Kurume, wrote that 61 percent had been involved in antisocial behavior. When this study is cited, it is usually implied that the author was dealing with people who repeatedly used large doses of the drug and under its influence committed major crimes. Noda, however, does not explicitly say this. Another study often referred to in a misleading way was conducted by T. Masaki, who found that of sixty murderers convicted in Japan during May and June of 1954, thirty-one had some unspecified connection with the use of amphetamine. He also noted that during this period 10,148 persons were taken into custody for offences against the Awakening Drug Control Law; 52 percent of them were found to be addicts. However, just as Masaki did not elucidate the connection in the murder cases, he failed to describe these "offences," and made no attempt to control for other variables. According to M. Nagahama, in 1955, 4,866 Japanese were "arrested for crimes directly or indirectly stemming from the use of stimulant drugs," but the nature of the relation (in particular, whether and in what ways it was causal) was not indicated.[10] Without more precise information one must be very cautious in drawing conclusions from these data.

United States government publications reveal a wide range of opinion on the subject. *The Task Force Report: Narcotics and Drug Abuse*, published in 1967 by the President's Commission on Law Enforcement and Administration of Justice, took the position that research contradicted claims linking amphetamine use to crimes of violence, sexual crimes, or accidents. Four years later the Select Committee on Crime presented the opposite view, claiming that testimony obtained from a number of physicians and social scientists showed a relationship between abuse of amphetamine-type drugs and violence and crime. The statement of Dr. J. C. Kramer is typical:

> From all evidence, amphetamines do tend to set up conditions in which violent behavior is more likely to occur than would be the case had the individual not used it. Suspiciousness and hyperactivity may combine to induce precipitous and unwarranted assaultative behavior. Under the influence of amphetamines, lability of mood is common, the user abruptly shifting from warmly congenial to furiously hostile moods for the most trivial of reasons.
>
> Most high-dose amphetamine users describe involvement, either as aggressor or victim, in episodes in which murder or mayhem was avoided by the slimmest of margins. There are, of course, instances in which violence actually occurred. From descriptions of a number of these events it is clear that they would not have taken place had it not been for the use of amphetamines.[11]

In considering the few studies analyzing the relation of amphetamines to violence and crime, two major points must be considered: Do amphetamines have the capacity to awaken or increase an individual's tendencies toward aggressive or violent behavior during a high, on a "run," or while "crashing"? If there is a connection between crime and the use of amphetamines, to what extent is it a direct consequence of taking these drugs rather than a function of unavailability (as in the case of heroin)?

Hostile or aggressive behavior was first systematically observed in the subjects studied for P. H. Connell's now famous 1958 monograph, *Amphetamine Psychosis*. Recent literature confirms and further documents his observations. In "A San Francisco Bay Area 'Speed' Scene," J. T. Carey and Jerry Mandel quote a law enforcement official's characterization of the problem:

> One of the main problems we've got to face is this damned aggressiveness—these amphetamine users, they're all this way. This is the common denominator. I've seen guys that would pop fifty ten milligram pills or shoot some Meth and they're just all over—they can't stand still—they just can't keep from doing things and they're jumping around all the time. If they've got something in their hand they'll hit you without realizing what they're doing—and they'll—if they've got a flashlight they're likely to go like that (swings) and hit you with it.

Carey and Mandel either observed or received firsthand reports of thirty violent incidents involving persons who regularly took daily doses of 100 to more than 1000 mg of amphetamines intravenously. These actions usually were not premeditated and often would seem motiveless to an outsider: for example, a man might strike his girlfriend, or a parent hit a child, for no apparent reason. "I let this couple crash at my house, and the next morning as I was about to say 'good morning' to her she put her head down and smashed into my stomach like a goat . . . It knocked me down. Then they grabbed their belongings and left . . . Two weeks later she appeared at my door with another friend, and just asked for a room they could stay . . . like nothing had happened, and she probably didn't even remember it."[12]

The authors note that as the dosage is increased beyond the usual "therapeutic" 10-15 mg, quantitative changes in behavior become qualitative. Alertness and energy are experienced as jumpiness. Awareness of immediate, close-range stimuli is enhanced, but very much at the expense of distant stimuli. In discussing how the extent and character of aggression may vary, they suggest that it has to do with whether the person is high or coming down, the duration of the particular run, and how long the run-crash-run cycle has been going on. During the coming down phase (crashing), the intensity of the the user's irritability may cause him to be intolerably selfish. Arguments are frequent, and although they occur over ostensibly insignificant matters they often degenerate into yelling and hitting. J. R. Tinklenberg and R. C. Stillman state that "It is during this period of 'coming down,' particularly after a prolonged run, that the user is most prone to assaultive behavior."[13] Carey and Mandel also observed that the extent and degree of violence increase with the duration of a run and with the number of consecutive runs made. They suggest that when heavy users keep their first five or ten runs under two days in duration, the incidence of violence may not be any higher than among a nonamphetamine-using sample.

The fact that massive doses of amphetamines often induce a form of paranoia has been discussed already. Although amphetamine-induced "paranoia" usually is not accompanied by the disordered thinking characteristic of the true paranoid schizophrenic, amphetamine-induced delusional beliefs may be persistent and long-lasting: "I finally decided last week (fifteen months after last shooting crystal) that I really had a delusion under speed. I saw a police car pull up in front of the house, two men get out and walk up the street. I ran to look out the rear window, and when they didn't show up in a minute or so, returned to the front window. There was the same car, only it wasn't a police car, in the same spot, and the same two men walking further up the street . . . only they weren't policemen either."[14] There is little doubt that this tendency to paranoid thinking significantly enhances the danger that the already volatile and impulsive amphetamine abuser will act out his irritability and aggressiveness in violently criminal behavior.

In a study of forty amphetamine users who regularly consumed at least 80 mg daily, Griffith describes some of the manifestations of aggression and even sadism which arise during so-called "drug parties," noting the reactions of three men who, while attending separate parties, after unrelated bouts of drinking, each received 75 mg of Methedrine in single intravenous injections: "Within minutes of the injection, each 'went crazy,' according to users. They became 'wild' and combative, would shout insults and accuse those about them of 'having it in for them' or, for a variety of reasons, 'planning to knife them.' Much that was said was incoherent. Abrupt changes in behavior in two individuals spontaneously subsided in approximately an hour. The third made his 'woman' (a prostitute), and inflicted numerous cuts and bruises."[15]

Numerous examples of the capricious manner in which a high dose amphetamine abuser may suddenly turn against both friends and strangers have been cited. In the cases of two patients who took doses larger than those usually prescribed:

> the assaults were particularly frightening because of their un-provoked, grossly psychotic quality: One patient while walking down the street and feeling like the "king of the universe" no-ticed a man walking near him. He had a fleeting idea that this stranger might be a homosexual but then his grandiosity reas-serted itself; "I decided he just didn't belong in my picture of things—so I took him out of the picture." He then explained that he did this by carefully waiting until he was just abreast of the individual and then spinning and hitting him. This was re-peated three or four times until he became frightened by what he was doing and came to Bellevue voluntarily. The second patient saw his roommate sleeping and felt that he "looked dead." He thereupon took a doorhandle and beat his head with it until restrained by a second roommate and taken to Belle-vue.[16]

There is a tendency to lash out uncontrollably with little warning and less provocation: "Overindulgence [in amphetamine use] renders the user incapable of logical or normal behavior. He ex-periences hallucinations and often lives in constant fear of other people. His suspicion that he is being followed, and the uncontrollable and abnormally aggressive nature characteristic-ally associated with overindulgence in the drug, sometimes drive him to unprovoked attack on others, some of whom may be inno-cent bystanders."[17]

Nevertheless, some authors contend that the actual incidence of crime and violence is no greater or more devastating among amphetamine abusers than in the general population. A fre-quently quoted report is that of P. D. Scott and D. R. C. Willcox, who in 1965 conducted a study of young people admitted to two London Remand Homes. They analyzed urine samples by the methyl orange test and by paper chromatography to identify the ones who had recently been using amphetamines. Table 6, showing the types of offenses committed, compares these youths with an equal sample (n=50) whose urine test on admission was negative, and a sample of youths admitted in 1949, when amphet-

Table 6.   Recent amphetamine use, as determined by urine test, of young people admitted by London Remand Homes by types of offense (percentage).

Test result	Acquisitive	Against person	Other
		Offense	
Positive	68	6	26
Negative	72	6	22
1949 sample	68	4	28

Source: P.D. Scott and D.R.C. Willcox, "Delinquency and the amphetamines," *Brit. J. Psychiat.*, 111 (1965), p. 872.

amine use was unknown in that age group. The authors state: "It is already apparent that positive urines in remand home boys do not correlate with very agressive offenses: no bodily harm was suffered by any of the very few victims."[18]

This study is objective and methodologically sound; however, its differences with the results of most other studies (many methodologically inferior) may be more apparent than real. Scott and Willcox acknowledge that "amphetamine, with its known tendency to produce a paranoid psychosis, may be particularly dangerous in an offender who is already inclined to feel persecuted. In such cases the balance may be tipped from aggressive defensiveness to murder." This statement prefaces the only three case histories which the authors present in detail. The first concerns an eighteen-year-old boy, not included in the sample, who committed murder during a robbery attempt. "A man shone a torch at him. The lad 'felt frozen' for a moment, then lashed out with his knife, killing the man with multiple stab wounds." He had regularly taken "purple hearts" (Drinamyl) to give himself the confidence to go to dances and talk with other youths, and just prior to the murder he had ingested ten of them. The authors admit that in this instance there is a "possible link between amphetamine-taking and murder." (Drinamyl contains 32 mg amobarbital for every 5 mg of dextroamphetamine, and barbiturates also can induce violent and impulsive behavior.) The second case involves a seventeen-year-old who had been taking purple hearts for six months. On the day he committed a murder he took twenty, ten of them before going to a dance hall and ten on arrival where the stabbing took place.

Note that the eighteen-year-old was too old for the sample, which ranged in age from twelve to seventeen years, and the seventeen-year-old was at the extreme end of the sample. We discuss in Chapter 9 the fascinating medical finding that amphetamines may have an *apparently* paradoxical effect on disturbed young children and adolescents, quieting them and so helping them to think more clearly and deal more effectively with their environment. These boys in Scott and Willcox's sample may have found the effect of amphetamines to be relatively benign. The two older youths probably had passed beyond the age during which the amphetamines are capable of exerting this apparent paradoxical effect, and therefore displayed aggressive and hostile behavior.

A startling paper by E. H. Ellinwood, "Assault and Homicide Associated with Amphetamine Abuse," recounts the histories of thirteen persons who committed homicide while intoxicated by amphetamines. The mean age of this group was 25.8 and the youngest was 18. In most instances the paranoid thinking, emotional lability, panic, and lowered impulse control induced by the amphetamines was instrumental in the homicide. The following excerpts illustrate the gradual development of paranoid delusions in a chronic amphetamine abuser. This particular user spent most of his time alone, and so had little opportunity for reality testing his delusional thinking.

Mr. B. was a 26-year-old man who had used amphetamines for more than two years and had gradually increased his dose to 500-800 mg. per day. Often he used barbiturates or alcohol to calm him down but he had had neither prior to the homicide. Although he obtained amphetamines from people in the drug subculture and obtained money for drugs illegally, Mr. B. was not extensively involved in the drug subculture. Essentially he was a loner who spent most of his time in his apartment.

"During the last three months, I got more and more fearful and suspicious." At first he knew he was "thinking crazy." "Then it became real, and it still feels so at times. I thought my neighbor was plotting with the Feds to get me." He took his apartment apart, including his furniture, trying to find microphones and "looking devices."

During the last three or four days before the homicide, Mr. B. did not sleep at all. He described a panic state over his ill-defined tormentors, who were sometimes thought to be federal agents and sometimes a gang that was after him because he had stolen drugs from one of its members. Thinking that his neighbor was one of "them" he waited and watched one evening until his neighbor returned. "I went to his door to listen. He heard me and opened the door and I shot him."[19]

Another case illustrates the more "rapid evolution of paranoid thinking after acute high-dose use." A young truck driver ingested 180 mg of amphetamines within a twenty-hour period in an effort to drive 1,600 miles nonstop. He began to suspect that his boss was trying to kill him with poison gas and shot him in the back of the head.

A third case illustrates "the intense ambivalence combined with emotional lability to which the individual may be reacting, while appearing to others to be bizarrely unconcerned about the violent act." This thirty-two-year-old woman shot her lover with a pistol during an argument over his possible involvement with another woman and the return of her husband from Vietnam. Over the previous eighteen months she had increased her daily dosage of amphetamines to 400-600 mg per day. Just prior to the killing she had reached a dosage level of 600-1200 mg per day, and she had not slept for four days. When her victim tried to flee, she shot him twice more, killing him, and then asked a passerby to "turn him over and take a picture of his pretty face." Shortly thereafter, in a police patrol car, she tickled the sheriff on the ear, asking him if it felt good, and later, while being interrogated, got up and announced she had to leave to go to the hairdresser.

A number of factors appear to have precipitated homicide in the cases reported by Ellinwood: (1) an acute large dose of amphetamines or a large increment over the amount usually used; (2) loss of insight into the delusional nature of thought, precipitated either by sleep deprivation or other drugs; (3) amphetamine-induced emotional lability and impulsiveness along with suspiciousness, delusions, fear, and panic; (4) a solitary life; (5) mutual enhancement of suspiciousness and paranoid ideas by association with other speed freaks;* (6) carrying a concealed weapon; (7) armed robbery as a means of obtaining the money for the drug; (8) conflict over drug dealings.

In cases of multiple drug abuse, one must be careful to qualify statements indicting amphetamines as the cause of any drug-related crime or violence. Because many high-dose amphetamine abusers also abuse other drugs, it is often extraordinarily difficult to determine the relative importance of amphetamines. Alcohol and sedatives, particularly barbiturates, used in combination with amphetamines cause loss of intellectual awareness and lower impulse control. Also, amphetamines increase the amount of alcohol or sedatives a person can consume before passing out.

An abuser who is involved in a particular speed culture often adopts a whole new set of mores and attitudes toward other people and their property. Aggressiveness, violence, and stealing may become culturally acceptable. During a visit to the Roschdale Free College in Toronto in 1970, one of the authors (L.G.) was impressed by the extraordinary policy which allowed anyone who wished to live at the college to remain there—except the speed freak. Even this extremely tolerant group of people conducting an unusual experiment in communal living could not put up with the unprovoked violence and "ripping off" of the amphetamine abuser.

The incidence of violence and crime rose dramatically in Haight-Ashbury after it became the "speed capital of the world" in 1968. The amphetamine abusers:

> suffered terrifying hallucinations, mistook their friends for police officers, and lashed out with murderous rage at any real or imagined intrusions . . . [Many] had to be segregated and restrained before they could do physical harm, especially if they were going up or coming down in crowded atmospheres.

Although these instances of violence were often precipitated and/or heightened by the pharmacological effects of amphetamine, they naturally differed according to the personalities of the young people involved. The hoodies, for example, rarely went on long drug binges or became seriously disoriented, primarily because they wanted to prove that they could control

---

*In a "crash pad," however, even individuals who are all equally deluded will sometimes point out each other's paranoid thinking.

themselves. Instead, they took speed to enhance their self-confidence, particularly if they had just been burned or ripped off by confederates, and went hunting with their dogs and their weapons for those who had humiliated them.

The more psychotic youths also created a serious menace, yet their violence was of a more random kind. The thinking of these young people was always disorganized, but they became inordinately disturbed and paranoid when they were strung-out on speed. . . . the majority of these [violent] incidents occurred in group situations where the young people consumed speed. While congregating in the dilapidated residences occupied by older and more habitual abusers, for example, the young adolescents often became tense and excited not only because they were inexperienced about the drugs they were taking but also because their courage was on the line.

If their passions were then ignited by some emotional spark, such as the presence of a persistent knick-knacker [one who fingers and walks off with whatever objects he happens to touch], the arrival of a suspected rip-off artist, or the appearance of a spaced out and sexually available girl, the novice speed freaks could become torn between their wish for peer group approval and whatever sense of conscience they possessed. As a result, they sometimes exploded into sudden savagery to release their accumulated tension and could end up assaulting the knick-knacker or the supposed thief, or raping and/or torturing the hapless girl. Roger Smith and those clinic physicians who were familiar with such turnouts and gang bangs explained to the police, yet did not excuse, the events in terms of the precipitous impulsiveness of the adolescents and the behavioral sink aspects of the district. But the police wanted no explanation. As far as they were concerned, the young people behaved like rats in a cage.[20]

Amphetamine's tendency to promote violence seems to be enhanced by crowding. L. H. Smith and his coworkers determined that the LD 50 of amphetamines (the amount required to kill half of a sample population of experimental mice) declines from 100 mg/kg to 25 mg/kg when the animals are crowded closely together:

simple aggregation of the animals increased the toxicity of the drug fourfold. In analyzing this phenomenon of aggregate amphetamine toxicity we found a polyphasic mortality curve. The mortality was high at the 25 mg per kg dose and then decreased, so that at 75 mg per kg the drug was less toxic than at 25 mg. It then increased again at 100 mg per kg where a second LD 50 appeared. In analyzing this polyphasic mortality curve we found that at the 25 mg per kg dosage, the animals were in a hyperexcitable and agitated state in which the mechanism of death was actually that of one animal killing another. As the drug dose was increased the animals became preconvulsive. The dose was not high enough to cause convulsions (the mechanism of death at 100 mg per kg), but the animals were so disorganized that they could not mobilize directive attacks at one another.

The Haight-Ashbury now has some resemblance to a giant mouse cage in that individuals are taking high-doses of central nervous system stimulants and interacting very often in a destructive fashion.[21]

Smith and Luce quote a police lieutenant's description of this Haight-Ashbury "mouse cage":

These kids have turned the Haight-Ashbury into a law-enforcement nightmare. During the first half of this year alone, eighteen murders, fifty-eight rapes, three hundred and seventy robberies, two hundred and four assaults and over sixteen hundred cases of burglary were reported at this station. The figures for this fall are already that high and should be much higher, since many of the victims were criminals themselves and would never report the damage done to them. The murder rate increases every day; three of our most recent ones occurred in one week, and drug dealers were involved in at least two of the fatal crimes.

But this is nothing. We get some incidents out here you simply wouldn't believe. A few weeks ago, my men picked up an eighteen-year-old kid and his girl friend on Haight Street selling military explosives out of a shopping bag. We get these people standing in the middle of the street shooting at anything that moves. We hear all the time about runaway girls coming to the area with no place to stay who get picked up by Negroes or bike riders on the street, locked in closets and raped for days at a time. Gang bangs and turnouts occur all the time, and burns are so common we should really list them in a separate category.[22]

J. R. Tinklenberg and R. C. Stillman believe the length of time an individual has used methamphetamine may be an important factor in the incidence of violence:

> The different rates of violence in long-term users as compared with short-term or infrequent users of mehamphetamine are striking. In our opinion this difference is clearly indicative of a cumulative amphetamine effect that predisposes the user toward assaultive behavior. We have observed in long-term users progressive deterioration of their ability to control their own behavior. This impairment may be severe and may result in sudden destructive acts, which the users may recognize as inappropriate but feel unable to curb.[23]

In considering behavior as complicated and multidetermined as most crime and violence, behavior patterns prior to drug use must be taken into consideration. Truancy, difficulties at work and in school, and infractions of the law were common among the patients of Angrist and Gershon even before amphetamine use. Thirty-five of their thirty-nine patients would have had police records even without drug-related arrests. Bell and Trethowan concluded that all their amphetamine-addicted patients "showed evidence of poorly integrated personalities" and had disturbed childhoods, "with a high incidence of alcoholism and other mental illness in their families."[24] Five of Ellinwood's sample of thirteen had histories of impulsive behavior quite apart from their use of drugs; five others were found to be schizophrenic after complete withdrawal from amphetamines. And in another study, in which he compared amphetamine addicts with addicts drawn from the general population at the Lexington Narcotics Hospital, Ellinwood noted that the "incidence of previous juvenile delinquency was higher" than in the general addict population, and the amphetamine addicts "had been more frequently admitted to reform schools."[25] Although we doubt the importance of personality predisposition in amphetamine addiction, it may be possible that character disorders involving abnormal aggressiveness, lack of impulse control, unstable object relations, or paranoid tendencies are exaggerated by amphetamines to the point of producing violence.

Finally, the need for amphetamine may lead to crime. The abuser's concerns "increasingly narrow into the immediate present of procuring and using drugs as he becomes separated from the past and unconcerned about his future. Any interference with these single-minded pursuits becomes an overwhelming threat, as his life has few other sources of satisfaction or meaning. Thus assaultive behavior becomes more probable as the inhibitions to immediate action that usually come from recalling past experiences or considering future consequences are minimized."[26] Many amphetamine abusers support their habit through petty theft or other minor crimes. Risking apprehension, they thereby increase the possibility that they will feel so threatened as to react violently. Even housewives who begin taking the drug for obesity or depression become technical criminals if they steal prescription pads from the family doctor.

One of the most common crimes committed by amphetamine users is selling ("dealing") the drug. Most is on a small-time street level basis, but some dealers go on to bigger things.

Three distinct career routes are observable in the speed scene: first, the majority remain on the street level, dealing small amounts of speed and other drugs, surviving on a day-to-day basis. They are subject to and perpetrators of violence, burglary, and armed robbery. Many are hospitalized by friends and relatives, many are arrested, some are killed. Many, however, are able to control the extent of drug use, develop reputations as trustworthy dealers, and eventually they can move into the upper levels of the speed marketplace, as distributors or chemists.

Finally, a startling number of speed users have progressed to the compulsive use of barbiturates and heroin. Such a conversion has obvious implications in terms of the kinds of criminal activites which are then required of them in order to survive. At the same time, few of these young people have the kinds of criminal skills which typify many of the heroin addicts now seen in institutions like Lexington or Fort Worth. As a result, there is very little money generated from without the scene through con games, burglary, bad checks, or credit cards. Those without skills resort to what one might call "low-level hustles," i.e., criminal activites in which little skill is required, the payoff is minimal, and the risks involved great. These would include homosexual prostitution, "burning" (selling an adulterant as a drug), "ripping" (robbing others in the speed scene of money, drugs, chemicals, weapons and the like), and frequently such low-level crimes as purse snatching or street mugging. These activities are perhaps responsible for the majority of violent acts which have occurred recently, with the drug effect playing only a secondary role.[27]

In the foregoing analysis, Dr. R. C. Smith underestimates the degree to which an amphetamine addict may have a compulsive need to obtain his drug. It is not necessary to invoke barbiturate and heroin abuse to account for this degree of compulsion. Furthermore, the low level of "criminal skills" may merely reflect the fact that amphetamines are more easily available and therefore less costly than heroin, or it may be the result of their ego-disruptive properties, which make it difficult to acquire *any* skills, criminal or otherwise. That chronic amphetamine abusers are not more often involved in premeditated crime may be explicable by M. O'Connor's hypothesis that their non-drug-abusing criminal associates consider them too irrational, unpredictable, and violent: "The usual behavior of the heroin addict is considered either logical or predictable by fellow users, or those familiar with addict characteristics. The abuser of amphetamines, on the other hand, is frequently suspected of being a 'kook.' His tendency to overindulge or use a combination of drugs having antagonistic physiological effects too often results in bizarre and unpredictable behavior. Consequently, the non-drug-abusing criminal is extremely cautious when dealing with these types."[28]

At least three distinct but mutually reinforcing psychopharmacological properties appear to make amphetamines uniquely criminogenic. First, high doses of amphetamines invariably cause a focusing of attention on immediate, close range stimuli. This often results in hair-trigger, reflexlike, and unpremeditated lashing out at innocent persons who have done nothing that could normally be construed as provocative. This "stimulus-bound" condition also reduces the user's ability to remember even recent events or to weigh consequences. The "present orientation" is strongly reinforced by speed culture mores. For many, sustained human relationships become impossible. The addict becomes even more apt to perceive anyone who seems to be interfering with his immediate drug-related pursuits as intolerably threatening, because he has lost most other sources of gratification. The result is a tremendously increased probability of antisocial behavior. By the time he has "progressed" to true speed freak status, his associations with others are characterized by a fundamental inconstancy and impermanence. The speed culture population turnover rate is high because of arrests, drug-related diseases, psychotic "freakouts," woundings, and even killings, as well as high mobility—addicts are continually moving to where the best (most "righteous") speed is available. The resultant lack of stability in the ever-narrowing world of the confirmed speed freak makes him a caricature of even the extreme "sociopath," whose only code is getting (or doing) what he wants, when he wants, with a minimum of effort or concern for the rights of others.

Amphetamine's second criminogenic psychopharmacological property is inseparable from its ability to enhance the abuser's immediate awareness of stimuli, sensory clues, and peripherally visible objects or persons. Often the abuser will interpret this "sensory flood" as an indication that he is the recipient of unlimited supplies of energy, ideas, and wisdom. But this amphetamine-induced overemphasis on the personal invariably creates a deep sense of conflict. Which information is to be trusted, and to whom can he safely give how much of what? In addition, the speed freak, who sees himself as the solipsistic center, the personal focus of universal energies, regards any perceived hesitations, obstructions, or interferences from others as critical—even life-threatening—dangers. After a few days of continuous "running," he is often so blatantly paranoid that he imagines that others are plotting against him and must be attacked first. This extremely distrustful and self-referential mode of thought persists even during crashing; in fact, as we have noted, many believe the speed freak is *most* prone to assaultive, homicidal, or suicidal behavior when crashing, especially after a run of five days or more. This "personal orientation" is, like the "present orientation," enormously reinforced by the typical interpersonal reactions (or lack thereof) occurring in the speed freak's "social" life. His primary and often exclusive concern is for the procural of *his* amphetamines; the suggestion of *sharing* drug

supplies is construed as threatening. Perhaps the single most
noticeable fact to an outsider is the almost complete absence of
cooperation, communication, or consideration in the speed
freak's general outlook. Indeed, the rare person in a speed culture who displays overt concern for others is usually ostracized as
a homosexual or sly opportunist. Suspiciousness, isolation, and
alienation pervade the speed marketplace. Because of the frequency with which rip-offs occur, especially thefts of the ultimate
commodity, speed, most drug transactions are carried out in
"neutral" settings like bowling alleys, and often the participants
bring along acquaintances for protection or carry concealed weapons. Even with these precautions, many buyers are ripped off by
accomplices of the sellers as soon as they are in vulnerable situations, and a number of these thefts are accompanied by violence.
Assaultive or murderous behavior occurs just as often among
speed abusers who are alleged "friends," where personal expectations are at least implicitly involved, and likely to be disregarded,
abused or frustrated—especially from the point of view of the
"maltreated" speed freak. When the speed freak's expectations,
even if grossly unjustified, are perceived as rejected, he generally
regards it as a personal affront, and vicious retaliation is common. Probably the most dangerous thing a speed user can do if he
is arrested or apprehended is to comply with the police in exchange for release or reduction of charges. Roger Smith has
quoted one user on the precariousness of the life of a "friend"
who "turned snitch": "A cat I knew fairly well, last time he got
busted he gave up 42 names. He's up in County right now giving
up every name he can think of. He got a lot of people some righteous time. If he does manage to get back out on the street, he's
dead this time. If he goes to the joint, he's definitely dead, without any hesitation whatsoever."[29]

The third and most acute criminogenic psychopharmacological
property of amphetamines is their psychomotor stimulating
effect. Under the influence of speed even the most normally leth-
argic person often *must* do something, even if it is as boring and
repetitious as stringing beads for hours. When such a deep and insistent need to do *something* is thought to be disapproved or
blocked, the speed abuser may attack the perceived thwarter with
murderous rage. Often such violent "retaliation" is intrinsically

rewarding because it relieves the abuser's feelings of pent-up psychological and muscular tension. Again, this tendency is strongly reinforced by speed culture mores. An addict who has been slighted, "burned" (sold bad or highly diluted speed), ripped off, or injured is expected to *over*-retaliate. The necessity of revenging genuine or imaginary wrongs is generally referred to as "making things righteous," an expression often reiterated among speed freaks. If the speed culture member does not live up to the expectations of his hypersensitive and hypervigilant associates, he risks becoming an outcast among outcasts; persons who do not retaliate immediately after the slightest imagined wrong become targets of ridicule. Accordingly, retribution accomplished by beatings, stabbings, shootings, and sometimes torture, becomes a way of life. In turn, the victims of these attacks generally retaliate as soon as they can. The endless cycle of revenge would wipe out speed colonies if the speed freaks were not so disorganized that they tend to forget even the sins of "snitchers" or get arrested in bungled attempts at revenge. But, because amphetamine-related crime occurs primarily within speed cultures, where it is largely ignored by the police, and because speed freaks rarely attempt any large-scale external crime, "official" crime rates for speed users are deceptively low.

If amphetamines, like heroin, were legally unobtainable, and if the cost of maintaining an amphetamine addiction were as high as that of maintaining a heroin addiction, it is likely that the crimes committed by amphetamine addicts would be much more violent than those now attributed to heroin addicts. The amphetamine addict does not have to steal $400 to $500 worth of goods each day to sell for $100 to a fence in order to raise the money needed for purchasing his drugs. Even if he is taking the drug intravenously in such huge quantities that he must obtain it on the black market, his addiction will be cheaper than a heroin addiction of comparable severity. For this reason we must be most careful in recommendations for a more reasoned approach to the question of amphetamine abuse. If we attempt to curb the aggressiveness and assaultiveness which *directly* derive from its use by instituting stricter legal penalties for the distribution and use of the drug, we run the risk of increasing the crime which inevitably results from the strict prohibition of any addictive drug.

The Place of Amphetamines in Medicine

"Amphetamines are 'magic pills'; their
effect is dramatic; they do make the
patient feel good. But administering
them in cases of mild depression only
masks the underlying problems
instead of affording the patient the
opportunity to attempt to
deal directly with his troubles. Most
patients complaining of fatigue, lack of
energy, nervousness, depression, anxiety,
or insomnia are really asking for a kind
of short-term psychotherapy from a person
they believe to be empathetic and
trustworthy. When a physician responds
with a pill, he is depriving his
patient of the service he ought to be
providing, and may be initiating or
perpetuating a malignant pattern of drug
use as a substitute for coping with
the emotional turmoil of daily life."

Amphetamine was first used effectively in the treatment of narcolepsy, a rare disorder. As with most new drugs, the amphetamines aroused great interest. W. R. Bett said, "it may be
doubted whether, with the possible exception of the sulphona-
mides, penicillin, and streptomycin, any therapeutic agent of
modern scientific medicine has aroused such vivid interest in professional circles and in the lay press as benzedrine sulphate." His
paper, published in 1946, shows what can happen when a drug is
prescribed on the basis of promotional campaigns and broad general assumptions, rather than adequate clinical research. It lists
an enormous number of uses for Benzedrine, all of which, with

few exceptions, have since been thoroughly discredited. Yet, "the great preponderance of competent clinical opinion favours the view that the incidence of undesirable reactions complicating benzedrine therapy in normal dosage range is negligible and that the few cases reported in the literature are usually traceable to indiscriminate or unsupervised use." Bett summarily disposes of the question of addiction: "addiction is very rare and only occurs in the severe psychopath who would have probably become addicted to some drug or other anyway."[1] (This led to the suggestion that Benzedrine might be used in the treatment of alcoholism and morphine or codeine addiction.) In recent years, the list of accepted medical uses for amphetamines has been reduced to the treatment of obesity, narcolepsy, depression, and hyperkinesis—and today even these are seriously questioned.

Obesity

Amphetamines have become the overwhelming drug of choice in the treatment of obesity. Practically all the drugs now used for appetite suppression are characterized by the presence of the phenylethylamine chain. In 1967, 14,500,000 new prescriptions for anorectic drugs were filled, in addition to 31,000,000 refill prescriptions, at a total cost of sixty-six million dollars. Other sources place the average annual expenditure at around one hundred million dollars. In cases of amphetamine psychosis, more patients cited weight-reducing than any other as their initial reason for using the drug. According to unpublished information supplied by a large pharmaceutical manufacturer in 1948, 92 percent of physicians were using amphetamines to treat obesity, and 65 percent of patients seeking help for this problem were receiving amphetamines. Their effect on appetite, called by some a "side effect" of the central stimulating action, has become the major medical rationale for overproduction.[2]

Expert medical opinion is gradually recognizing that obesity is not a somewhat humorous cosmetic difficulty, but a complex, long-term problem involving critical psychological and social determinants. No one really knows its causes. It is defined as a state in which fat accumulates because food intake (in terms of caloric content) is greater than energy output. About 20 million people in the United States are obese, and 25 percent of them are 20 percent or more above optimum weight. Genetic, glandular, and other physical and physiological causes play a statistically small role in obesity (probably in less than 10 percent); usually, the obese person simply overeats. According to one study, only 12 percent of ninety-six very obese patients attributed their condition to "glandular disease"; the rest admitted that overeating was the cause and referred to psychological factors like nervousness, family difficulties, and ingrained habits.[3] Many investigators suggest that obese patients need psychotherapy; otherwise, no dietary regimen or chemotherapy will rectify or control their excess eating.

Apart from uncommon metabolic aberrations, the principal factors governing appetite are social and psychological. Some people are trained in childhood to overeat; others move in social and business circles where food and alcohol are present in abundance and one is expected to partake. With effort, habits can be broken and living circumstances altered. Emotional problems are far more difficult to deal with. Chronic tension and depression, unusually strong oral drives, low capacity to delay gratification, and the substitution of food for other forms of pleasure—all common in cases of obesity—increase the likelihood of becoming dependent on drugs, including amphetamines. Most troubled obese patients will not persist in their efforts to diet. The few who do and lose some weight, regain it. A drug that reduces appetite without requiring solving the patient's emotional problem seems a reasonable alternative to what would otherwise be the almost certain failure of these individuals to lose weight if they were to depend solely on will-power. But the wisdom of such a solution must be examined. Do clinical and experimental studies reliably establish that amphetamine and its congeners have a measurable anorectic effect? If so, are the benefits great enough to justify their use despite the long-term adverse effects?

There is still no real understanding of how amphetamine reduces appetite. Experiments with animals have demonstrated that it is not a function of local effects on the gastrointestinal tract. There is some evidence that lesions in the hypothalamus may result in a substantial increase in appetite. If some obese people actually have a dysfunction of the hypothalamus, it is possible that amphetamines reduce appetite by their effect on this area of the brain. However, if this mechanism exists at all, it is probably secondary to the central stimulating effect. It has been suggested that diuresis may cause some of the weight loss associated with the use of amphetamine. Both diuretic and antidiruetic effects have been reported, however, and the role of diuresis in true weight loss is far from clear.[4]

In 1938 a research group led by Poul Bahnsen compared one hundred normal subjects receiving amphetamine with an equal number receiving placebo. Nineteen of the active drug group and one control reported a reduction in appetite. The first attempts to apply these observations to the clinical management of obesity were made that same year by M. F. Lesses and A. Myerson, and by P. Rosenberg in 1939; both papers reported favorable results.[5] Since then a long series of reports and clinical studies has agreed with them. For example, S. C. Harris, A. C. Ivy, and L. M. Searle found that seven obese patients lost more weight when taking amphetamine than when taking placebo. Those who lost most were the ones who ate least, so the main cause of weight loss was apparently suppression of appetite rather than something like higher activity level. Harris also conducted another experiment in 1947 to investigate the possibility that weight can be lost with amphetamines even when caloric intake is maintained. Ten volunteer medical students agreed to eat 3,000 calories per day. During weeks one and two, the students received no medication, and during weeks three and four, they received placebo. During this control period totaling twenty-six days, there was an average weight loss of 0.7 pounds. This the authors attribute to the fact that for some of the subjects a 3,000-calorie diet was inadequate to maintain body weight. For study weeks five to thirteen, half of the students received 10 mg of dl-amphetamine before each meal, and the other half received 5 mg. During week five, the subjects in both groups lost an average of one pound. However, the amounts leveled off quickly, and the total average loss for the active medication phase was only 1.85 pounds. The authors concluded that reduction of caloric intake, not increase in motor activity or metabolic rate, is the essential variable in weight loss from amphetamines.[6]

These studies suggested that by reducing appetite somewhat, amphetamine might make it easier to adhere to a dietary regimen that demanded even less food consumption than the dieter would normally desire while taking the drug. In fact, much of the controversy related to the clinical studies deals with the importance of dietary restriction as a treatment adjunct. In a twelve-week study by W. H. LeRiche and A. Csima, 171 patients were placed on a high protein diet of 700 calories per day and randomly assigned to drug A (placebo) or drug B (15 mg dextroamphetamine sulfate and 7.5 mg prochlorperazine [Eskatrol Spansule] daily). After two weeks, drug A patients were switched to drug AA (the active medication), and drug B patients to drug BB (remaining on active medication). During the first two weeks of treatment the placebo patients lost an average of 3.5 pounds, and the amphetamine group an average of 6 pounds, indicating that the effect of the protein diet was enhanced by the amphetamine. The importance of tolerance in connection with the anorectic effect is also shown in this study. In the second phase (ten weeks in duration), the drug AA patients lost an average of 8.4 pounds, as compared with 5.2 pounds for drug BB patients. The research design had provided the subjects of the latter group with two more weeks of medication, and they had therefore presumably built up a greater tolerance to its anorectic effects.[7]

Another useful study was conducted by D. Adlersberg and M. E. Mayer on 299 obese patients who were being treated in a clinic of a large general hospital. Treatment groups were arranged as follows: Group A patients were treated with dietary restrictions alone; Group B began with this, but after two to five months oral thyroid medication (2-3 grains desiccated thyroid daily) was added; and Group C, after three months of dietary restriction, received amphetamine sulphate (5 to 10 mg twice daily, one to two hours before lunch and dinner). Although all three groups lost weight, Group C (diet plus amphetamine) was the most successful. However, dosages had to be increased over time to maintain weight loss and overcome tolerance. A useful contribution of this study is the authors' attempt to differentiate between long- and short-term results. The most impressive weight losses for all three groups occurred in the first one or two months. Overall, amphetamines emerged as superior to the thyroid regime; but interestingly, in the long run diet alone compared favorably with diet and amphetamine. Further data on tolerance are supplied by Gelvin and McGavack, who studied twenty-seven obese patients attending the Welfare Island Dispensary. They took an initial dose of 15 mg Dexedrine per day (rapidly increased to a maximum of 30 mg) and were permitted to eat as they pleased. After eight weeks, 47 percent were maintaining a weight loss of one pound per week; after twelve weeks, only 23 percent continued to lose even that much. Twenty weeks after the beginning of treatment only one patient was still losing weight.[8] Obviously, if it is necessary to increase the dosage continually to maintain the appetite-inhibiting effects, there is considerable risk of addiction.

The use of amphetamine to correct faulty eating habits has been suggested, but studies with animals have shown how difficult this is. Harris gave intramuscular injections (2.5 to 20 mg d-amphetamine sulfate) to dogs one hour before feeding, with the result that food intake was substantially decreased. In the case of one dog (16 kg in weight) who was given injections of 10 mg per day, food consumption was reduced by 87 percent and body weight by 27.4 percent within thirty-two days. After thirty days, an injection of saline solution was substituted for the amphetamine. The animals' appetite immediately increased greatly; obviously conditioning by the amphetamine regime could not be sustained without the anorectic effect of the drug itself.[9] Similarly, the experience of most physicians treating patients for obesity suggests that little long-term learning effect can be attributed to the amphetamine regime; most patients, once they stop using amphetamines or become tolerant to them, resume their former eating habits.

A second series of papers on obesity and amphetamines emerged in the 1950s, heralding the use of combination drugs in which amphetamine was supplemented with a barbiturate (in most instances amobarbital). The advantage was reported to be an easing of the emotional extremes found in obese patients. These studies, most of them uncontrolled and methodologically unsound, stated that patients lost weight, as with amphetamine alone, but also improved in mood. No data indicated that the combination drugs were any more effective than amphetamines alone. The FDA has at long last acknowledged this, stating that combination drugs differ neither in efficacy nor "in the incidence of adverse side effects from anorectic drugs alone."[10]

In the late 1950s a third series of studies began to appear, dealing with the effectiveness of new amphetamine congeners or new forms (for example, "timed-release" packaging) of already existing amphetamines. These drugs all share the same basic chemical skeleton and have effects, including adverse ones, very similar to amphetamine sulfate, although it was claimed for one drug after another that it had fewer "side effects." W. Modell writes that: "it seems unlikely that any minor structural change in this group which continues the same theme will separate the effect on appetite from the other effects of the central stimulant action that may be clinically undesirable. Yet it is precisely this which is inferred from many claims made for these drugs, namely the recurrent claims for reduced incidence of insomnia, anxiety, and nervousness, with potent anorectic effect."[11] Still, they were sometimes compared with dextroamphetamine or a combination drug and found superior. I. H. Kupersmith conducted what he termed a "comparative clinical investigation" in which he employed ephedrine-ethylenediamine complex, d-amphetamine sulfate, d-amphetamine sulfate with a barbiturate, and placebo. The weight changes per month in descending order were -11.3, -7.7, -3.0, and +1.2 pounds. In their eagerness to establish the superiority of the new amphetamines many authors failed to build even minimal controls into their research designs. The Kupersmith data come from three different groups of subjects at different times and places. The only demographic data he includes are that they were "overweight subjects" or "overweight patients."[12] From such data it seems likely that the most important independent variable was the researcher's desire for the results to come out as they did.

A 1959 article by S. C. Freed and E. E. Hays on the drug Ionamin is representative of the kind of anorectic drug evaluation reports that have appeared in reputable medical journals during the last thirty-five years. The authors do not indicate how their subjects were selected, but it is apparent that they did not use any nondrug, placebo-administered, or even dextroamphetamine-treated control group or attempt to follow up their patients after cessation of Ionamin treatment. Furthermore, the data they present are sparse and incomplete; they do not even provide information on how obese any of their subjects were before beginning their drug and diet regimens. From the limited data they supply, we can calculate that one group of sixty patients treated with fairly high (30 mg daily) doses of Ionamin lost an average of less than seven pounds over the one-month period. This is not very convincing when one considers that the weight of many people who are not taking any drugs or making any effort to lose weight may fluctuate almost as much as this in a month and still be well within normal limits.

The authors also minimized the "side reactions" to Ionamin, asserting, for example, that the insomnia often experienced was "somewhat different from that occurring during amphetamine therapy," in that their patients "reported a wakefulness which was not unpleasant, compared to the nervous overexhilaration which [has] . . . prevented sleep following amphetamine treatment."[13] If this statement deserves any credence—not that it necessarily does—it suggests that Ionamin is more likely to lead to drug abuse than racemic amphetamine; people generally do *not* persist in taking drugs they consider unpleasant.

Freed and Hays claim that Ionamin is "chemically and pharmacologically different from amphetamine." However, the following year W. Modell emphasized that: "Phenyltertiarybutylamine resin . . . advertised as not being an amphetamine drug, is a carboxylic acid-type of exchange resin which contains substituted phenylbutylamine moieties that are released in the gastrointestinal tract. As shown in the formulas, the amine itself clearly belongs to the amphetamine series." Ten years later, he devoted only two brief sentences to the alleged unique mode of action and value of Ionamin in his comprehensive and objective edition of *Drugs of Choice*: "All systemic effects, therefore, stem from an amphetamine-like action. There is no good evidence that this is in any way a superior member of the group."[14] Not suprisingly, the drugs used by Freed and Hays were supplied by the manufacturer.

The vast majority of the clinical investigations on the anorectic effects of amphetamines yield, to one degree or another, favorable results. This judgment must be qualified, however, because excellent results are obtained in the early stages of almost all types of treatment because of the initial willingness of subjects to cooperate with a new physician and the psychological impact of a new therapy. But even if we consider amphetamines generally useful in this respect, we must still come to grips with the question of adverse effects. Much of the obesity literature minimizes the number and severity of these effects or actually states that there are none. Finch, for example, claims that "dexedrine sulfate is a nontoxic safe drug which may safely be used in obstetric patients to aid them in preventing excessive gain of weight." Studies like his have led to large-scale prescription of amphetamine to pregnant women when there is evidence that it may be a teratogenic agent.[15] An amphetamine derivative called fenfluramine, sold in the United Kingdom, Europe, and Australia as "Ponderax," seems to be a highly specific appetite suppressant with low CNS-stimulating and euphoric properties and low addictive potential. Even so, Oswald and his coworkers cautiously conclude only that it *may* be preferred to other amphetamines. They emphasize that "most slimming pills are also 'pep pills' and invite abuse. Past experience leads to scepticism when claims are made that a new appetite-reducing drug does not affect alertness or mood."[16]

Other clinicians, mindful of amphetamines' potential for harm, assert that in weight reduction the exposure is limited to a relatively short period. But, though this may be the intention, it often does not turn out that way. People who have problems controlling their need for constant gratification, as indicated by compulsive eating, find it hard to put aside a medication that makes them "feel good." What is more, many patients consider their attempt to lose weight doomed to failure once they have lost this "magic" potion that protects them from themselves. When the drug is discontinued, a psychological vacuum is created which has to be filled with food. On occasion, patients have gained back even more weight than they lost, a condition commonly known as the "rebound phenomenon." So, although short-term use of the drug causes a short-term weight loss, it also helps the patient avoid the issue of changing his eating habits. The following personal account given to one of the authors (L.G.) is typical:

> What do you say about a 25-year-old girl who is fat? Not a great deal. She said even less about herself, until one day, after she had convinced herself that her problem was basically metabolic, she announced that she was going to a doctor.
>
> Not particularly sympathetic about her weight problem, the doctor told her she had to diet, but to help her, he would prescribe an appetite depressant, dexedrine, to be taken before breakfast.
>
> That was in November, and thus began my own experience with amphetamines.

I was convinced, because I was not told otherwise, that these magic little pills would solve my weight problem, which was substantial, amounting to an excess of 50 pounds. I left the office, confident that if I followed the regimen and exercised will power, I would eventually be thin. I filled the prescription and the next morning took the first pill. Granted I was not hungry, but fat people often don't eat because they are hungry—they eat because they are unhappy and there is nothing else to do; they eat because it is raining; or because it is a beautiful day. The day passed uneventfully and so did the evening (fat girls don't go out), and then I got ready to go to bed. And couldn't. What's the sense in going to bed if you can't go to sleep, and that is what eluded me. I was so "high" that my mind was running circles around itself. My thought patterns resembled Joyce's stream of conscious technique; I could not concentrate on any thought for more than a matter of seconds and then my mind would dart to something else, seemingly unrelated. To say the least, I was disconcerted because I had no control over my thoughts. I tried all the standard remedies for insomnia; none worked—I could not even count more than half a dozen sheep. Finally around 4:00 A.M., I dozed off.

The next day was little better but eventually, as I recall, my tolerance built up quickly, and I did not have night-time "highs" after a couple of weeks. My weight problem was much more persistent. I found that dexedrine did depress my appetite as long as my will power was in high gear; when I slipped, I became a compulsive snacker, eating literally anything and everything I could get my hands on. When will power took the reins again, I would manage to drop a few pounds.

Weeks and months passed, and I remember thinking that the pills were no longer doing their job. I experienced a craving to take more than my one pill a day, but never quite had the courage to do so. I also found myself becoming jittery and jumpy. Minor things would unnerve me and I tended to want to be alone more and more. I became progressively unhappy and would burst into tears over the most trivial things. I remember a period of strange, weird dreams, where I was thin, lovely, and the center of attraction. Then I would wake up to fat reality.

After six months, I began to question the validity of continuing; I wasn't losing weight, and I was miserable in the bargain. Interestingly enough, my friends had begun to question long before, seeing sometimes subtle, sometimes obvious personality changes in me. I was far more irrascible than usual and developed a temper that was out of character. I am a fairly even-tempered person, not given to moods, or highs and lows. However, I became alternatively moody, euphoric, depressed. I would snap at people for no reason at all, and was generally "bitchy" to those around me.

In April I decided to stop taking "the magic diet pills." I had taken my last pill on Thursday, and on Friday, went to work as usual. By 2:00 P.M. my solicitous boss told me I looked awful and asked what was wrong. I told him nothing, really, except that I felt as if the Boston Celtics were using me as their basketball. As the afternoon wore on, I wore out, and felt as if the players had let the air out of the basketball. The boss told me to go home. I did. And went to bed. Until late Sunday afternoon. My mother's repeated attempts to rouse me met with no success. Each time I tried to get out of bed, I fell back exhausted. When I finally managed to get downstairs, I explained that I had stopped taking the dexedrine on Thursday, and could only attribute the events of the past several days to its side-effects. We both agreed that the rest of the pills should be flushed down the toilet. They were.

What can you say about a 32-year-old girl who's thin? A lot, and she does. After the dexedrine, her personality took about a month to return to what it was. She slipped back into her old eating habits, but after a while, decided the time had finally come. She joined Weight Watchers and she lost 52 pounds, without so much as an aspirin to help her.

The FDA recently reviewed studies of anorectic drugs and the records of more than nine thousand patients, and found that "the amount of weight loss associated with the use of anorectic drugs varied from trial to trial. The increased weight loss appeared to be related in part to variables other than the drug, such as the physician-investigator, the population treated, and the diet selected." It concluded that "all anorectic drugs including amphetamines and methamphetamines have a limited usefulness in the treatment of obesity, and because of their significant potential for dependence and abuse should be used with extreme care."[17]

The FDA now requires labeling for these drugs stressing that they are indicated only in short term (a few weeks) treatment and in conjunction with dietary restrictions. It finds even this treatment acceptable only if alternative methods have proved ineffective.

These recent developments apparently have had some effect on prescribing habits. A newly published survey of 450 physicians shows that the number of renewed prescriptions for amphetamine has declined. A growing awareness of the dangers of amphetamines is evident; 73 percent of the doctors in this sample rated their abuse potential as "very high." In contrast to the 1948 estimate of 92 percent, the present survey indicates that about two-thirds of the doctors prescribe them for obesity. Most (69 percent) rated their effectiveness only poor to fair, but considerable amounts are still prescribed.[18]

We doubt the wisdom of using amphetamines for weight reduction under any circumstances. Although they can cause a three to four-week euphoric "high" that may have as one of its "side effects" a diminished food intake and consequent weight loss, after this period they are no longer effective as anorectics unless the user increases the dose, thus initiating a pattern of abuse. And after use is discontinued, the average person quickly gains back the weight he lost—or more.

Narcolepsy

First described in the medical literature ninety years ago, narcolepsy is marked by an uncontrollable desire for sleep or sudden attacks of sleep. Onset usually occurs between the ages of ten and twenty, and it never completely remits. Opinions on its incidence vary widely. The report of the Select Committee on Crime (1971) stated that probably no more than two-hundred persons in the United States are afflicted with it. A. Goldstein, Chairman of the Huntington, Long Island, Narcotic Guidance Council, reported that none of the physicians in Huntington (population 200,000) had seen a single case of narcolepsy in at least a year, and that two cases had been reported for Suffolk County, New York (population one million), in two years. He estimated the number of narcoleptics in the United States to be about 20,000. However, V. Zarcone recently estimated that there were about 66,000 narcoleptic persons in the country, and in fact, eighty cases were located in a short time in San Francisco simply by advertising in one newspaper and by word of mouth. R. E. Yoss and D. D. Daly found about one hundred new cases each year at the Mayo Clinic.[19]

Whether or not narcolepsy is a rare disease, it is certainly a complicated one. It may involve either REM sleep or non-REM sleep, and either type of sleep attack may be complicated by cataplexy (a partial or complete loss of muscle tone), sleep paralysis (which may be a variant of cataplexy because it is characterized by a loss of muscle tone during the transition from sleeping to waking or vice versa), or hypnagogic hallucinations (a sort of drifting semidream state which occurs spontaneously and is characterized by a stupor or daze). Some narcoleptics suffer from none of these complications; others experience various combinations of them. The drug of choice in the treatment of cataplexy, sleep paralysis, or hypnagogic hallucinations is the antidepressant imipramine (Tofranil), which eliminates these three symptoms with few adverse effects and without risk of dependence. This drug does not, however, eliminate the sleep attacks themselves. In most cases no brain pathology is evident, and some physicians think heredity may be a factor. In 1942 Krabbe and Magnussen reviewed all the literature and found that fifty-four of the reported cases were concentrated in nineteen families. In 1959 Daly and Yoss reported a family in which twelve cases of narcolepsy appeared in three generations. They suggest that the disorder is transmitted by a single dominant factor with relatively slight penetrance.[20] It has also been suggested that narcolepsy serves a defensive function against feelings such as anger, guilt, or sexual impulses which are unacceptable to the patient, and in which the narcoleptic sleep and cataplectic attack serve as regressive aids to repression. Another hypothesis is that narcolepsy is the result of a pathophysiologic disorder of the reticular activating system, perhaps related to a neurohumoral deficiency.[21]

Before the advent of amphetamine, ephedrine sulphate, first used for the treatment of narcolepsy in 1931, was usually prescribed. It produced marked improvement in the symptoms of the disease, but was discontinued because of deleterious effects. After a favorable report by Myron Prinzmetal and Wilfred Bloomberg in 1935, amphetamine was welcomed as a replacement. Reports in 1936, 1937, and 1940 were equally encouraging, and it seemed reasonable to conclude that amphetamines presented no problems or complications whatsoever for the narcoleptic patient. In a more recent report D. M. Williamson details the case of a fifty - five-year-old coalminer with a diagnosis of narcolepsy with cataplexy who was treated "very successfully" with dexamphetamine sulphate (10 mg twice daily). Again there were no apparent adverse effects worth reporting.[22]

For a narcoleptic whose work is as dangerous as coal-mining dextroamphetamine or methylphenidate (Ritalin) may have to be prescribed, but most can perform very well without drugs if they take at least one nap a day. Even if a patient is suffering from sleep attacks alone, and not the other three symptoms of narcolepsy, the risk of addiction, toxic physiological reactions, and psychosis must be weighed against the advantages of a drug-induced maintenance of uninterrupted wakefulness. While sleep researchers continue to work on narcolepsy, one thing that can be done to help narcoleptics is to distribute more information about the disorder.[23] Many patients report that physicians to whom they turn for help do not understand the problem or have never heard of it. Employers may fire seemingly lazy or irresponsible employees who could perform adequately if they were granted one or two short naps a day. Narcoleptics themselves should understand the nature of their illness. They are greatly relieved to learn that they are suffering attacks of normal sleep and are not psychotic, epileptic, or abnormal in some very strange way.

Depression

Next to boredom, depression is probably the most common complaint of adults. Unfortunately, the word has been applied to so many mood alterations, symptoms, and syndromes of varying severity and etiology that it is difficult to establish a clear diagnostic classification. Sadness and a sense of fatigue are common to all the clinical states generally referred to as depression. More severe cases may be characterized by feelings of hopelessness, helplessness, worthlessness, and guilt; suicidal thoughts; psychic and motor retardation; sleep disturbances; and anorexia. Depressed patients also often exhibit anxiety and hostility. In fact, recent researchers have stressed the importance of recognizing the coadunate manifestations of anxiety and depression, particularly since there is now some evidence that different types of patients respond to different treatments.[24]

Historically amphetamines were one of the first classes of drugs to be used in the chemotherapeutic approach to depression, thus heralding the era of the modern antidepressants. E. Guttman first commented on the mood-elevating effects of Benzedrine in 1936, while administering the drug in an attempt to determine the connection between mental phenomena and blood pressure alterations. His observations stimulated further experimentation with the drug on various kinds of depressions, and the same year, he and S. A. Peoples listed some of the striking effects they observed in depressed patients, ranging from increase in motor activity to change in mood, generally in the direction of euphoria. They concluded that "this drug is certainly effective and a promising therapeutic ally, but one cannot make use of it until it is known whether permanent administration produces anything like adaptation, habituation, or even addiction." A year later, however, in a study with W. Sargant, Guttman reported that, though patients with mild depression accompanied by retardation were favorably influenced by Benzedrine therapy (in oral doses of 10 to 30 mg per day), the drug produced or intensified anxiety in severely depressed patients.[25]

In a more thorough but not well-controlled study that same year (1937), D. L. Wilbur and his coworkers found that Benzedrine exaggerated symptoms of anxiety and restlessness of thirty-five psychoneurotic patients, and it therefore was not recommended. Among thirty-two patients with chronic exhaustion, however, 78.1 percent improved, with marked exhilaration reported by most. The results were similar in thirty-three patients suffering from "mood disorders," including ten depressed manic-depressives and twenty patients with "simple and reactive depression"; 70 percent experience "marked relief."[26] This means little, however, since it approximates the reported rate of spontaneous improvement. Later researchers have stressed the need for carefully controlled studies, since the clinical symptoms of depression show a strong trend toward spontaneous remission.

Even at the early stage of clinical experimentation there was doubt about the efficacy of amphetamines in treating severe depressions. In 1939 E. Davidoff and E. C. Reifenstein tentatively concluded that amphetamines had not been shown to be of value in the depressed phase of manic-depressive illnesses, and that they were ineffective in other severe depressions. P. G. Schube and colleagues found that none of eighty psychotic patients improved when given Benzedrine, 10 mg daily, for thirty days. (Fourteen became worse, and ten had to discontinue treatment because of adverse reactions ranging from increased nervousness to suicidal drive.) Early studies of less serious depressions, while demonstrating some therapeutic utility for amphetamine, raised questions about the consequences of use. M. H. Nathanson observed that although many patients suffering from "nervous exhaustion" improved when given 10 mg of Benzedrine twice daily, it was necessary to weigh the benefits against harmful effects including the possibility of habituation and abuse. It was also noted that the intensity of the euphoric response to amphetamines surpassed the response to morphine, heroin, and pentobarbital, making them prime candidates for abuse.[27]

In spite of these warnings W. R. Bett asserted a decade later that "a large number of clinical observations both from general practitioners and from specialists testify to [amphetamine's] immediate, and often dramatic, value in breaking the stranglehold of depression, restoring 'energy feeling,' and renewing optimism, self-assurance, increased initiative, appetite for work, and zest for living." He passed along Gorrell's suggestion that physicians take the drug when attending seriously ill patients and obstetrical and surgical cases in order to allay fatigue. Even more astonishing was C. D. Leake's chapter on therapeutic uses in his authoritative book, *The Amphetamines*, published in 1958. His list of beneficial effects was even longer than Bett's; for example, contrary to previous evidence, he reported that d-amphetamine had been successful in treating psychotic depressions, and suggested that amphetamines "may relieve the trend toward suicidal tendencies." But as early as 1937 Schube mentioned the possibility that Benzedrine increased the risk of suicide by increasing emotional energy, and N. H. Johnson later postulated that amphetamines provided some depressed patients with enough mobility to increase the danger of suicide.[28] Furthermore, suicide attempts may occur during the severe depression that often follows withdrawal. This alone is sufficient reason for caution in treating depressed patients with amphetamines.

As the adverse CNS-stimulating effects of the amphetamines, particularly insomnia and anxiety, became more apparent, interest developed in their conjunctive use with sedatives like sodium amytal, which had been known since 1931 to have a temporary ameliorating influence upon the symptoms of depression. A. Myerson began using amphetamine sulfate to counteract the disagreeable symptoms of barbiturate sedation in 1936, advocating "judicious use of barbiturates or other sedatives towards night, and of amphetamine sulfate aided by small doses of caffeine or strychnine in the morning" to re-establish a "normal cycle." He claimed to have obtained a "marked change in mood and an incomplete approximation to normal feeling and activity" with 200 mg sodium amytal plus 5 to 10 mg of amphetamine sulfate administered orally two or three times a day, stating that "the combined drugs do not cure the depression, but keep the patient comfortable while Nature is bringing about the cure."[29]

J. S. Gottlieb, in a series of uncontrolled studies, found that when the two drugs were administered together, the analeptic effect of amphetamine reduced the hypnotic effect of sodium amytal, so that the combination was more potent and more lasting than either drug individually. He reported that about 90 percent of depressed patients responded positively to this treatment, but noted that "those who improved, had the medication instituted near the terminations of their current attack." Hence, it is not clear whether the favorable effects were actually due to the drug combination, or, again, simply reflected the natural course of the illness. In 1952, with F. S. Bobbitt and A. W. Freidinger, Gottlieb studied the reactions of depressed and schizophrenic patients to the combination and decided that the value of the drugs might be limited in relieving depression, and that other related drugs might prove more effective.[30] Both Myerson and Gottlieb conceded that many patients did not improve and recommended that, especially because of the suicide danger, the drugs be discontinued if no response was observed after a few days. Recognizing the hazards of amphetamines and barbiturates, they stressed the need for limiting their availability and for careful supervision of their administration.

Later researchers cast further doubt on the efficacy of this combination. In an excellent double-blind study involving four hundred general practitioners from all parts of the British Isles D. Wheatley compared dextroamphetamine to placebo, and in a separate trial compared a combination of 5 mg dexamphetamine plus 65 mg amobarbital to its individual components. The study showed that there was no difference between dextroamphetamine and the combination for primarily depressed patients, and also no difference between dextroamphetamine and placebo. Wheatley concluded that amphetamines, whether alone or combined with barbiturates, had no place in the treatment of depression. But drug companies, recognizing the financial potential of combining the two drugs, began to market them under trade names such as Dexamyl and Ambar. The combinations attempted "to hide or mask the alerting and nerve irritating properties of the medication [amphetamine] thereby inducing patients to abandon their natural healthy caution against a toxic substance by adding another toxic and habit-forming substance such as a barbiturate."[31] Physicians and the pharmaceutical industry must bear a great deal of responsibility for the fact that the dual abuse of barbiturates and amphetamines in England is much more prevalent than the abuse of heroin, and the situation appears to be about the same in the United States and Canada.

In response to the growing awareness of the adverse effects of amphetamines, by the 1950s the drug companies had developed some amphetamine congeners they declared to be "non-amphetamines." One such product was methylphenidate (Ritalin) which was supposed to elevate the mood of depressed patients without inducing insomnia or anxiety. Typically, the drug was at first praised by many researchers. Studies by Natenshon (1956), Jacobson (1958), and Landman, Preisig, and Perlman (1958) reported that it produced good results when administered to mildly depressed patients.[32]

F. J. Ayd, on the other hand, had little success with this drug in treating depressions. Although he noted that methylphenidate was a safe analeptic, he found it to be of little value in treating endogenous depression. His results agreed with those of A. A. Robin and S. Wiseberg, who found in a controlled, double-blind study of patients suffering from moderately severe depressive reactions that methylphenidate in doses of 10 to 20 mg twice daily was no more effective than the placebo. Nathan Thal also reported that, although methylphenidate may be useful in mild exogenous depression, the results of his study did not justify its use as an antidepressant in severely depressed patients.[33] Thus, the published evidence is at best equivocal, and it appears that methylphenidate's usefulness is limited at most to the treatment of some mildly depressed patients and possibly to that of elderly or medical patients where other drugs are contraindicated.

The development of two new classes of drugs, the monoamine oxidase (MAO) inhibitors and tricyclics, revolutionized the treatment of depression. One current theory is that some, if not all, depressions are related to a deficiency of catecholamines, particularly norepinephrine, at adrenergic receptor sites in the brain.[34] The hydrazine derivatives, such as iproniazid (Marsilid), are thought to relieve the symptoms of depression through their MAO-inhibiting properties, which increase the level of serotonin and norepinephrine in the CNS. Imipramine (Tofranil), the prototype of the tricyclic derivatives, was developed as an antipsychotic tranquilizer but soon found to be useful as an antidepressant. The tricyclic derivatives are thought to potentiate the effects of norepinephrine and other biogenic amines; they are believed by many to be the most effective of the somatic approaches to depression, rivaled only by electroconvulsive therapy (ECT) in their efficacy.

A number of methodologically sound studies comparing the new antidepressant drugs to the amphetamines and/or placebo have found amphetamines to be ineffective, if not harmful, in the treatment of *all* types of depressions. Thal compared the amphetamines (including methylphenidate) to various MAO-inhibiting compounds in severely depressed patients with a history of suicidal attempts. The drugs were administered to groups of nine patients each. A control group of nine received only "the usual doctor-patient relationship, with no formal attempt at psychotherapy"; two recovered spontaneously. Another group of nine patients was treated with ECT; eight recovered. Amphetamines only aggravated the depression; phenelzine (Nardil) was the most useful of the MAO inhibitors. E. H. Hare and his associates, in another controlled trial, found phenelzine significantly better than dextroamphetamine or placebo in reducing agitation and anxiety. J. W. L. Doust and his colleagues compared the effects of imipramine, dextroamphetamine, iproniazid, and placebo in a double-blind crossover study of twenty-four carefully selected, therapeutically recalcitrant, chronically depressed patients, and found that none of the three drugs demonstrated marked or predictable clinical responses in the group taken as a whole, although several patients were helped by either imipramine or iproniazid. In a more comprehensive study, J. E. Overall and others evaluated the efficacy of imipramine, isocarboxazide, dex-amphetamine-amobarbital, and placebo, and found imipramine significantly superior to the other three drugs.[35] All of these later studies were controlled, but their patient populations and experimental designs were dissimilar, which may account for the incongruence of some of the results. Nevertheless, in none of them were amphetamines found to be of value.

More recent studies have stressed the capacity of the stimulants to potentiate the effects of the tricyclic antidepressants. The efficacy of the tricyclics depends on their steady-state levels in the bloodstream, which are determined in part by the rate of hepatic drug metabolism. Methylphenidate has been shown to inhibit drug metabolizing enzymes in human subjects, thereby elevating imipramine levels in the bloodstream. These higher levels were associated with clinical improvement. H. Lal and his associates have reported that dextroamphetamine also inhibits hepatic drug-metabolizing enzymes in animals, though to a much lesser extent than methylphenidate.[36]

In 1971 a study was made of the effects of methylphenidate on the steady-state blood levels of imipramine in seven patients with recurrent refractory psychotic depressive illnesses. Patients served as their own controls because their histories of refractory depression diminished the possibility of spontaneous recovery: four had received multiple courses of ECT, and three others had been admitted for this type of treatment after antidepressant drug therapy failures. The patients were given imipramine for approximately three weeks until steady-state blood levels were reached; then they received 10 mg methylphenidate twice daily in addition to imipramine, for a period ranging from ten to twenty-one days. Imipramine alone was then continued in the same dosage for several more weeks. The results were striking: five of the seven patients had prompt, complete clinical remissions, concomitant with a rise in blood levels of imipramine. These levels continued to climb even after methylphenidate was discontinued.[37]

Similar findings were reported in another study by the same group. The imipramine blood levels of two severely depressed patients receiving 150 mg imipramine plus 20 mg methylphenidate daily were reported to be almost as high as those obtained with 450 mg imipramine alone. Clinical improvement was found to be correlated with blood levels. One patient receiving 150 mg imipramine plus 10 mg dextroamphetamine also exhibited high blood levels.[38]

Such combination therapy may offer several advantages. The lower doses of imipramine required to achieve the clinical goal may decrease the incidence of adverse imipramine reactions. The mild stimulation of methylphenidate or amphetamine may help to counteract some of the initial sedative effects of the tricyclic antidepressants, and this immediate response may encourage patients to continue taking imipramine. In fact, some clinicians have recommended amphetamine therapy simply to tide the patient over until the tricyclics begin to have a clinical effect, a period of about three weeks. Combination therapy with tricyclics is now possibly the only justifiable use of the amphetamines in the treatment of depressions.

A 1962 survey disclosed that 52 percent of general practioners' prescriptions for amphetamines were written for persons complaining of depression, fatigue, and/or anxiety.[39] Most physicians know that reassurance and even superficial exploration of the patient's concerns are usually effective with a mildly depressed patient. But this seems to require more time, or more skill, sensitivity, and patience than most doctors have. Instead, they promote the idea that amphetamines and other psychoactive drugs should be used to relieve "illness" that is often indistinguishable from the tensions of everyday life. Amphetamines are "magic pills"; their effect is dramatic; they do make the patient feel good. But administering them in cases of mild depression only masks the underlying problems instead of affording the patient the opportunity to attempt to deal directly with his troubles. Most patients complaining of fatigue, lack of energy, nervousness, depression, anxiety, or insomnia are really asking for a kind of short-term psychotherapy from a person they believe to be empathetic and trustworthy. When a physician responds with a pill, he is depriving his patient of the service he ought to be providing, and may be initiating or perpetuating a malignant pattern of drug use as a substitute for coping with the emotional turmoil of daily life.

The Treatment of Hyperkinetic Children

"Considering the confusion within the medical community about hyperkinesis, the self-assurance with which educators and the drug industry have promoted the use of amphetamines in schools is frightening."

Hyperkinesis

Amphetamines are widely used in schools to control a syndrome referred to by physicians as "hyperkinetic behavior disorder" or minimal brain dysfunction," and, by parents and teachers, as "hyperactivity." These stimulants have become established as the preferred treatment even though doctors are unsure of the nature and etiology of the disorder. Public attention was drawn to this issue when, on June 29, 1970, a sensational article appeared in the *Washington Post*, claiming that from 5 to 10 percent of the 62,000 elementary school children of Omaha, Nebraska, were being treated with "behavior modification drugs to improve classroom deportment and increase learning potential."[1] This proved to be a great exaggeration—5 to 10 percent was the estimated prevalence of learning disabilities and not of amphetamine use—nevertheless, the article aroused interest and concern about the increasingly widespread and largely unexamined practice of prescribing drugs for behavior control.

The response to the *Post* article made it clear that the practice was not limited to Nebraska, and a congressional hearing held on September 29, 1970, disclosed some disquieting facts: 150,000 to 200,000 children, according to the testimony of Dr. Ronald Lipman of the FDA, were then being treated with stimulant drugs, and the number was expected to increase. In fact, an article published in the *Christian Science Monitor*, October 31, 1970, reported a National Institute of Mental Health estimate that "there are up to 4 million 'hyperactive' children in the United States who could benefit from these drugs."[2] The use of amphetamines was growing, despite an appalling lack of follow-up studies on their long-term effects. Until that time only one such study had been undertaken. Preliminary results were reassuring; the children who had been diagnosed as hyperkinetic and had received amphetamines showed a low incidence of psychiatric disorders in adolescence. But Congressman Cornelius Gallagher, who chaired the hearing, was justifiably appalled at the fact that after thirty-five years only one study (involving sixty-seven cases) could be adduced to demonstrate the absence of harmful effects. Clearly this was too small a sample by which such a widespread practice could be justified.

The drug industry has continued to promote the use of amphetamines for disturbed children and is largely responsible for extending the practice. Nat Hentoff reported in May 1972 on some remarkable items from a 1971 CIBA territorial sales report, in which an executive was urging his salesmen to become "more effective pushers": "Your ingenuity," the report says, "in the promotion of RITALIN FBP (Functional Behavior Problems) is becoming more apparent."

> Item: Mr. X, CIBA representative in Paducah, Kentucky, reports having a community of approximately 10,000 that has established a screening program of pre-school children to identify as early as possible those children who would most likely have learning disabilities. This is the only city known where an entire school system will be engaged in such an endeavor . . .
>
> Mr. Y of South Bend, Indiana, reports that at an inservice meeting of special education personnel . . . a physician brought two hyperactive children to use in a demonstration of the basic symptoms of Functional Behavior Problems. That's getting involvement, folks.

Hentoff also quotes a CIBA man from Kansas City, reminding his colleague:

> about a few people whom we frequently overlook when making presentations and contacts on functional behavior problems in children. Two in particular are the juvenile court officers and

probation officers. The juvenile court system comes in contact with children of all ages but their primary value in this situation would be to discuss Functional Behavior Problems with teachers and school officials with whom they are in contact. [Our man in Kansas City] points out that juvenile bureaus connected with local police are prime targets; even though they are in contact with older children they can spread the word.[3]

Children with learning and behavior difficulties should be identified and given attention. However, when the medical profession does not yet understand the use of amphetamines with problem children, salesmen from drug companies are hardly the appropriate people to institute screening program information or advise juvenile court officers.

In many cases, educators have been strong proponents of stimulant treatment for problem students. In New York the mother of a child labeled "hyperactive" by his elementary school teacher received an ultimatum from the teacher: "put the child on drugs or we will not be able to keep him in school." A southern California mother was reported as saying, "We've been harassed and pressured by the school for four years now to put our 9-year-old on medication—for hyperactivity—and we've refused for four years. Two family doctors have backed up our decision." A Colorado mother told how she had reluctantly "caved in to the combined requests of the school nurse, the school psychologist, principal, and teachers" that she put her six-year-old son on medication to treat his "learning disability." Another California mother complained that the school would not accept a "no" from a family physician. "Most every parent who has an overactive child in the school is told to go see the same pediatrician," she reported, "because that doctor knows what the school wants."[4]

Even if parents do not resist, the question remains whether educators should have the authority to make such recommendations. In Baltimore the use of amphetamines to treat unmanageable children in the city school system had reached such proportions by 1970 that Dr. H. M. Selznick, then school system superintendent of special education, had to acknowledge that guidelines and controls on responsibility for the administration of the drugs were sorely lacking. His apology continued, "We do not want teachers administering the drugs since they are not medically trained. But, it is our suspicion that some teachers who have had 'wall climbers' do assume this responsibility.'' Eric Denhoff, a pioneer researcher on the use of amphetamines for "problem" children, recognized this abuse as recently as 1971 in an editorial published in the *Journal of Learning Disabilities*: "In the 1950's, educators learned about [the] . . . psychopharmacological aspect of behavior modification, and began to encourage parents to seek such help from the child's physician. Soon it became evident that these drugs were being used indiscriminately—prescription would depend mostly upon a description of behavior by a teacher or parent."[5] While psychiatrists estimate the incidence of hyperkinesis among elementary school children at 4 to 10 percent, educators' estimates range as high as 15 to 20 percent.

By 1974 not much has changed. The issue is emotionally charged and reliable information is still scant and hard to locate. What, more than expressing acceptance or indignation, can citizens do? What would be an enlightened policy?

Historical Background

The therapeutic use of amphetamines in the treatment of hyperkinetic children dates back to 1937, when Charles Bradley observed that Benzedrine produced "spectacular" effects on a number of children displaying disturbed behavior in school. Their disorders ranged from specific learning disabilities, through aggressiveness associated with epilepsy, to withdrawn schizoid behavior. Thirty children were observed within a residential treatment setting; with drug therapy, fourteen showed a marked improvement in school performance, as indicated by an increase in drive, interest, accuracy, and speed of comprehension. On another dimension of change, fifteen of the thirty became "distinctly subdued in their emotional responses," manifesting an increased sense of well-being approaching mild euphoria, diminished mood swings, a more easygoing attitude, and an increased awareness of and interest in their surroundings. (Seven children were common to both these groups.) The remaining children showed lesser responses of varying degrees: only one became more hyperactive, although three seemed to cry more readily, as if their emotions were more easily aroused. All effects of amphetamine disappeared as soon as the medication was discontinued. "It appears paradoxical," Bradley commented, "that a drug known to be a stimulant should produce subdued behavior in half of the children. It should be borne in mind, however, that portions of the higher levels of the central nervous system have inhibition as their function, and that stimulation of these portions might indeed produce the clinical picture of reduced activity through increased voluntary control."[6] It is also possible (and this will be discussed later in a different context) that the subdued behavior might very well be an "artifact of observation" (as C. K. Conners pointed out), reflecting not gross body movement and activity level as such, but the way in which activity is organized in relation to the social demands of various situations. In other words the amphetamine-treated subjects mights have been expending the same amount of energy (and perhaps even more) as before they were given the medication, but because they were channeling it into more socially acceptable activities, their behavior *appeared* subdued. Bradley himself, after twelve years of observing the effects of racemic amphetamine and dextroamphetamine on a total of 388 children, suggested that the effects might not be as paradoxical as they appear.[7] Despite this disclaimer, research has proceeded largely on the assumption that amphetamines do produce a "paradoxical" calming effect on children, and subsequent developments have been very much influenced by this assumption.

The same year (1937) Bradley reported his results, findings by M. Molitch and J. P. Sullivan independently suggested that Benzedrine had a positive effect on test scores. Using 96 boys between the ages of ten and seventeen, who had been committed by the courts as juvenile delinquents, and were considered to have behavior problems, Molitch and Sullivan devised a double-blind experiment to determine the relative efficacy of placebo and Benzedrine on New Stanford Achievement Test scores. Basal test scores were determined for each boy, after which the subjects were given either placebo (46 subjects) or 10 mg Benzedrine (50 subjects) and retested. The average differences between initial scores and treatment scores definitely favored the amphetamine group, but since no statistical analyses were made, the precise significance of the results is not clear.[8] The authors recognized the preliminary nature of their findings and suggested that further research was indicated.

Bradley, too, found evidence of a stimulating effect on school achievement in almost 50 percent of the children; the improvement was observed in all subjects, arithmetic in particular.[9] So, even in the very first experimentation with amphetamines on disturbed children, two avenues of research were suggested: the "calming" effect on observed behavior and the stimulating effect on school performance. By 1950, when Bradley published his summary of studies on 388 Dexedrine- and Benzedrine-treated disturbed children, representing over a decade of observation and thought, many other studies supported or amplified his original findings. These studies dealt with a variety of diagnostic categories, although not specifically with hyperkinetic behavior disorders. In 1940 Cutler, Little, and Strauss, employing a double-blind experimental technique to determine the effects of small daily doses of racemic amphetamine on mentally retarded children, found that neither behavior nor academic performance was affected by daily doses of 5 to 7 1/2 mg over a period of six months. However, when a subsample was given 10 mg Benzedrine "as sudden stimulation," their performance on psychomotor tests was favorably affected and there was a tendency toward improvement on the New Stanford Achievement Test. Though findings were inconclusive, this suggested a dose-related effect. Bradley and Bowen studied the effects of Benzedrine on one hundred children being treated for a variety of behavior disorders. (Those of psychogenic origin were most numerous, but there were also cases of convulsive disorders, schizoid personality, structural neurological defect, deficiency in intellectual functioning, specific reading disability, and post-encephalitic behavior disorders.) Although most of their observations were in accord with Bradley's earlier findings, a significant minority, nineteen, responded with increased affect and energy, exhibiting increased alertness, initiative, interest in their surroundings, and aggressiveness in competitive activities. In almost 65 percent of these "stimulated" children, the response was clinically an improvement, since they had originally been shy, withdrawn, and underactive.[10]

Further insight into the effects of stimulant drugs on disturbed children was provided by Bender and Cottington who studied twenty-eight boys and twelve girls, ranging from five to thirteen years, who were treated with Benzedrine in the Psychiatric Division of Bellevue Hospital. Diagnoses included neurotic behavior disorders, psychoneuroses, "psychopathic personality," schizophrenia, and organic brain disease, with the first two comprising

75 percent of the sample. In general, the least neurotic children responded with an increased sense of well-being which enabled them to make a less fearful, more positive adaptation to the therapeutic environment, and they could more freely express and hence work through their feelings in both the therapeutic and group situations. Many of the more severely neurotic manifested a decrease in hyperactivity and an increase in attention span; but they also became more evasive and resistant to dealing in therapy with their deeper conflicts, as though their new sense of well-being made this unnecessary. Those with organic brain disease and schizophrenia showed no response whatever to the drug, and the effects on children with "psychopathic" personalities were so unfavorable that medication had to be discontinued. The authors explained that, while the disturbed behavior of the neurotic children may simply have indicated conflict within basically integrated personality structures, the disturbed behavior of the "psychopathic" children may have been part of an ego structure developed to mask a basic lack of emotional integration. The drugs may have facilitated the neurotics' integration, while reinforcing the "masking" behavior of the "psychopathic" personalities. In contrast, S. R. Korey reported that four of seven "psychopathic" juvenile delinquents showed favorable responses to the administration of amphetamine over a six-week period. No unfavorable responses were noted except as toxic reactions to the drug, and as soon as dosage was adjusted to a toleration point, such reactions reportedly disappeared.[11]

The effect of amphetamine on behaviorally disturbed children with EEG abnormalities was investigated by B. Pasamanick. Four of the ten children studied responded quite favorably to the administration of 20 to 25 mg daily of Benzedrine, where anticonvulsant drugs had failed; of the remaining six, however, three showed no change and three became worse.[12] These results suggested that EEG abnormality is not a predictor of response to amphetamine. It is likely, moreover, that the behavior problems of some of these children were associated with something other than the EEG abnormalities.

While early investigations of the effects of amphetamine on children's behavior disorders were being conducted, other events were leading independently to the development of the notion of the "hyperkinetic impulse disorder." In 1934 E. Kahn and L. H.

Cohen noted that a deviant behavioral syndrome, which often occurred as a sequela to encephalitis, could also be observed in people with no known brain damage. In all subjects the symptoms—hyperkinesis, inability to maintain attention and quiet attitudes, lack of coordination, and impulsiveness—were associated with neurological signs of central nervous system (CNS) dysfunction. On the basis of this association, and because the behavior appeared to be involuntary, the authors concluded that it was determined by a dysfunction of the brain stem and labeled it "organic drivenness."[13]

A similar syndrome had been observed in children who had been brain-injured from causes like anoxia or head injury during the perinatal period. The long-standing historical association of hyperkinesis with brain dysfunction led M. W. Laufer in 1957 to delineate a new diagnostic category:

> It has long been recognized and accepted that a persistent disturbance of behavior of a characteristic kind may be noted after severe head injury, epidemic encephalitis and communicable disease encephalopathies, such as measles, in children. It has often been observed that a behavior pattern of a similar nature may be found in children who present no clear-cut history of any of the classical causes mentioned.
>
> This pattern will henceforth be referred to as *hyperkinetic impulse disorder*. In brief summary, hyperactivity is the most striking item . . . There are also a short attention span and poor powers of concentration, which are particularly noticeable under school conditions. Variability is also frequent . . . The child is impulsive . . . irritable and explosive . . . [and manifests] low frustration tolerance.
>
> Poor school work is frequently quite prominent. The previously described behavioral items in themselves create a pattern which makes it very difficult for the child to participate in the work of a school room. In addition there is often visual-motor difficulty which, combined with the other difficulties described above, makes for poor work in arithmetic and reading. In writing and reading "reversals" are frequent and the handwriting is often crabbed and irregular.[14]

Laufer did more than define a new diagnostic syndrome: he also postulated an organic determinant which, though never conclusively shown to exist, became part of its definition. He chose two groups of subjects from a home for emotionally disturbed children solely on the basis of whether or not they manifested the clinical syndrome of the "hyperkinetic impulse disorder." A history of factors considered capable of producing brain damage was not included in the criteria of selection, and, in fact, of the children identified as hyperkinetic, only 34 percent had such histories. Metrazol, a drug used to test the presence of brain dysfunction, was administered to each, and the amount necessary to evoke EEG spikewave burst and a myoclonic jerk of the forearms in response to a stroboscope was determined. The amount for the hyperkinetic children proved significantly less, regardless of whether their histories showed evidence of brain damage. Using Gastaut's evidence that a low photo-Metrazol threshhold indicates dysfunction of the diencephalon, Laufer concluded that the "hyperkinetic impulse disorder" has an organic determinant, specifically a dsyfunction of the diencephalon. Amphetamine administered to the hyperkinetic children raised their threshold to the level characteristic of the nonhyperkinetic group. Unfortunately, the effect of amphetamines on the photo-Metrazol thresholds of the *non*hyperkinetic children was not determined, nor was any effort made to correlate changes in photo-Metrazol threshold with changes in behavior. Thus, though impressive, the findings are inconclusive.

Diagnostic Confusion

For educational psychologists who realized that many disturbed children might not respond to psychotherapy, and for educators interested in learning disabilities and their relation to behavioral disturbances, medical science had provided a new diagnostic category, the hyperkinetic syndrome, along with evidence of its responsiveness to amphetamine treatment. But further findings have been inconclusive despite several systematic investigations carried out since the 1960s. In general, these studies have raised more questions than they have answered. For one thing, the subject populations in these amphetamine experiments have been heterogeneous in clinical diagnoses, reasons for referral for treatment, and types of learning difficulties. Many of the studies do not deal specifically with hyperkinetic children, and among those that do there is no general agreement on criteria for selection. Nor are the studies comparable in rating instruments and measurements used. So, although statistically significant findings abound, it is difficult to assess their meaning.

Significant improvement in symptoms as judged by parents, teachers, and caretakers is the most consistently reported result, although this is somewhat equivocal because of the possibility of rater bias. G. Weiss and his colleagues reported significant symptomatic improvement in a 1968 uncrossed double-blind study of thirty-eight public school children (thirty-two boys, six girls) between the ages of six and twelve. The pupils, selected on the basis of chronic, severe, and sustained hyperactivity or motor restlessness at home and at school, had IQ's of at least 80 and were free of overt physical or neurological disease. None were psychotic or epileptic; in a small, "though not inconsequential number" of these children (not precisely reported), there was psychopathology other than the hyperkinetic syndrome. The results indicated that dextroamphetamine administered for three to five weeks up to a maximum dosage of 20 mg daily was significantly more effective than placebo in producing an "overall" improvement in the children as perceived by their mothers. The rating instrument was designed to assess four behavioral dimensions: hyperactivity, excitability, distractibility, and aggressivity. In contrast to mothers' ratings alone, when ratings of mothers, psychiatrists, psychologists, and teachers were pooled, only hyperactivity and distractibility showed significant improvement in the drug group. The possibility of rater bias on the basis of expectancy cannot be ruled out, since 35 percent of the dextroamphetamine-treated children experienced loss of appetite at the beginning of treatment, which might have signalled the presence of drugs. Moreover, as the authors point out, the reliability of the findings is uncertain because of the difficulty of assessing conditions like "distractibility" with a questionnaire.[15]

Still, these findings accord not only with Bradley's early clinical descriptions but with several other recent methodologically sound studies. For example, a 1965 double-blind study by Eisenberg, Conners, and Sharpe employed the same selection criteria as the Weiss study, except that children with "psychopathic" personalities and those requiring immediate institutional care were excluded. Eighty to ninety subjects were divided into two approximately equal groups. One received either 5 mg of dextroamphet-amine or 15 mg of methylphenidate twice daily; for purposes of analyzing the results, these treatments were considered identical since no statistical differences between them were found. The other group was given placebo. The treatment continued for eight weeks. Clinicians' judgment of improvement, based on the school reports, mothers' reports, and psychiatrists' estimates of the children's behavior in the clinic, showed a statistically significant difference favoring the stimulant-treated groups. Teacher ratings definitely favored the stimulant-treated group in five categories—academic performance, classroom behavior, attitude to authority, attitude to peers, and overall behavior.[16] Aggression scores also showed a significant reduction in the stimulant-treated children, with statistical significance constituted as much by an increase in the scores of the placebo subjects as by a decrease in the scores of the drug subjects—which calls into question the meaning of the finding. These subjective evaluations could represent a rater expectancy effect based upon actual improvement seen only in some areas of behavior; however, improvement on objective performance tests supported them.

In 1968 a group headed by L. C. Epstein performed a double-blind crossover study with ten children (nine males, one female between the ages of 5.75 and 9.5 years) selected on the basis of hyperactivity, short attention span, poor concentration, and associated inadequate school performance; five showed evidence of injury to the CNS. The subjects were used as their own controls and each received dextroamphetamine and placebo for two weeks in doses ranging from 10 to 20 mg daily. Statistical analyses of effects on behavior reported by parents and psychiatrists were not done, but the impressions reported are noteworthy. The "organic" subjects were deemed markedly improved by both parents and psychiatrists: "the children were able to sit longer and concentrate better, and nervous mannerisms were sharply curtailed"; they were better able to "carry on a discussion, and better understand what was said to them"; "they were more apt to take the time to answer questions verbally instead of just shrugging their shoulders."[17] In contrast, only one child in the nonorganic group was judged by his parents to have improved markedly on the drug and even this was not unequivocally corroborated by the psychiatrist. There was differential responsiveness of the two groups to dextroamphetamine in objective measures too, but the differences were not consistently in the same direction. It is interesting that the organic group tolerated a higher dosage (20 mg average daily) than the nonorganic group (15 mg daily) and suffered fewer adverse effects; this may be related to the more rapid urinary excretion (and hence amphetamine excretion) reported for the organics. These findings seem to support the hypothesis of Kahn and Cohen (1934) and Laufer (1957) that "real" hyperkinesis is not just a symptom complex but is organically based. Laufer, however, defined organicity on the basis not of a history of possible damage to the CNS but of a photo-Metrazol threshold below the norm. Yet many of his subjects who exhibited the symptom complex had a low threshold despite the absence of evidence of brain damage. Thus, it is not possible to compare the two studies.

Epstein's findings are perplexing, since amphetamines have so often been reported to improve gross symptomatology in diagnostic categories apparently unrelated to brain damage. Bradley reported improvement in children with behavior disorders of psychogenic origin and with schizoid personalities as well as in children suffering from what might have been organically based behavioral difficulties. Bender and Cottington reported symptom improvement in neurotic children. More recently, a number of investigators have found that amphetamines improve the symptomatology of juvenile delinquents, of "disturbed children" in a residential psychiatric setting and in a group foster care institution (diagnoses undelineated), and of children with undifferentiated learning difficulties with associated behavior problems. In a well-controlled double-blind study of "most difficult" institutionalized delinquent boys, house parents and schoolteachers noted a significant decrease of disturbing, antisocial, aggressive, and hyperactive behavior in the dextroamphetamine-treated group over placebo and control groups, particularly when the dosage reached 30 to 40 mg daily.[18] When caretakers' ratings of disturbed children in a residential psychiatric treatment setting and in a group foster home were analyzed in combination, a significant decrease in those outwardly directed symptoms disturbing to caretakers was noted in the group treated with 20 to 60 mg daily of methylphenidate over the placebo group, although large individual differences in responsiveness to the drug were reported.[19] In a study of children with learning disabilities, with or without associated behavior problems, parents' ratings showed a significantly greater reduction in "hyperkinetic symptoms" (poor attention span, restlessness, impulsiveness, and temper outbursts) for the group treated with dextroamphetamine than for the placebo group. Almost no differential change between groups was noted on "neurotic symptoms" such as shyness, anxiety, and withdrawn social behavior,[20] which suggests that stimulants affect certain dimensions of behavior regardless of the diagnosis of the patient.

Symptoms

What sorts of behavior are altered by amphetamines in a way that accounts for the impression of improvement so often reported? Findings on the actual amount of physical activity are not consistent. R. L. Sprague and others in 1970 found that methylphenidate significantly reduced activity level as measured by a stabilimetric cushion. Yet J. G. Millichap and his associates found that, although methylphenidate tended to reduce motor activity as measured by an actometer (an activity-watch worn on the wrist which measures locomotion on a horizontal plane), so did placebo. In another study by Millichap and E. E. Boldrey, actometer-measured motor activity actually *increased* when subjects were treated with methylphenidate for one day, even though parents and teachers perceived improved motor coordination and reduced impulsivity. T. R. McConnell and R. L. Cromwell reported similar findings, but their subjects were retarded, which may account for the difference in their reactions from hyperkinetic children of average intelligence. All this contradictory evidence suggests that the subjective rating scales and objective instruments are measuring very different aspects of activity, and that the paradoxical calming effect may be an artifact of observation, reflecting the organization of activity in relation to social demands.[21]

An important controlled double-blind crossover study was carried out by Conners and his associates on a group of fifth- and sixth-grade learning and behaviorally disabled black children, "not specifically selected because of psychiatric or neurologic impairment." Ten mg of dextroamphetamine were administered daily to each subject for a month. In a factor analysis of objective personality and performance tests, dextroamphetamine had no significant effect on ability and performance, but produced a highly significant improvement in assertiveness, drive for achievement, and vigor of response. These factors have been reported to correlate with competence, efficiency, and determination. Despite the mixed findings on objective tests, teachers' symptom ratings as well as their general global ratings indicated improvement for the drug-treated subjects in classroom performance and in the three rated categories of behavior, attitude toward authority, and attitude toward peers.

As the authors note, the effect seems motivational. Through its CNS-stimulating properties, the drug may allow the children to make use of previously dormant abilities. This would parallel Bradley's earlier clinical descriptions of increase in children's drive and interest in their surroundings. Conners concludes: "Despite the finding of rated improvement in three areas of classroom behavior, attitude toward authority, and group participation, it seems doubtful that the medication specifically affects these areas. Rather, it would seem more plausible to assume that teachers observe the calmer, [because] more determined behavior of the pupils, and tend to generalize the benefits to all three areas of rated performance."[22] The increased determination and vigor of response and the perceived symptomatic improvement may simply reflect more organized goal-directed behavior and closer approximation to social norms. Activity level may be only indirectly affected by the drugs. Where great mental effort is required, for example, increased vigor of response might result in greater concentration and a concomitant decrease in motor activity; in a freer "play" situation, increased vigor of response might result in an actual increase in motor activity as a result of the child's involvement in his social environment. But in that case a higher actiivity level would not be disapproved.

Independent findings in other areas support the interpretation put forth by Strauss and Kephart, that short attention span, distractibility, and hyperactivity all refer to the same thing. It has been reported that attention, as measured by a variety of objective tests, is enhanced by the administration of amphetamines. D. H. Sykes and colleagues demonstrated this with the use of H. E. Rosvold's Continuous Performance Task (CPT). Forty chronically hyperactive children (thirty-four boys, six girls) between the ages of five and twelve, who attended normal classes, were subjects for a double-blind study. Specifically excluded were psychotic, epileptic, or grossly brain-damaged children, or children whose behavior problems were clearly emotionally based; IQ's were 80 or above. Methylphenidate was administered to half, with dosage adjusted to individual tolerance. Most children received 30 to 40 mg daily for five to seven weeks. The drug-treated subjects did significantly better than the placebo subjects, making not only more correct responses but also fewer errors (responses to insignificant stimuli).[23]

Stimulant-related increase in attention is also suggested by results produced by other methods, notably the Porteus Maze Test, an objective measure of planned, organized, and particularly impulse-inhibited behavior.[24] Quantative improvement on this test was demonstrated in Eisenberg's 1965 study. A highly significant improvement in Porteus Maze performance was reported for stimulant-treated subjects, while only minimal improvement, perhaps resulting from practice, occurred in the placebo-treated children.[25] A study of disturbed children by Conners and Eisenberg suggests a possible relation between drug effect and intelligence. Maze tests administered under treatment conditions showed a significant difference between drug- and placebo-treated subjects in the two lowest IQ groups (65-79 and 80-91), but none for the high-IQ (94-135) subjects.

There are two possible explanations for the lack of significant differences between high-IQ treatment groups. One is based on the observation that many of the subjects referred to the medication as "smart pills," and had high expectations of becoming happier and calmer and better on tests. Such expectations might have provided the more intelligent and insightful placebo subjects with motivation enough to balance the benefit the stimulants provided for the drug subjects. A second possible explanation is that the Porteus Maze, developed originally as a tool for classifying mentally retarded children, is not sensitive enough to make fine distinctions for those well above average in general intelligence.

In the Conners study, children with learning problems were given dextroamphetamine and placebo. Both groups showed similar improvement on the Porteus Maze Test after the first two weeks of the study; only after the last two weeks was improvement more marked in those treated with the drug.[26] This could have been the result of increasing the daily dosage in the last two weeks from 15 mg to 20-25 mg, or of the cumulative effect of treatment.

Although some early studies suggested that amphetamines enhanced cognitive and intellectual functioning, more recent, methodologically sound ones have resulted in apparently contradictory findings.[27] In 1972 Conners, questioning inconsistencies in a series of studies conducted by himself and his associates on children diagnosed as suffering from minimal brain dysfunction (MBD, the most recent term for the hyperkinetic impulse disorder), selected those which had employed common pre- and post-drug measuring instruments, and developed a profile analysis in order to achieve as much diagnostic homogeneity as possible. A group of 178 previously treated subjects (78 on placebo and 100 on drugs) were accepted for this study. Conners found that they could be distinguished in terms of seven different patterns of baseline performance on psychological tests, and that their response to stimulant drugs differed widely and depended on their initial profile of abilities as represented by the seven patterns. The sample, though all diagnosed as MBD in accordance with the official definition, was heterogeneous in its profiles, and changes under drug therapy differed accordingly. These preliminary studies are not yet useful diagnostic tools, but they indicate that some of the apparent inconsistencies in the literature can be understood if initial profiles of abilities and deficiencies are taken into account. Conners suggests that there is "no single syndrome of hyperkinesis [which] is uniquely responsive to [drug] therapy, . . . and several [discernible] patterns of change of perceptual and cognitive abilities may result from drug therapy."[28]

Site of Amphetamine Action

How are these differing patterns of change brought about by amphetamines? Their mechanism and site of action are poorly understood in adults and all but unknown in children. The work of Laufer and his associates with Metrazol is still the best documented pharmacological study of the action of amphetamines in hyperkinetic children, although even this study was merely suggestive, and no one has tried to replicate it. Their work suggested that hyperkinesis results from a diencephalic dysfunction. Normally, the diencephalon, thought to be the rostral component of the reticular activating system (RAS), serves to sort, route, and pattern impulses from sensory receptors before they are amplified at higher levels of the brain. It inhibits irrelvant stimuli and keeps them from "flooding" the cortex. The presumed diencephalic dysfunction could result from a structural impairment of the brain stem or the diencephalon itself, exposing the cortex to irrelevant stimuli, or to a maturational imbalance in which a relatively underdevelped cortex cannot meet the demands of a normally functioning diencephalon. In either case, Laufer thought that amphetamines stimulated the inhibitory functioning of the diencephalon in such a way as not to overwhelm the cortex.[29]

This reasoning was partly based on animal experiments, especially those of P. B. Bradley, whose work with cats suggested that "the site of action of amphetamine may be related to the brain stem reticular activating system of Magoun."[30] But if studies done not specifically on hyperkinetic children can be brought to bear on the issue, then those such as Bradley's make it just as plausible that amphetamines act in hyperkinetic children by increasing general alertness through stimulation of the reticular activating system in the brain stem. The action of amphetamine is related to that of norepinephrine, which is concentrated in the brain stem, and it is generally believed that influences of the brain stem reticular formation on the cerebral cortex is responsible for the maintenance of alertness. Amphetamines appear to increase alertness through the mediation of the influence of the brain stem reticular formation on cortical arousal mechanisms. They may also decrease the threshold for arousal responses produced by direct stimulation of the reticular formation. This would explain the behavioral changes in hyperkinetic children as normal, not "paradoxical," effects of amphetamines. An increase in general alertness could cause an increase in focused attention and a decrease in responses to interfering stimuli. On the other hand, even if the hypothesis of a diencephalic dysfunction is accepted, a nonparadoxical interpretation is still suggested, since the brain stem reticular formation functions both to maintain the cortex in a state of alertness and to regulate incoming stimuli reaching the cortex. Thus, if the brain stem is an important site of action of amphetamine, its stimulating effects would both increase alertness and prevent interfering stimuli from reaching the cortex, reducing the need to attend to diverse stimuli and enhancing the possibility of sustained attention to one thing at a time. This, too, would accord with the behavioral findings reported.[31]

Some scanty evidence, based mostly on animal studies, suggests the cortex as a possible site of amphetamine action. Prefrontal lesions in monkeys have been shown to release hyperkinetic behavior which is significantly reduced by stimulants; on the other hand, cortical lesions have lowered convulsive thresholds to amphetamine, and in the rat, cortical lesions have sensitized the animals to drug-induced hyperkinesis.[32] Interestingly, what evidence there is of direct cortical response to amphetamine relates primarily to motor activity (which is mediated by the cortex). Yet, as we have pointed out, the motoric element of the hyperkinetic syndrome is one of the less important ones and might in fact be an artifact of observation, reflecting attentional difficulties mediated primarily by the reticular activating system. Thus, although there may be a form of hyperactivity mediated by a cortical dysfunction, no consistent evidence shows that it responds to amphetamines. Moreover, other specifically cortical funtions, particularly perceptual and cognitive, have not been consistently responsive to amphetamines. It is more likely that where the hyperkinetic syndrome is responsive to amphetamine treatment, this responsiveness is mediated by the direct effect on the brain stem reticular formation. In the absence of any evidence to the contrary, it is parsimonious, as Conners points out, to assume not that amphetamines have paradoxical pharmacological effects on hyperkinetic children, but that through the mediation of the RAS they "produce more organized perceptual response . . . for a variety of children [as well as adults], with effects being more dramatically noticeable in children with diencephalic lesions or other forms of imbalance between cortical and subcortical mechanisms."[33]

Adverse Effects of Amphetamines

Although statistically significant results in favor of amphetamine have been obtained fairly consistently on certain measures, much variability has also been reported, and the results are not as spectacular as they might appear. Not all hyperkinetic children improve on the drug, and some get worse. Bradley reported that of 275 children treated with Benzedrine, almost 11 percent showed an exaggeration of all the original symptoms as well as increased agitation, tension, and anxiety; of the 113 children treated with Dexedrine, almost 16 percent exhibited a similar exaggeration of symptoms. Sol Levy reported similar findings. A few dramatically adverse reactions have occurred: Mattson and Calverly reported amphetamine-induced dyskinesia in three young children; H. H. Eveloff reported a similar finding in an eighteen-year-old girl; P. G. Ney presented a case of amphetamine-induced psychosis in an eight-year-old hyperkinetic boy.[34] A. R. Lucas and M. Weiss recently reported hallucinosis among the reactions of three young patients to methylphenidate hydrocholoride. The dosage of a six-and-a-half-year-old girl had been gradually increased from 5 to 15 mg per day over a nine-day period. Regression and withdrawal associated with bizarre mannerisms became pronounced. Although she did not report hallucinations, her behavior indicated that she was experiencing them. A ten-year-old boy received a cumulative dose of only 40 mg over a five-day period. On day five he had received two 10-mg doses. He felt great power and strength and saw a rainbow and a whirlpool of colors with lions, tigers, and marching elephants. In the third case, a fifteen-year-old girl had been taking 20 mg twice a day since the age of nine for hyperactivity, distractibility, and short attention span. Visual hallucinations developed when she took 60 mg to relax after an upsetting argument with a friend and continued for two days until she ceased taking the medication.[35] Such cases, though very rare, merit attention.

Toxic effects like anorexia, insomnia, gastrointestinal distress, dizziness, fine tremor and coldness of the extremities, and pallor usually occur even in children who are benefited by amphetamines. They are rarely severe enough to require discontinuance of treatment, and most gradually diminish or disappear after the first week; when they persist, they are usually minimized or eliminated by adjusting the dosage or time of administration. However, significant weight loss has occasionally been reported with continued use of amphetamines, despite the adjustment of dosage. In general, methylphenidate has fewer toxic effects than racemic amphetamine or dextroamphetamine; the principal one is a mild and usually transient insomnia.[36]

A study by Safer, Allen, and Barr, published in 1972 and since replicated, raises the question of long-term deleterious effects.

Nine children who had been taking stimulants for two years or more were compared in changes of height and weight with seven children who, although referred for stimulant treatment, had not been treated because of parental objections. Eight of the stimulant group showed less than expected annual weight gain, and in seven percentile weight continued to decrease for the second and third years on medication. Five of the nine showed a similar decrease in percentile height over the period of long-term medication. Although the decrease in percentile height (as opposed to weight) was not statistically significant when compared with baseline percentiles, it was highly significant when compared with the height changes in the control group, for whom percentile height actually increased.[37]

Another set of data amplified these findings. Twenty hyperactive children who had been taking dextroamphetamine or methylphenidate daily for the nine months of the school year were studied. All were white middle-class children, 80 percent of whom were receiving special educational instruction for learning disabilities. Seven also received stimulants for the three summer months; thirteen did not. Although the children gained weight over the nine-month period on medication, the amount of gain was less than normal; the effect was statistically significant with dextroamphetamine and higher doses of methylphenidate (20 mg and above daily). The children taken off stimulants for the summer gained more weight than would normally be expected for children of their age; those who remained on stimulants continued to gain less. Nevertheless, the large weight gain by those taken off medication did not quite compensate for the suppression of weight gain during the previous nine months. Admittedly, complete compensation might have been achieved if the children had remained off medication for more than the three months. In fact, in an unpublished study by Kenneth Zike, recently cited by Eisenberg, a group of 83 drug-treated hyperkinetic children who were followed for a period of one to eleven years showed no evidence of suppresion of growth. In particular, one subgroup of thirty-one methamphetamine-treated subjects (average dose, 20 mg per square meter of body surface area) showed a growth curve above the 50th percentile on the Iowa grids.[38] Such contradictory findings leave the issue unresolved; however, Safer's results do signal caution.

Diagnostic Confusion and the Use of Amphetamines

If the layman is confused by developments in the use of amphetamines for hyperkinetic children, it is because the experts have come to no agreement about the facts the public is being asked to accept. There is no consensus about the nature of the hyperkinetic syndrome or how to diagnose it. It is still no better understood than it was when Laufer and his associates defined it and postulated an organic basis for it. This ignorance is underscored by the fact that the importance of the assumed brain dysfunction has now been subtly reduced by adding the qualifier "minimal." S. D. Clements has officially renamed the syndrome "minimal brain dysfunction [MBD] syndrome" and defined it as follows:

> The term "minimal brain dysfunction syndrome" refers . . . to children of near average, average, or above average general intelligence with certain learning or behavioral disabilities ranging from mild to severe, which are associated with deviations of function of the central nervous system. These deviations may manifest themselves by various combinations of impairment in perception, conceptualization, language, memory, and control of attention, impulse or motor function.
>
> Similar symptoms may or may not complicate the problems of children with cerebral palsy, epilepsy, mental retardation, blindness, or deafness.
>
> These aberrations may arise from genetic variations, biochemical irregularities, perinatal brain insults, or other illness or injuries sustained during the years which are critical for the development and maturation of the central nervous system, *or from unknown causes.* [39]

This is merely a sophisticated statement of ignorance about a rather vaguely defined symptom complex.

In "Hyperactivity and the CNS: An Etiological and Diagnostic Dilemma," C. J. Weithorn discusses with refreshing logic and clarity the difficulties of characterizing and diagnosing hyperkinesis. She suggests that there may be two distinct forms: "one, a motor hyperactivity (due to defective inhibitory mechanisms in the cortical motor system), and the other, a generalized hyperreactivity (due to defective inhibitory mechanisms in the sensory sphere)." And, "application of this formulation to the behavior of hyperactive children would indicate that there is a distinction to be made between a motorically restless child and one whose movements are in response to a multiplicity of stimuli."[40] We noted earlier that attentional, rather than motor, impulsivity seems to respond to amphetamines. It is possible that distinct forms of the hyperkinetic disorder respond differently to drugs, which could account in part for the confusion in terminology.

The blurring and confusion of the various diagnostic categories meant to differentiate hyperkinetic, perceptually handicapped, and emotionally disturbed children is indicated by Barbara Fish in "The 'One Child, One Drug' Myth of Stimulants in Hyperkinesis." She believes that lack of agreement about the use of terms like minimal brain dysfunction and hyperkinesis has "created the misinterpretations of the literature on stimulants in children that still plague us."[41] Laufer reported that dextroamphetamine is more effective in treating children with behavior disorders of organic etiology, whereas Bender and Fish reported that *neurotic* children are more responsive to the drug.[42] Yet, in fact, Laufer's population was a heterogeneous mixture of personality disorders found in psychiatric treatment settings, and it was only on top of these diagnoses that the label "hyperkinetic syndrome" was superimposed. It had already been postulated that the syndrome had an organic basis, specifically a diencephalic dysfunction. Moreover, of those categorized as hyperkinetic, only 20 percent had been diagnosed as having chronic brain syndrome and/or convulsive disorders. Among those categorized as nonhyperkinetic, the same diagnoses applied, although there were proportionally fewer cases of organic brain syndrome and convulsions, and proportionally more cases of anxiety reaction. Since many of the children categorized as (organically) hyperkinetic were also diagnosed as having behavior disorders of psychogenic origin, it was logically incorrect to conclude that behavior disorders with organic components are more responsive to amphetamines than behavior disorders of psychogenic origin.

More recent studies have shed no further light on the variables which best predict stimulant response in children. As Fish notes, although the 1969 study by Conners and Eisenberg demonstrated no change in neurotic symptoms with the use of stimulants, no analysis was done to determine whether hyperactivity symptoms in children diagnosed as "neurotic" were stimulant responsive.[43]

Furthermore, because heterogeneous samples were used in so many of the later studies, and individual variability was so common within significantly improved drug-treated groups, it is impossible to determine which variables respond to amphetamine treatment. This impossibility was well documented by Conners and his two colleagues, who pointed out that students who were *not* labeled "hyperkinetic" nonetheless improved markedly while on amphetamines.[44] If the investigators had not taken extreme care to emphasize that there was no reason to suppose the existence of any organic damage or even deep-rooted psychiatric problems, this study quite possibly would have been cited as further "evidence" for the effectiveness of amphetamines in improving the school work and general behavior of hyperkinetic children.

A recent study by J. H. Satterfield and others on EEG and neurological correlates of stimulant response in MBD children is open to a similar misinterpretation. Each of fifty-seven children diagnosed as cases of MBD by two independent psychiatrists was given an extensive neurological work-up; EEG's were performed, and several psychometric tests were administered. Methylphenidate and placebo were given in a double-blind experiment for three weeks, in dosages adjusted for good clinical response subject to individual tolerance. When teacher-rating scales were analyzed, it was found that the children with both an abnormal neurological examination and an abnormal EEG responded significantly better to methylphenidate than those with normal neurological examination and normal EEG. Ninety percent of the former group showed 30 percent or more improvement; this suggests that a combination of abnormal EEG and neurological examination predicts good response to stimulants. But 60 percent of the group with normal EEG and neurological examination also showed 30 percent or more improvement.[45] Had Satterfield not carefully pointed this out, his study too could have been cited as further "evidence" for the organic dysfunction theory.

The hyperkinetic syndrome needs reconsideration. There may be a higher incidence of brain abnormality among children diagnosed clinically as MBD than among "normal" controls, although the evidence so far is unclear. Satterfield and his coworkers found evidence to support this contention, but Werry and Sprague point out that when the criterion is intensive neurological

examination rather than observations of behavior, hyperkinesis
does not occur any more often in an "organic" group than in a
"normal" (non-brain-damaged as measured by neurological testing) control group. Fish insists upon the necessity of a logical system of diagnosis that distinguishes "between diagnoses of mental
disorders which define the level and type of total personality disorder and terms which define major developmental symptoms."
She concludes that the usefulness of amphetamines in treating
"children with behavior disorders is [not] limited . . . by the
presence or absence of overt anxiety or hyperactivity, nor by the
presence or absence of minimal brain dysfunctions, . . . but the
critical controlled study . . . has yet to be done."[46]

The Role of Educators

Considering the confusion within the medical community
about hyperkinesis, the self-assurance with which educators and
the drug industry have promoted the use of amphetamines in
schools is frightening. An interesting treatment of the situation
appeared in the *Saturday Review* on November 21, 1970. First, a
thoughtful and well-organized article by E. T. Ladd, entitled
"Pills for Classroom Peace?," pointed out major dangers involved
in the administration of amphetamines to schoolchildren diagnosed as hyperkinetic, and discussed them one by one. Second
came a brief insert (less than a page of the Ladd article), written
by C. Ellingson, entitled "The Children with No Alternative."
According to this, children who need some kind of "replacement
chemotherapy" are not "normal, active, ebullient youngsters who
are chafing under the restraints of classroom discipline," but
ones whose central nervous systems are not functioning normally,
so that they are the "victims of forces they cannot control."[47]
Ellingson claims that modification of their behavior is not the
primary aim of drug administration. It is merely one of the anticipated results of a correction of some specific but still undefined
(hypothetical) chemical imbalance. Ladd, however, points out
that forcing young children to take any kind of medication may
constitute an infringement of their civil rights, no matter how
expedient such measures appear to school personnel trying to
cope with disruptive behavior. He emphasizes that the only ob-
jectionable behavior a school has any legal right to control or
modify is that which it *must* police in order to "accomplish its job

and protect persons and the institution." When the aims of education are as ill-defined or as poorly articulated as they seem to be in most of our schools today, there is too much latitude for administrators and teachers to decide what kind of behavior is incompatible with the school's "job."

Even Ladd's article is misleading in some ways. He mentions the risk of physiological damage, including addiction or long-term and even permanent organic changes, then dismisses them, claiming that amphetamines are not physiologically addictive for children, that physicians prescribing these drugs for elementary students are especially cautious, and that in any event the situation is being "policed" by the FDA. These arguments are questionable. It is not at all clear that some children may not suffer subtle adverse physiological effects that may not become evident for many years. We have mentioned the Safer study suggesting that growth may be adversely affected. Ladd himself entertains the possibility that administering amphetamines to children may subtly condition or dispose them eventually to joining the "drug culture." And the FDA is notoriously an ineffective watchdog. Ladd's faith in physicians is also misplaced. Many do not rely on their own clinical tests or even on firsthand observations, but prescribe amphetamines solely on the basis of teachers' and school administrators' reports of "deviancy" which may be nothing more than healthy but active curiosity or a lack of interest in what the teacher is saying. Ladd realizes that using drugs to "modify" classroom behavior subverts desirable educational goals. If we want our educational institutions to help young people deal with and learn to regulate "self-destructive" or "antisocial" tendencies, it makes no sense to give them drugs as soon as they exhibit restless or unruly behavior. They deserve educational environments designed to help them "come to grips with their natural dispositions and learn to use in a certain way what Philip Jackson at the University of Chicago has nicely called their own 'executive powers.' Any form of intervention that relieves a restless or unruly child of the need, or deprives him of the opportunity, to use his executive powers deprives him to that extent of the chance to develop insights and skill in self-control."[48]

The divergent opinions reflected by Ladd and Ellingson suggested a need for "official" federal clarification, so the United States Department of Health, Education and Welfare called a conference on The Use of Stimulant Drugs in the Treatment of Behaviorally Disturbed School Children. On January 11 and 12, 1971, fifteen specialists from the sciences and social sciences were summoned to discuss the matter and arrive at conclusions about the current status of knowledge on the subject and about the conditions under which the drugs should be given to children. (Any adequate accomplishment of the first task would have precluded a clear resolution of the second.) The Report of the Conference was worded so as not to offend anyone, particularly the drug industry, whose vested interest in the existence of hyperkinesis is great. A statesmanlike document, written cautiously and persuasively, it managed to arrive at two fundamentally opposite sets of conclusions. First it stressed the difficulties in diagnosing hyperkinesis, and the lack of adequate research on the long-term effects of stimulants adminstered to young children. But then it endorsed the use of amphetamines in the medical treatment of what was now officially defined as "minimal brain dysfunction," even though no research had been able to establish the nature of this presumed organic malfunctioning or deficiency. The HEW Report took a naively optimistic stand, urging all who were "benefiting" from drug treatment to act ethically and show restraint and good judgment. The drug companies were requested not to send any more representatives to schools to "seek endorsement of their products by school personnel."[49] The media were urged not to be sensationalistic. Teachers and parents were asked to try affection, psychotherapy, and simple patience before resorting to a medical "solution." Doctors were reminded that they should be certain that their diagnoses were accurate.

The most disturbing aspect of this report was not what it said or did not say, but that it has been used to justify the existence of hyperkinesis as an established disease and the overprescription of stimulants to treat it. It has been mailed to various persons described in a flattering cover letter as being "in a position to be concerned, and to influence others concerning the management of hyperkinesis in the schools."[50] It has been cited in the press as an endorsement for the use of stimulants by "leading experts in medicine, welfare, and education." In direct disregard of its content, it has been used by drug companies in advertisements recommending stimulant products. One critic of the report has correctly remarked:

The diagnostic tools cited, such as patient histories, psycho-metric tests and various mechanical devices measuring just how much a child fidgets do no more than restate what has already been observed: that the child is restless, inattentive, etc. They do not in themselves confirm the hypothesis that these kids are "brain damaged." A comparable situation, from a medical point of view, would be, if a doctor told you that you were suf-fering from a kidney disease that could only be detected by the fact that you beat up your wife, cut yourself when you shaved and felt tense and angry at work; and who then proceeded to confirm his diagnosis by finding out how long you had beaten your wife and measuring just how hard you hit her![51]

The behavior taken to be a sign of minimal brain dysfunction is real enough! Restless, angry, disturbed, and inattentive students are a major problem for many parents and teachers. It may also be true that some children exhibit such behavior because of or-ganic brain damage or neurohormonal deficiencies. But it is hard to believe that the 200,000 or more schoolchildren who are now routinely given stimulants are *all* suffering from organic brain damage or deficiencies in CNS chemicals. Nor is the fact that am-phetamines sometimes reduce disruptiveness and increase at-tention any reason to suppose that they affect some organically based hyperkinesis; as we have seen, they can influence behavior and learning problems generally recognized to be of psychogenic and environmental origin in much the same way that they affect problems presumed to have an organic basis.

Effectiveness of Amphetamines

Even in instances that may be considered true cases of minimal brain dysfunction, stimulants are not always the drugs of choice, and drugs are not always useful. R. D. Freeman has reviewed the literature to 1969 on the efficacy of amphetamines in reducing hy-peractivity, distractibility, alleged hyperkinesis, or MBD, and has concluded that the shortage of controlled objective and scientific studies, together with the strong possibility of a placebo effect resulting from eagerness on the part of children to please—and teachers or physicians or drug companies to be pleased—has made it nearly impossible to determine with any accuracy whether amphetamines specifically alleviate even the symptoms alleged to be those of hyperkinesis. He has warned that one should be especially careful in judging the efficacy of a drug with such varied and powerful effects on a set of disorders as ambiguously defined as learning disabilities. Furthermore, the phenothiazines have proven more useful than stimulants in some cases, and some very positive results have been demonstrated with imipramine (although the safety of the latter has been called into question by some recent reports of seizures in children).[52] In any case, in a review of the literature on hyperkinetic symptoms, H. S. Novak finds that "comparative results indicate that medication, when and where effective, produced immediate and beneficial control of the behavior of [only] about 15 to 20 percent of the populations tested."[53] And there has been no way of predicting beforehand which students will profit from which, if any, drugs.

Even for those children who initially seem to profit from medication, long-term benefits may be insignificant. Aside from the preliminary study reported by Laufer, the only two published follow-up studies on the long-term effects of amphetamines on hyperkinetic symptoms in children are not reassuring. One was conducted by Weiss and her associates on a group of children who, on initial interview five years earlier, had been diagnosed as severely hyperactive. All sixty-four had been treated with chlorpromazine (Thorazine) for one to two years, and then, if the original medication was ineffective, with dextroamphetamine, methylphenidate, or thioridazine (Mellaril). At the time of follow-up, when most were adolescents, it was found that, although the more pronounced manifestations of restlessness had diminished, attentional handicaps persisted. Underachievement in school and general academic difficulties were evident in 80 percent of the children, although they were of at least average intelligence; 70 percent were judged to be emotionally immature; and many suffered from low self-esteem and feelings of hopelessness. This study did not employ amphetamines in a systematic way, and it is not possible to draw sound conclusions about their relative efficacy. But the results do indicate that amphetamines and other drugs were not particularly beneficial in this group.[54]

The other study analyzed more systematically the effects of dextroamphetamine on eighty-three teenagers. Of those studied, 92 percent had initially been treated with dextroamphetamine or methylphenidate; of these, 60 percent had shown improvement for at least six months. At the time of follow-up, although about half of the sample were rated as showing some overall improvement, over 75 percent still manifested poor concentration, impulsivity, and defiance, while 25 percent were involved in antisocial activities that suggested that they might develop serious pathology as adults.[55] Most continued to have serious difficulties with schoolwork and suffer from feelings of low self-esteem and worthlessness, probably resulting from a cycle of low motivation, failure, and discouragement.* It appears that, despite the excitement about the potential of amphetamines for treating hyperkinetic children, they cannot perform miracles.

Alternatives to drug therapy are now emerging which are safer and may be more effective in the long run. In 1971 Alvin Toffler reported to the American Psychological Association on the results of a series of experiments using easily learned classroom behavior modification techniques on hyperactive children with either normal or abnormal EEG tracings. After twenty-four hyperactive elementary schoolchildren with normal IQ's had been administered complete EEG'S, they were given simple reinforcement for attentiveness to an academic workbook task in an experimental classroom environment. Their rates of attentiveness, cooperation, and accuracy were measured before, during, and after the application of simple positive reinforcement techniques of praise and reward for even trivial successes. Both normal and abnormal EEG groups showed significant decreases in hyperactivity, and the improvements carried over into their regular school environments. One of the more interesting findings was that the abnormal-EEG group showed even greater decreases in hyperactivity and increases in overall classroom performance than the normal-EEG group. No improvement was noted in a nontreated control group of similarly "disturbed" or hyperactive children (with or without normal EEG's). Toffler concluded that simple behavior modification should be attempted first for even the most severely agitated hyperkinetics, since it is by their *behavior* that they are being judged "sick," "deviant," or "deficient." This conclusion is supported by the Werry and Sprague recommendation that drugs "should not be used as the

---

*Although it is often stated that hyperkinesis is outgrown by adolescence, it turns out, that, whatever hyperkinesis may be, many of its symptoms persist. If restlessness and poor attention appear to diminish, it may be that the child has developed less disturbing ways of manifesting his problems.

only or even the primary treatment, except where circumstances preclude behavior modification procedures."[56]

Behavior modification techniques are no panacea, and they, too, have a significant potential for abuse. But they do have the virtue of requiring a sensitivity to the child's needs, talents, and preferences. Instead of simply making a child more manageable, they may bring out his best qualities; they allow him to discover his impulses and use his own capacity for self-control in dealing with them instead of just eliminating temporarily the more disturbing impulses. Besides, behavior learned through the use of such techniques can be generalized beyond the specific situation in which it was originally produced. By contrast, drug-facilitated learning is not only not generalized to a broad spectrum of situations but possibly forgotten quite readily.[57]

A drug may make a child more attentive and manageable in the short run but in the long run leave him with a sense of failure and worthlessness, by giving him a false sense of well-being that prevents him from developing his own capacities for coping. Interestingly enough, despite many reports by *children* who have been administered stimulants of an increased sense of well-being, it has been insisted in the literature that "euphoria" is never a "side effect" of these drugs in children. This presumed absence of euphoria has been used as an argument supporting the notion that amphetamines have very different (paradoxical) effects on children than on adults and may, therefore, be considered safe for them. But there is no reason to believe that what a child considers "feeling better" is any different from what an adult experiences. It is no better for a child than for an adult to be dependent on a sense of well-being induced by a potentially damaging drug.

Our society has been undergoing a critical change in values. Children have seen claims to authority and existing institutions questioned as an everyday occurrence. The classroom has become a stage on which this value upheaval is played out. Teachers no longer have the authority they once had in the classroom, and they often have no other well-defined way of relating to children. The child, on his part, now demands, often through his behavior, to be acknowledged as a person and treated with concern. "Hyperkinesis" has sometimes been used as a convenient label with which to dismiss this phenomenon as a physical "disease" rather than treat it as a social problem. Where hyperkinesis actually exists, it is hard to distinguish from other disturbances expressed in similar behavior patterns. Accordingly, symptoms, not causes, have become the focus of treatment, and a significant potential for abuse arises. Amphetamine treatment for these symptoms is, in the long run, not very effective, and may be detrimental in the same ways it is for adults.

Living with Speed

> "To put it quite simply: our
> culture influences, encourages, and
> sometimes causes people to use
> amphetamines; and their behavior
> under the influence of these
> drugs often constitutes a caricature
> of the very society that produced it."

Among the commonly used psychoactive drugs, the amphetamines have one of the most formidable potentials for psychological, physical, and social harm. Although they may be safely used in small doses over limited periods of time, many people risk serious dependency. There is danger of cell damage in several organs, including the brain, and chronic high-dose use will almost without exception produce short- and possibly long-term psychoses. Even brief episodic consumption of moderate to high doses involves a risk of physical disorders and psychoses. It has not been conclusively established, but there is strong suspicion that prolonged high-dose use may lead to a global deterioration of mental functioning. Also the high-dose amphetamine abuser may commit impulsive, destructive and often outrageously antisocial acts.

Drug Advertising

The fact that most introductions to amphetamines come through doctors' prescriptions suggests that physicians are not well educated about this class of drugs. The average physician gets most of his information on drugs not from objective, balanced, professional reports of controlled, comparative experiments but from hard-sell drug advertisements or pharmaceutical company traveling salesmen, euphemistically called "detail men." Some physicians have sharply criticized members of their own profession. Dr. Walter Modell states that: "One area of medical knowledge given the least expansion in the third and fourth years of medical college is pharmacology and applied pharmacology. I think it is anticipated that it will be 'picked up' by the student in internship. But I'm afraid by that time the blandishments of the detail men become attractive to the busy intern." Dr. Louis Lasagna has also expressed concern: "The physician leaving medical school is lucky if he is well-versed in the use of the increasingly large numbers of 'standard' drugs used most often in practice." And Dr. W. B. Bean is even more out-spoken: "In recent years we have seen post graduate medical education nearly taken over by the siren song of advertising with illustrated brochures, wholesale distribution of samples of power-ful drugs, and the ventriloquism of the detail man spouting his spiel like the barker at Madame Snakehair's sideshow. The detail man is a lineal descendent [sic] of the medicine man of pioneer days."[1]

Surveys of physicians' prescribing habits have supported these charges. Such studies, however, are open to criticism: the samples were not always large enough to eliminate chance variation; the doctors may not always have recalled correctly or admitted the real sources of their drug information; the ways in which the questions were worded may have influenced replies. But, inaccu-rate as they are, they probably underestimate the doctors' reli-ance on drug advertisements and detail men. And they do give at least a rough idea of the important influences on physicians' judgment. More significantly still, the studies agree in all im-portant respects.

Table 7 compares the results of three studies in which phy-sicians were asked where they first learned about a new drug. The detail man was the initial source for 31 to 52 percent; direct mail advertising for as many as 22 percent; and medical journals only 9 to 25 percent. Apparently from half to almost three-quarters of the time a physician's first information about a new drug comes from advertising promotion.

Even more important is the source that persuades a doctor to prescribe a new drug. Table 8 shows some dissimilarity in re-sponse, but this may reflect the ways the questions were phrased. In the Coleman survey, 21 percent of the doctors admitted that they had finally been persuaded to prescribe a drug on the basis of direct promotion by the pharmaceutical company (detail men, 5 percent; advertisements in medical journals, 2 percent; and di-

Table 7. Initial source of drug information according to physicians (percentage).

Source	Study		
	Caplow and Raymond	Ferber and Wales	Coleman et al.
Detail men	31	38	52
Medical journals	25	25	9
Direct mail advertisements	16	19	22
Colleagues	14	6	10
Medical meetings	7	4	3
Other	7	8	3
Number of doctors answering	182	328	87

Sources: T. Caplow and J.J. Raymond, Jr., "Factors influencing the selection of pharmaceutical products," *Marketing*, 19 (July 1954), 18–23. R. Ferber and H.G. Wales, "The effectiveness of pharmaceutical promotion," *University of Illinois Bureau of Economics and Business Research Bulletin 83* (Urbana, 1958), p. 22. J.S. Coleman, E. Katz, and H. Menzel, *Medical Innovation: A Diffusion Study* (Indianapolis: Bobbs-Merrill, 1966), p. 59.

rect mail advertising, 14 percent), and another 21 percent because of what they read in a drug firm's periodical. Ferber and Wales found that at least 39 percent of the doctors they polled were first induced to use a drug by the seller (in the form of detail men or direct mail), and the corresponding Gaffin total was 67 percent. In the latter, when the 1,011 doctors were asked which two or three sources they considered the most important and reliable for securing information about a new drug before prescribing it, 68 percent mentioned detail men, 25 percent direct mail advertisements, and 22 percent free samples. Thirty-one percent named medical meetings, 24 percent conversations with colleagues, and 40 percent medical journal articles. In a survey conducted by the Pharmaceutical Manufacturers Association in 1960, 62 percent of the physicians polled listed the drug industry as their preferred source of information in deciding whether to use a new drug, while 35 percent mentioned medical journals (which could still mean advertisements) or meetings and conversations with colleagues.[2] Apparently doctors considered advertising promotion twice as important as information reaching them through professional associates.

Table 8. Source of information convincing physicians to prescribe a drug for the first time (percentage).

Source[a]	Study		
	Coleman et al.	Ferber and Wales	Gaffin
Detail men	5	21	41
Medical journals	42[b]	28	15
Direct mail advertisements	14	18	26
Colleagues	28	13	7
Medical meetings	8	4	2
Other	3[c]	16	9
Number of doctors answering	87	328	1,011

[a]Some doctors named more than one source. Percentages have been adjusted to 100 percent.

[b]Including professional journals (21 percent) and periodicals published by drug companies (21 percent).

[c]2 percent composed of advertisements in medical journals.

Sources: J.S. Coleman, E. Katz, and H. Menzel, *Medical Innovation: A Diffusion Study* (Indianapolis: Bobbs-Merrill, 1966), p. 59. R. Ferber and H.G. Wales, "The Effectiveness of pharmaceutical promotion," *University of Illinois Bureau of Economics and Business Research Bulletin 83* (Urbana, 1958), p. 24. *Attitudes of U.S. Physicians toward the American Pharmaceutical Industry* (Chicago, Ben Gaffin and Associates, 1959), p. 21, C-13.

In his defense, it should be pointed out that the tremendous advances in medical technology have made it a truly Herculean task for the harried and overworked physician to learn all he should know about the flood of new techniques and drugs inundating him. The recent wave of "mood" drugs is just part of this deluge of new treatment modalities, and the average doctor is more than glad to accept any drug and prescribing information, even if it originates from the manufacturer. The question is the accuracy and reliability of such information—and the answer is not reassuring. The pharmaceutical industry is concerned with profits first, and its drug information is designed primarily to convince doctors to prescribe brand-name drugs, many of which are significantly more expensive than their generic-name counterparts. Pierre Garai, an advertising man, admitted in 1964 that:

approximately three-quarters of a billion dollars is spent every year by some sixty drug companies in order to reach, persuade, cajole, pamper, outwit and *sell* one of America's smallest markets—the 180,000 physicians . . . And it is not too much to say that perhaps no other group in the country is so insistently sought after, chased, wooed, pressured, and downright importuned as this small group of doctors who are the *de facto* wholesalers of the ethical [i.e., prescription] drug business . . . Why all this drum-beating? The answer is quite simple. One, the drug companies cannot compete effectively without it. Two, it works . . . Effecive promotion, heavy promotion, sustained promotion has carried the day. The physicians have been sold. So has the country.[3]

According to the former Food and Drug Commissioner, J. L. Goddard, the drug industry spent $750,000,000 for advertising and promotion in 1966, at least $3,000 for every physician in the United States. As long ago as 1958, the twenty-two largest drug companies alone spent more than $580,000,000 on promotion; this was 24 percent of their gross receipts from sales of drugs, compared with 6 percent for research and development. Whether corporate profits are measured in terms of percentage of total sales, percentage of invested capital, or percentage of stockholders' equity, in the decade between 1956 and 1966 the drug industry consistently ranked highest among manufacturing industries.[4]

According to a study published in *Advertising Age* in 1963, "the average doctor today is exposed to more than four times the number of medical journal advertisements he was exposed to 10 years ago." As early in the drug explosion as 1958, the director of advertising and promotion for Detroit-based Parke, Davis estimated in a speech to the American College of Apothecaries that the prescription drug industry has turned out 3,790,908,000 pages of paid journal advertising (the equivalent of four million Bibles, or 158,000 complete sets of the *Encyclopedia Britannica*). *Advertising Age* also reports organized medicine's vested interest in the economic well-being of the pharmaceutical industry: "In the case of the American Medical Association, more than half of its total revenue is derived from the pharmaceutical advertising placed in its various publications. *The Journal of the American Medical Association* now carries nearly 6,000 advertising pages a year, a volume exceeded by only one other weekly periodical in the country, *Oil and Gas Journal.*"[5]

The AMA has asserted that it is the largest publisher of prescription drug advertisements in the world. The amount it receives from advertising has increased tremendously since the first rumblings of the psychoactive drug explosion in the early 1950s. Up to 1950 the AMA's total revenue from advertising was around $2,500,000 per annum. During this period the organization was still a champion of the people: around the turn of the century it had vigorously battled the home-remedy nostrum swindle; it was instrumental in establishing food and drug legislation designed to protect the consumer in 1906 and again in the 1930s. But by 1955 its drug advertising income had increased to over $4,000,000[6] and its policies had changed. It had dropped its influential Seal of Acceptance drug evaluation program (there was no point in needlessly antagonizing its primary source of income) and had stopped publishing three books which had been of great assistance to physicians who needed sound, unbiased medical information on drugs: *Useful Drugs, The Epitome of the U.S.P. and National Formulary,* and *Glandular Physiology and Therapy.* It had also stopped requiring that drugs be advertised in its publications by generic names only, and it had ceased supplying medical students with the drug handbook *New and Nonofficial Remedies.* In 1957 the publication of this annual volume was discontinued; its replacement, *New and Nonofficial Drugs,* was killed in 1964, the same year that the AMA-USP Committee on Nomenclature met the fate dealt out in 1956 to the AMA Council on Pharmacy and Chemistry.

A recent chairman of the AMA Council on Drugs (the impotent substitute for the once zealous and effective Council on Pharmacy and Chemistry) admitted:

Regulation seldom if ever succeeds by persuasion alone; some kind of club is needed. In the case of drugs the Seal of Acceptance was that club. It had helped to keep the big companies in line, while the smaller companies scrambled to be in the ranks with them. The club was not big enough, but it could have been made larger. The club was there if the AMA wanted to swing it.

Finally, a program of regulation takes cash and lots of it, and the lack of cash may be the real rock on which the seal program foundered. In 1955 the AMA had just come through the searing experience of being prosecuted for a criminal violation of the antitrust laws, and had been convicted. The fine it had to pay was trivial, but the costs of the legal battle had not been. Moreover, the AMA was mounting a costly campaign to prevent government payment for medical care. And the accusation by the government that the AMA was restraining trade might well be echoed by some drug company whose products were not approved by the AMA, and this would cost more money! Added to this was the glimpse of that hoard of gold representing potential advertising from which the AMA was barred by the seal program. What could be simpler than to cut the Gordian knot, abolish the seal program, and with one bold stroke cure all these financial ills?

Whatever the real reasons for the abandonment of the seal program, it is apparent that the zeal that had in the past generated consecration, crusading, and consistent pressure was gone, that the cash draw was low and might get lower. And so the club was thrown away.[7]

By 1956 the AMA had almost abandoned its program of grants for therapeutic research and had begun to cut the budget of its increasingly ineffective Council on Drugs, although appropriations for its Department of Public Relations had begun to rise steeply. Moreover, it had begun to oppose much-needed legislation in a covert alliance with the drug companies. The reason for the AMA's turnabout was financial: its revenue from drug advertising continued to rise spectacularly. By 1957 its income from the drug industry exceeded dues and subscription revenue. In 1960 it received $8 million from drug advertising and almost another $2 million for releasing its mailing lists to drug companies. By 1963 AMA advertising income exceeded $10 million. In 1966 it approached $13.3 million. In 1971 the organization is believed to have grossed over $15 million from advertising. This income is, incidentally, free from taxation on the grounds that it is substantially related to the AMA's professed purpose of promoting the "art and science of medicine and the betterment of public health."[8]

A profitable accommodation for the drug industry, the AMA's membership list is leased directly to drug manufacturers for use in mailing advertising materials to doctors through AMA-franchised mailing-list houses. The volume of such advertising is as imposing as that of medical journal advertising, and mailings are often elaborate and sophisticated folders, booklets, and brochures. An editorial in the *New England Journal of Medicine* in August 1963 noted that in the year beginning May 1, 1962, one not atypical general practitioner received 3,636 separate mailings of advertisements and free samples of 604 different drugs. According to another source, the physician receives more than 4,000 pieces of pharmaceutical literature annually.[9] Like journal advertising, direct mailings are increasing every year. According to the calculations of one physician as long ago as 1959, American doctors received nearly 80 *tons* of direct mail drug advertising *per day*: "It would take two railroad mail cars, 110 large mailtrucks, and 800 postmen to deliver the daily load of drug circulars and samples to doctors if mailed to one single city. Then after being delivered, it would take over 25 trash trucks to haul it away, to be burned on a dump pile whose blaze would be seen for 50 miles around."[10]

Drug advertising can be misleading, inaccurate, or downright false. Students in a pharmacology course at the Albany Medical College studied drug advertisements, met with detail men and sometimes pharmaceutical company executives, wrote letters to the companies, and checked the claims made in advertisements by studying the articles cited in them. At the end of the course, 74 percent of the students thought the drug manufacturer had exaggerated the value of the drug 80 to 100 percent of the time, and 70 percent thought the advertisements misleadingly minimized undesirable "side effects" at least 80 percent of the time.[11]

We hear frequent complaints about the drug advertisements' "Madison Avenue" slickness and hard-sell techniques—as any layman who glances through a medical journal while waiting in a doctor's office will understand. Their often offensive tone and poor taste are only minor matters. The catchy names and slogans, three-dimensional cartoon and human figures, and inane messages spouting reassuring blather in technicolor on almost every other page of many medical journals are an insult to intelligence and sensibility. Yet the American people, overexposed to similar examples of hard sell by detergent, automobile, and other advertisements, are relatively immune if not completely cynical when confronted by this kind of attempted intellectual rape. The real objection to such drug advertising is its underlying assumptions about human existence and human dignity. Consider the following "case" from a medical journal:

POOR YARDLEY—"This suburban living isn't all it's cracked up to be," he moans, "Just one headache after another, especially with my lawn. Insects and weeds everywhere . . . the neighbors' kids trampling down my grass . . . dogs and cats ruining my shrubs . . . and those pesky beetles chewing away on my prize begonias. . . . All this plus commuting forty miles a day, soaring taxes and trouble with my car. . . . To make matters worse my stomach bothers me a lot. It aches and rumbles so much I don't enjoy my meals like I used to. Could it be nervous indigestion?"

On the opposite page, "Yardley Crabgrass" is depicted as a cowering catatonic schizophrenic besieged by giant insects, howling monsters, and motorized demons. But, the reader is informed in a conversational (and condescending) tone, he can be saved by modern medicine. His gastric distress is:

. . . functional, no doubt nurtured by his constant concern over his grass and flowers. You solve one of his most gnawing problems by giving him your secret formula for wiping out Japanese beetles. You also suggest a pair of stereo earphones to silence those English Beatles. Then you write him a prescription for Donnazyme. It provides belladonna alkaloids to quiet his gut, phenobarbital to calm his nerves, plus digestive enzymes and bile salts to supplement a possible deficiency and thereby aid his digestion.

He's a "natural" for DONNAZYME antispasmodic/sedative/digestant. Each tablet contains . . . [12]

The basic philosophical premise of such advertisements seems to be that human life itself is a drug-deficiency disease. An editorial in the *New England Journal of Medicine* expressed long-overdue outrage:

physicians are encouraged to use these [psychotropic] drugs as "treatment of choice" for what are problems of everyday living —not traditional mental illnesses. We see pictures and captions of women distressed by washing dishes or giving a child a bath, of athletes who must be quickly returned to the game, of men who are irritated by environment noise, etc.—conditions hardly psychiatric diseases. Other advertisements are directed to resonate with and to reinforce male prejudices—i.e., chronic, always female, complainers who upset the physicians' office routine as well as husbands' sleep. In the pages of this very *Journal*, we have seen advertisements urging physicians to use a tranquilizing agent "for the anxiety that comes from not fitting in"—for "the newcomer to town who *can't* make friends. The organization man who *can't* adjust to all the status within his company. The woman who *can't* get along with her new daughter-in-law. The executive who *can't* accept retirement! . . ."

Rather than circumscribing and limiting usage, the editorial continues:

drug companies seem intent on widening indications [for drug use] into areas of human experience that might call for social action and psychologic insight as well as the time-honored virtues of endurance, patience, and mastery. Surely, we are not ready to accept passively the chemical solution to all problems as the ads would have us do. Psychoactive drugs are not innocent even when not toxic. Their use, in addition to creating a dependence or worse, tends to undermine confidence in personal mastery. Rather than adjunctive, they are frequently antithetical to psychotherapy since the temporary euphoria and feeling of well-being that they give may discourage the work of personal exploration and problem solving. Similarly, on a broader scale, the use of drugs may serve to vitiate the engagement and action that are currently so urgently needed to deal with our pressing social and worldly concerns.[13]

Despite the strong opposition of the AMA, a federal law passed in 1963 now requires that all contraindications of drug use, together with drug "side effects," be published in every advertisement in "brief summary" form. As applied to drugs, the quasi-medical term "side effects" is a euphemism invented by advertising agency copywriters: " 'Side-effects' is a fashionable expression, consoling in its implication of something relatively unimportant . . . What are side-effects? This expression . . . was not used until about ten years ago . . . the suggestion is that, by a heaven-sent providence, the main effects of drugs are all therapeutically desirable and the side-effects are unwanted but happily (being only side-effects, after all) irregular in appearance and relatively insignificant."[14] The term "side effects" avoids acknowledging the fact that toxic or adverse effects may be as powerful as the "therapeutic" ones. Often the boundary between toxic ("side") effects and the action for which the drug is used is vague. In the case of amphetamines, effects originally considered undesirable came to be advertised as "therapeutic."

Drug advertising copywriters display a good deal of creativity in inventing evasive literary techniques to satisfy the legal requirements which require warnings of "side effects" while allaying the suspicions of physicians. "The 'side-effect' flimflam currently used in some drug advertisements to befuddle doctors can be summarized briefly: 1. Start with a disclaimer of innocence. 2. Put the inconsequential side effects first to set a mild tone. 3. Vigorously point out any lack of proof-positive, even if all indications point to the drug's involvement. 4. Remember that all reactions are 'rare.' 5. Bury the worst side effects any way possible, especially by jamming them into a parenthetical phrase. 6. Utilize obfuscation and sophism to increase confusion. 7. Keep the paragraph as a whole from sounding the way it should sound—like unadulterated *danger*."[15] Another critic has noted the way the warning section of a drug advertisement can be effectively hidden or buried:

Many a three-page display provides an example with which we are all familiar. Striking scenes, agonized faces—including, in observance of current fashion, a sprinkling of those that are black—and succinct captions rivet the eye on the center spread where a drug is extolled by its catchy and most pronounceable trade name. If you bother to turn the page, you will find, in due conformity with the law, a mass of information, including a long list of precautions, contraindications, and toxicities, all in such congested fine print as to discourage reading, and often enough with the untoward effects listed under a drug now identified by its jaw-breaking generic name.[16]

Some of these minor masterpieces read less like warnings than reasons for prescribing! One of the oldest and most reputable pharmaceutical companies for an amphetamine-barbiturate combination warns that "excessive use of the amphetamines by unstable individuals may result in psychological dependence . . ."[17] This misleading disclaimer lulls the physician into a false sense of security. Most doctors who prescribe amphetamines and other psychotropic drugs are not psychiatrists. They have little or no basis for determining whether or not a patient, whom they may see only once for a very brief time in an office setting, is likely to abuse a drug. Perhaps the favorite advertising ploy is the use of words like "rare" or "isolated cases" "In isolated cases some rare side effects of a reversible nature have occasionally been reported." It should also be pointed out that although new drugs may be heralded as being "relatively" (or "almost completely") free of any "side effects," serious and life-threatening adverse effects often do not necessarily become apparent in the short period of clinical testing before clearance of a new drug by the Food and Drug Administration; often it takes years for the evidence to accumulate gradually. One physician has pointed out that:

> one should not make definite claims in the first six months or even year of working with the drug because many of the side effects, sometimes the most dangerous complications and side effects of drugs, appear only after the drug has been in use for a year or more. So to make the statement that a drug is not addiction forming or doesn't produce any dangerous side effects within the first year is really quite preposterous and rather meaningless for anyone who knows the field. For a physician who is not a specialist in the field, it may be simply misleading.[18]

Printed advertisements are subject to at least some restrictions, but no one has any way of controlling the tongue of the detail man once he gets inside the doctor's door. The AMA-sponsored Gaffin study found that 48 percent of the physicians polled reported that the detail man was their earliest source of information about a drug which they subsequently prescribed, and 67 percent considered him their most important source of drug information.[19] These pharmaceutical traveling salesmen usually do not sell directly to the doctor, although they may dispense free samples. Their role is unique in American industry, since the "buyer" rarely uses the product and is not much concerned about the price. Their primary job is to establish a close and friendly personal relationship with the physician and give him "information" about new drugs. Some companies have formal training programs for their detail men; others simply have a sales manager spend a few weeks with the new recruit. Although the pharmaceutical companies try to attract knowledgeable people for this kind of work—graduate pharmacists and sometimes medical students on vacation—given the estimate that there are "somewhere between 20,000 and 50,000" detail men,[20] it is likely that many have had no formal training in medicine or pharmacology.

A pharmaceutical executive has described the detail man's role this way: "You see, we believe in the preeminent importance of detailing. We believe that our trained, highly professional sales representative is the most capable medium we have of persuading the physician to prescribe our products and the pharmacist to stock them . . . Being experts in professional relations, they instinctively act so as to please the physician."[21] They are so eager to please that, according to one veteran detailer, they avoid being messengers of bad news: "The detail man is told exactly what he can speak about, and he's not expected to be expert in how to use the product. Under the old laws, promotional literature did not necessarily contain mention of side effects. They do today, but detail men don't go out of their way to bring it up. Dealing with the doctor is not easy. Status and ego is his whole way of life. He doesn't like to admit that he's ignorant about anything. He wants to pick up the information about the new drug from us but he doesn't want to show that he needs it."[22]

The pharmaceutical industry tries to reach the physician through the patient as well as through direct advertising and promotion. According to one physician, formerly on the medical staff of Pfizer Laboratories:

> It is an unfunny joke in the medical profession that the very latest information on new advances in medicine most often appears in the eminent medical journals such as *Reader's Digest, Time,* and *The Wall Street Journal.* Some of this is legitimate good reporting. However, much of what appears has in essence been placed by the publications relations staffs of the pharmaceutical firms. A steady stream of magazine and newspaper articles are prepared for distribution to the lay press. These may take the form of so-called informative or background articles on conditions such as allergies or edema. Buried within the article, there is often a brief paragraph mentioning that a great drug has been discovered and manufactured by company X, and the name of the drug is given. The article does not say that the reader should rush to his physician and de-

mand the drug, but the implication is usually clear. And, of course, there is nothing to show where the article originated.[23]

The Doctor's Role

Although doctors occasionally find articles on new drugs in the popular media helpful, they rarely find the few examples of excellent medical reporting representative. They deplore the inaccuracies, omission of qualifications, promotion of renamed or slightly altered old drugs as new, and sensationalism in mass media drug articles. They are also disturbed by premature publicity, which may involve the release of drug news to the public before it has been communicated to the medical community. In some cases new drugs have received wide publicity even before they have been approved by the FDA for general medical use.[24]

Physicians are becoming increasingly aware that much drug advertising is misleading and stultifying. Unfortunately, most have discovered that the American public has been trained to expect only good from drugs, especially new drugs, and many doctors either capitalize on this situation or fail to resist its pressures. They are particularly apt to prescribe psychoactive drugs even when no definite indications for *any* drug treatment exist, and sometimes even when such therapy is contraindicated. It is discouragingly clear that many physicians prescribe psychoactive drugs without making any attempt to achieve an adequate diagnosis and without taking even minimal testing or precautionary measures. Their reasons range from indolence to the desire to give a patient who appears to be suffering from no organic disorder some tangible indication that the doctor cares. A common example is the case of the housewife who seeks medical help because she is "feeling down," sleeps a lot, and lacks energy. Rather than attempting to determine the basis for what is usually a mild depression and recommending or attempting psychotherapy (even very brief and supportive), her doctor may find it easier to prescribe a drug like Dexedrine. He knows that an amphetamine will probably make the patient feel better almost immediately and that therefore she will think she has gotten her money's worth from him.

Since the early 1950s the medical profession's eager, often unprofessional, acceptance has legitimized psychoactive drug use to the point where anyone who actually refuses to take such drugs is considered an anomaly if not a deviant. Yet most people who regularly or periodically take psychoactive drugs are not suffering from any organic or serious functional disability or illness. The medical use of these drugs is more often justified by the patient's feelings of dis-ease than by the existence of any recognized disease process. Social and cultural stresses are the important factors initiating drug use, and often there is no real distinction between the so-called "medical use" of psychoactive drugs and behavior that is generally recognized as drug misuse or abuse. There is really not much difference between the hippie or the Hell's Angel popping a handful of Dexedrine pills and the housewife or businessman who "just doesn't feel right" without the same drugs. The hippie may honestly admit that he is taking the drug to get high or to feel good, while the housewife or businessman is likely to pretend that he or she takes the drug only because it has been prescribed. The doctor is not only an "expert" on drugs but a figure in whom people place great trust. In a recent public survey physicians were rated highest among twenty major occupations for truthfulness, competence, and altruism (clergymen were second).[25] The physician in our culture plays the role of informal sanctioning agent; "doctor's orders" effectively relieve many people of doubt, misgivings, or guilt in connection with their habitual self-medication.

Drug Education

Since drug misinformation is common among the public as well as among physicians who have been "educated" by the pharmaceutical companies, drug education programs are often promoted as a solution to the problem of abuse. No doubt the honest presentation of information about the relative potential of various drugs for good and harm is important, but there are many reasons to doubt the usefulness of drug education in preventing abuse. In the first place, people who associate their use of drugs with opposition to the established social order are likely to resent and mistrust campaigns directed against the drugs by the institutions of that social order, even if they are ostensibly "educational" rather than punitive. They suspect that anything the government and the schools are so insistent about preventing must be especially threatening to the powers that be. "Scare" publicity, even intelligent "scare" publicity, often only increases the attractiveness of the forbidden. And there has been so much misinformation propagated in the guise of "drug education," especially about marihuana, that many young people are as skeptical about warnings against drug use as they are about commercial advertising. They have been told too many things that they know from their own experience to be false. So the natural rebelliousness of the young hardens into a conviction that what "official" authorities say about drugs is either deliberately deceptive or simply inane, and in either case is an insult to their intelligence.

Surveys of high school students' opinions reveal that, whatever the "facts" about a drug, the older a student is, the less likely he is to consider it dangerous and the more likely he is to disagree about it with his parents, the school, and the law. For example, in a study on student drug use in the Boston suburb of Brookline, 25 percent of the high school students, 47 percent of the elementary school (grades 6 through 8) students, and 63 percent of their parents thought that "any person who uses drugs for nonmedical purposes probably has serious psychological problems." (Alcohol and nicotine were apparently not counted as "drugs.") Thirty-nine percent of the parents and 37 percent of elementary students but only 5 percent of high school students considered smoking cannabis often to be "very dangerous." Occasional use of amphetamines was considered "very dangerous" by 59 percent of the parents, 48 percent of the elementary students, and 32 percent of the high school students. The older students may be underestimating the dangers of amphetamines, just as their parents and the younger children overestimate the dangers of marihuana; in both cases, the social attitudes of an age group rather than some "objective" or "unbiased" knowledge seem to be critical in shaping opinion.

Most of the students had taken a "drug education" course, but accurate knowledge of the properties of various drugs was limited mainly to those who actually used them. Only 6 percent of nonusers but 44 percent of multiple users correctly answered ten of sixteen true-false questions. Fifty-one percent of the nonusers thought cannabis was "physically addicting," while only 17 percent of those who had smoked it held this erroneous opinion.[26] It is hardly surprising, except in the context of the myth of "seduction of the innocent" and "pushers" preying on ignorant adolescents (another idea young people no doubt consider an insult to their intelligence), that the people who actually use a drug are the ones who have taken the trouble to learn something about it. Af-

ter all, it matters more to them. This situation suggests that informal education about drugs by fellow-users is more reliable or
at least more effective than formal school and government programs. It also suggests that knowledge of the psychopharm-
macological properties of drugs may be the opposite of a deterrent
to their use.

Drug information rarely has the properties of being officially
propagated, honest, accurate, and believed by the public it is
addressed to all at once. But even when it does, its usefulness in
preventing abuse is doubtful. The main case in point is the Report of the Surgeon General's Advisory Committee on Smoking
and Health of January 11, 1964. Within a few days of its publication, many people gave up or cut down on cigarette smoking.
The number of taxed packages soon fell 15 to 20 percent, and it is
believed that this represented a 25 to 30 percent decline in the
number of smokers. But this "Great Forswearing" of January
and February 1964 was followed by the "Great Relapse" of
March 1964, and soon almost as many people were smoking
cigarettes as before the publication of the report.[27] It is not that
the report and the sustained educational campaigns of such organizations as the American Cancer Society did not succeed in
instructing people about the dangers of smoking. A 1966 United
States Public Health Service Survey, for example, found that 71.3
percent of male smokers agreed that smoking is dangerous to
health, 55.2 percent believed that cigarette smoking is a cause of
lung cancer, and 33.4 percent believed it to be a cause of coronary
heart disease. The percentages for women were slightly higher. It
appears that awareness of the dangers is not enough, at least in
the case of a drug which has such a high potential for producing
dependence as tobacco or amphetamine. Many teenagers are well
educated about the dangers of tobacco, but think they will smoke
just for a short time, not realizing how hard it is to stop. Similarly, young people may decide to use amphetamines just to get
through examinations, and then find that giving them up is a
problem.

Prohibition

Where education is inadequate, prohibition sometimes seems a
solution. It could be argued that there should be a total ban on
the production of amphetamines, since they have a formidable

potential for abuse and increasingly limited therapeutic use-fulness. There are, however, several deterrents to this approach. First, while the present justifiable use of amphetamine as a medicine is quite circumscribed—and we believe will become more so in the future—there remain some legitimate therapeutic uses, and such a ban would impose a hardship in these cases. What is more, while we see the prescription of these drugs for the treatment of obesity and the symptoms of mild depression as medically unsound, many physicians, particularly overburdened general practitioners, would vigorously defend not only their right to prescribe amphetamines and to be the final arbiter of what is good or bad for their patients, but also the medical soundness of these practices.

The history of punitive-repressive measures to discourage the use of psychoactive drugs does not support those who think the best way to deal with the "drug problem" is through draconian legislation. The spread of tobacco during the sixteenth and seventeenth centuries was the most dramatic "epidemic" of drug use in recorded history. The "foule weed" was adopted by cultures so varied that cultural and social determinants must have played little part in its spread. Prohibitive laws failed, whether they were justified on grounds of health, religion, good taste, or the danger of criminal acts.

Repressive measures may actually do more harm to the individual and society than the original "evil," by causing drug abusers to resort to more dangerous substances. Opium smoking is on the decline around the world, but in parts of Asia where it has been outlawed, heroin has become the far more dangerous substitute. In India the government has been implementing laws to control cultivation and distribution of cannabis, but has not banned it entirely; a slow reduction in use has been reported, but it has been accompanied by a rise in the use of alcohol. At the end of the nineteenth century Ireland tried to suppress the use of hard liquor through temperance campaigns and strict enforcement of the tax laws. The Irish reduced their intake of alcohol and switched to ethyl ether, which provided a short-lived intoxication involving a "hot all the way down" sensation, followed by thunderous flatus, and, within ten minutes, a "high," which could be repeated without a hangover. In one area of Ulster an eighth of the population was labeled "etheromaniacs." Alarm over the ether "epidemic" became so great that the groups which had promoted the campaign changed their policy, and the Irish returned to the use of whiskey.[28]

A total ban on the production of amphetamines probably would not be effective anyway. Rather, it would greatly increase the production and smuggling of illicit amphetamine and so increase the risks of use, particularly where intravenous preparations are concerned, because of the greater likelihood of contamination with toxic impurities, viruses, and bacteria. Presently, amphetamines are not very difficult to obtain, legally or illegally. With a ban on legal production the supply would be scarcer and the price higher. If this happens, is there not more likelihood that organized crime will become involved in its distribution? The main reasons why so much crime, mostly against property, is associated with heroin use are that heroin is addictive, its use is illegal, it is expensive (on the streets), and distribution is controlled by organized crime. While amphetamines have a formidable potential for addiction, their use is not illegal, and they are not particularly difficult to obtain and are therefore relatively inexpensive. Consequently, organized crime is not as interested in them as it would be if there were a total prohibition on their use and manufacture. With the imposition of such a ban amphetamine would probably approach heroin in its potential to produce crime. In fact, given the capacity of high doses of amphetamine to produce violent assaultiveness and paranoia, there might be more to fear from a prohibition of amphetamines than there is with heroin.

Some believe the way around the problem of "kitchen" amphetamine is to ban the major chemical precursors of amphetamine as well as the drug itself. This would be impossible. As W. E. Doering puts it:

> Attempts to control amphetamines by banning their manufacture in the chemical industry might lead to an increase in their price, but not in their availability to sufficiently motivated persons. These are among the simpler organic molecules the synthesis of which present no difficulties which could not be overcome by determined graduates of the first college course in organic chemistry.

Several different types of synthesis can be used and many of these start with materials so commonly available and so indispensible to a wide variety of legitimate purposes that their removal from the market would not be practical or thinkable.

The amphetamines in general, and certainly methamphetamine in particular, are ideally suited to garage manufacture through the simplicity of their structures and the variety of readily available materials from which they can be made. Forced underground, these chemicals would be synthesized easily, perhaps at the increased price normally associated with illegal activities and with less concern for the quality of the product.[29]

If all amphetamine production in the United States were eliminated, it would be smuggled across the borders. Recently the Government Accounting Office stated in a report to Congress that trying to intercept the ten to twelve tons of heroin entering the country every year was like trying to find the needle in the haystack. The GAO estimated that only 6 1/2 percent of the total contraband was seized in 1971.[30] There is no reason to suppose that customs officials would be any more successful in interdicting amphetamines.

Treatment

If education is insufficient and prohibition usually fails, what are the possibilities for treatment and "rehabilitation" of amphetamine abusers? Bejerot, exploring new approaches to the Swedish amphetamine problem, has suggested "treatment villages" on islands or in "depopulated" rural areas for chronic users who regularly relapse into intravenous abuse. "The most important condition is that they are cut off geographically and thereby receive the relative isolation which the therapeutic villages need." He recommended that "all forms of medication should be avoided in the villages," including alcohol. But, although he has been one of the strongest opponents of amphetamine "maintenance," he admits that it might be necessary to establish separate "speed colonies":

If careful studies proved objectively that certain chronic amphetaminists really functioned better socially on a fixed dose of central stimulants, perhaps they should receive daily doses of repository type (durette-coated) slowly absorbed methamphetamine granules suspended in juice, on the same indications. From theoretical, physiological, pharmacological, and psychiatric angles, however, the treatment problem appears extremely dubious as *central stimulants are not normalizing but intoxicating.* This question should -be the subject of penetrating pharmacological and psychiatric research before this proposal is accredited much practical value.

"The proposal," Bejerot writes:

is perhaps controversial both medically and politically and may be so for quite different reasons among addicts; but it is a serious proposal on my part. If the drug dependence is as fundamental as the chronic user declares and the clinical picture shows, the patient himself must surely be grateful to be allowed to live in peace with his addiction in a pleasant and protected place. Healthy friends and relatives should, of course, be allowed to live there too and possibly receive remuneration for attendance on the sick. Even if such a drug colony would be an expensive affair for society the price would be low compared with all other possible solutions. The value of eliminating the risk to society of a number of chronic infectious foci is very great, and the arrangement is probably inevitable if we are to break the evil circle without filling prisons and mental hospitals with chronically sick and therapy-resistant cases. The measures are, however, almost worthless if they are not taken as part of a wider attack on a broad front againt the whole epidemic.

Before we scoff at Bejerot's notion as misguided and unfeasible, or label it a reactionary idea that would violate the civil rights of addicts, we might consider that in fact we already have "drug colonies," where medically sound or rational drug use is notably absent and living conditions unbearably degrading. Indeed, Bejerot's suggestion might have been derived from the recognition that "drug colonies" like those in Haight-Ashbury or parts of Manhattan already exist. How can the American addict break away from the subculture that may reinforce his drug-taking almost as much as the drug's pharmacological properties and psychophysiological effects? Under Bejerot's system, "for the chronic patient who wishes to try to return to the ordinary society again assistance would of course always be available. The drug-free villages could act as intermediary stations." Bejerot asks us to think about the "logical alternatives" to his suggestion:

"these are (a) to hold these highly contagious chronics responsible under the Dangerous Drugs Act and let the penal services take care of them; (b) to provide long-term treatment on closed wards in mental hospitals; (c) to provide them with a license to use dangerous drugs on their own and be content to study how many new victims they drag along into addiction; and (d) to close our eyes to the problem and pretend it does not exist."

"The last alternative is the easiest," he points out, as well as:

the one that has generally been practised. The defeat of the rapidly expanding intravenous abuse of central stimulants in Sweden is now mainly a political and moral problem. If mass spread of this serious form of addiction is recognized as an illness of epidemic type, the scientific solution is as clear as can reasonably be expected with the methods of actions and treatment as yet known. Most of those who describe regular epidemic control programs in this field as "reactionary" know very well that a situation of this type would never be permitted to arise in Eastern Europe or China. Is a society more progressive and humane the more down-and-out addicts it is prepared to tolerate?[31]

Bejerot's question is intended to be rhetorical, but actually it has no easy answer. The restrictions on civil liberties implied by a program like his or the parallel proposals for "civil commitment" of narcotics addicts and alcoholics in the United States are obvious. To treat drug dependence as an "epidemic disease" could create even worse injustices than treating it as a crime. The use of a drug spreads voluntarily or semivoluntarily, by speech and example, not through exposure to a virus or bacteria as with an infectious disease. If it is an unwarranted restriction on liberty to force someone to take treatment "for his own good," it is also wrong forcibly to prevent what is in effect a process of persuasion by locking up the potential persuaders.

The same problem of a contradiction between the dictates of humanity and freedom arises with prohibition. We have emphasized the failures of repressive legislation, but there have been some notable "successes" as well. Opium smoking has been all but eliminated in China by the Communist regime. Elimination resulted, however, not only from threats of punishment but also from a revolutionary change in social values and behavior patterns. Restrictions imposed by the Soviet Union have made the abuse of amphetamines impossible. Of course, the successful prohibition is associated with an omnipresent police state and a severe restriction of free choice for most people. Alcoholism remains an enormous problem in the Soviet Union. There has been no change in cultural patterns great enough to make possible the reduction of alcohol consumption by prohibition without the creation of a serious disruption of the social order.

However, elimination or reduction of the use of a psychoactive drug need not require revolutionary change or a police state or both. In 1955-1956 Japanese restrictions on amphetamines cut down greatly the abuse of the drug. Another example is America's prohibition of alcohol from 1918 to 1933, often cited as an example of the failure of repressive legislation. Everyone knows about the deaths from wood alcohol, the overburdening of the criminal justice system, and the efflorescence of organized crime. What is not so well known is that Prohibition drastically reduced the total consumption of alcohol, and with it much alcoholism and its attendant horrors as well as the incidence of a serious disease like cirrhosis of the liver. The social costs and benefits of our present narcotics prohibition are comparable in some ways: there is no doubt that consumption of opiates in the United States is much lower than it was at the turn of the century. Since the opiates are less toxic, potentially debilitating, and socially disruptive than alcohol, the argument in favor of prohibition and criminalization of them is actually less convincing. In any case, the point is that prohibition *can* reduce the consumption of a dangerous or addictive drug: the question is what price society is willing to pay.

In the United States, as in most nations today, we have decided, in effect, that we are willing to tolerate the sometimes horrifying physiological and social consequences of alcoholism for the sake of the enjoyment most of us derive from a few drinks. Of course there is more to it than that: the use of alcohol is traditional and widespread; it is deeply embedded in our cultural patterns, playing important symbolic roles. The use of opiates in the West has much shallower cultural roots, so prohibition, in spite of its social costs, does not arouse the kind of public outrage produced by the Volstead Act. Asian countries trying to stamp out the use of opium are engaged in a symbolic "Westernization," a repudiation of the old ways. It is unclear to what extent "rational" calculation of benefits and dangers goes into these considerations about prohibition of drug use, or even what rationality means in this context, since what a society regards as reasonable is unavoidably (and not irrationally) inseparable from its traditions and self-image.

Although prohibition sometimes works and forced treatment can mitigate some of the damage produced by drug dependence, a price is paid in the loss of freedom or relatively harmless pleasures. There is simply no easy answer to the question of what a free society can do about a drug that is obviously attractive and obviously dangerous. One recourse is what E. M. Brecher has called "domestication."[32] Caffeine is a stimulant drug that has some of the same psychopharmacological properties and some of the same dangers as amphetamines, although it is much milder. It is taken daily by millions of Americans in the form of coffee and tea and even given to children in soft drinks, apparently without doing much physiological damage (though this has been denied) and certainly without destroying the users' lives and disrupting society. It arouses little hostility among the public and no legal repression. It is taken in small doses, usually with meals, and, like the less successfully domesticated alcohol and tobacco, is not regarded by most people as a "drug" at all. Other drugs are adaptable to this pattern: for example, the use of alcohol in Italian and Jewish communities, and possibly the chewing of the coca leaf (cocaine) among the Andean Indians or opium-smoking in the western United States at the end of the nineteenth century.

It might be best if this compromise solution could be adopted for all drugs. Unfortunately, domestication cannot be instituted by decree. Certain properties of the drugs themselves and their manufacture are relevant: caffeine usually produces too many immediately unpleasant effects when taken at dangerous dosages to be a temptation; alcohol was not so great a problem when it was not available in great quantities or in the concentrated form of distilled liquor. Besides, history and cultural tradition determine whether a drug can be "tamed" by a society as much as they determine whether it can be effectively prohibited.

To what extent is it possible or desirable for amphetamines to be domesticated in the United States, either in the guise of a stimulant frankly taken for pleasure or in the guise of medicine? It is

...le. Amphetamines do not seem to have the pro-
...ant" effects of caffeine (which no one, for ex-
...ntravenously for pleasure) and have not been in-
...domestic ritual in the same way. However, abuse
of amp... e does not have cultural roots as deep as abuse of
alcohol, simply because this drug is relatively new. But certain
features of our society make amphetamines particularly attractive
and particularly difficult to use with moderation.

Mirror-Image

There is a curious mirror-image relation between cannabis and
amphetamines. Marihuana is not addicting, and there are no
serious sequellae upon cessation of chronic use; the amphetamines have a withdrawal syndrome which often includes severe
depression. Cannabis does not damage tissue; amphetamines
may. There are no well-documented cases of death from marihuana; speed can kill. Marihuana is not criminogenic and being
high on it probably diminishes the likelihood of violent or criminal acts; just the opposite is the case with amphetamines.
Cannabis in very large (usually ingested) doses can produce
toxic psychoses and in smaller smoked doses may in rare instances precipitate functional psychoses in people who are already
vulnerable, that is, people in whom psychosis might be precipitated by such events as an alcoholic debauch, an automobile
accident, a surgical procedure, or a death in the family. It has
been demonstrated that a psychosis which is all but indistinguishable from a schizophrenic reaction can be induced with
amphetamine in "normal" subjects in the laboratory, and
paranoia is common among speed freaks on the street. Amphetamine leads to the use of other psychoactive drugs; cannabis does
not. The risks involved in using marihuana (excluding those
which derive from its legal status) are of a different order of
magnitude from those which arise from the psychopharmacological properties of amphetamines. In fact, the dangers mythical-
ly attributed to use of cannabis are more appropriately associated
with amphetamines. Yet there has been an enormous concern
and near hysterical outcry over the use of marihuana, while public, governmental, and medical attitudes toward the use of amphetamines have ranged from enthusiasm to complacency; only
recently has there been some degree of concern.

To gain some understanding of how attitudes toward these two classes of psychoactive agents became so divergent and so incongruent with their actual relative potentials for harm, we must review some aspects of the drugs' social histories. Cannabis has a long history as a medicinal agent; its first recorded use is to be found in the Chinese *Herbal*, an ancient pharmacopoeia, written about 400 to 500 B.C. (often, probably erroneously, dated at 2737 B.C.). Its entry into Western medicine occurred in 1839 when W. B. O'Shaughnessy at the Medical College of Calcutta reported on his experiments in treating patients with rabies, rheumatism, epilepsy, and tetanus with tincture of hemp. He found it to be an effective analgesic with impressive anticonvulsant and muscle-relaxing properties.[33] Western physicians proceeded to explore the potentialities of cannabis, and in the next few decades scores of papers on its usefulness appeared in the medical literature. Before long it was widely used in the United States in the treatment of a variety of ailments which were symptomatically benefited by its analgesic and soporific effects.[34] But there were major limitations on its usefulness: it was not soluble in water and therefore could not be given parenterally; and cannabis indica (the alcoholic tincture of cannabis, the form in which it was dispensed as a medicine) was unstable, so physicians could never be certain of dose. In the second half of the nineteenth century it was superseded as an analgesic by the opiates, and with the development of synthetic analgesics like aspirin, and synthetic hypnotics like the barbiturates, physicians lost interest in cannabis indica. Its use as a medicine declined rapidly in the early decades of the twentieth century; the end came with the passage of the 1937 Marihuana Tax Act.

Curiously, during the American heyday of the use of cannabis as a medicine there was very little awareness that it could be used as an intoxicant. Among the few who knew this were the intellectual and literary-minded readers of those French Romantic writers who comprised the mid-nineteenth-century Le Club des Haschischins. The two most important of these writers, where cannabis is concerned, were Theophile Gautier and Charles Baudelaire. Their effusive accounts were very influential, even though Gautier was actually describing a toxic psychosis induced by large doses of ingested hashish, and what Baudelaire described as hashish experiences may in fact have been the effects of chronic use of laudanum (a mixture of opium and alcohol) on a fertile and imaginative mind influenced by the writings of Thomas de Quincey. The American counterpart of these authors was Fitz Hugh Ludlow, whose book *The Hasheesh Eater: Being Passages from the Life of a Pythagorean* was published in 1857. As with Baudelaire, there is some question of contamination of the descriptions by De Quincey's influence, but there can be no doubt that Ludlow's book was a success and excited the interest of intellectuals—not, however, to such an extent that large numbers of them actually used cannabis. One way in which Ludlow differed from his European counterparts was that, while they used hashish as a source of the drug, he obtained it from his "friendly apothecary" in the form of "Tilden's Extract" or some other brand of cannabis indica. Ludlow's writings provided one of the few connections in the mind of the American public (and a small part of it at that) between cannabis the medicine and cannabis the intoxicant. To the extent that general knowledge of the relation between the medicine and the euphoriant had existed at all, it practically vanished during the half-century that passed before cannabis in a different form (what we now know as marihuana, grass, dope, pot—the dried leaves and flowering tops of the Cannabis plant) began to come into this country from Latin America.

A good deal of mystery surrounds the "reefer's" debut in the United States. It is generally assumed that in the early decades of this century the custom of smoking the weed in cigarette form traveled with itinerant Mexican workers across the Texas border into the southwestern and southern states. Although marihuana use attracted official interest in most of the states west of the Mississippi, concern appears to have been most intense in New Orleans. Supplies of marihuana came occasionally from Texas and more often by boat from Havana, Tampico, and Vera Cruz. Using New Orleans as a distributing center, enterprising sailors became traffickers. It is said that by 1930 there was no major city without at least a coterie of marihuana smokers. Use of the drug was closely identified with Mexican-Americans in the West and with blacks in urban centers, and the early fury it aroused can be attributed in part to the fact that it was considered alien and un-American. Reflections of this attitude were found even in the medical literature, as illustrated by the following, published in the *New Orleans Medical and Surgical Journal* in 1931: "The debasing and baneful influence of hashish and opium is not restricted to individuals but has manifested itself in nations and races as well. The dominant race and most enlightened countries are alcoholic, whilst the races and nations addicted to hemp and opium, some of which once attained to heights of culture and civilization have deteriorated both mentally and physically."[35]

So marihuana, no longer recognized by the public as a medicine, was identified with Spanish-speaking and black people, and became tinged with racial and ethnic prejudice. It was easy for the public to displace some of its anxieties about minority groups onto the drug they used and to associate marihuana with crime, violence, sexual excess, and personality deterioration. Such bigotry is still an important force in society, and it is difficult for people to give up their false beliefs about marihuana. Today of course marihuana is identified with hippies and rebellious youth more than with racial minorities, but the displacement of social anxieties about "outsider" groups onto the drug continues.

In 1930 (less than two years before the Benzedrine inhaler first became available to the public) the Federal Bureau of Narcotics was founded. This bureau, under the leadership of its first director, H. J. Anslinger, undertook an "educational campaign" which magnified a regional, often nonchalant concern about marihuana into alarm over a "national monster." Before 1931, only twenty-four states (mostly in the West) had laws prohibiting the nonmedical distribution of marihuana. By 1937, nearly every state had adopted legislation outlawing the drug, and Congress had passed the Marihuana Tax Act. The lay press, with the help of the Bureau, contributed to the campaign by publishing alarmist stories of violent behavior, usually of a sexual nature, resulting from use of the weed. By 1950 the Bureau, which had heretofore denied that the use of marihuana led to the use of opiates, had embraced the so-called "stepping-stone hypothesis," soon to become the major argument against liberalization of the marihuana laws.

During that same period, the AMA was undergoing a remarkable shift in attitude toward cannabis. Before the 1937 Marihuana Tax Act, the American medical establishment had been quite knowledgeable about cannabis as a medicine and sensible about its capacity for abuse. Because of the difficulties imposed on its medical use by the Tax Act, cannabis was removed from the *U.S. Pharmacopoeia* and *National Formulary* in 1941. This set the stage for doctors to become ignorant about and change their attitudes toward the substance. In protesting the impending 1937 Marihuana Tax Act legislation, members of the Committee of Legislative Activities of the AMA had written: "Cannabis at the present time is slightly used for medicinal purposes, but it would seem worthwhile to maintain its status as a medicinal agent for such purposes as it now has. There is a possibility that a restudy of the drug by modern means may show other advantages to be derived from its medicinal use."[36] Thirty years later a *Journal of the American Medical Association* position paper, written by men who had apparently had little if any experience with the use of cannabis drugs and as little familiarity with the medical literature, asserted: "Cannabis (marihuana) *has no known use in medical practice in most countries* of the world, including the United States."[37]

This remarkable change in attitude is illustrated by the AMA's editorial policy. In September 1942, the *American Journal of Psychiatry* published a paper by S. Allentuck and K. M. Bowman entitled "The Psychiatric Aspects of Marihuana Intoxication" in which, among other things, they asserted that habituation to cannabis was not as strong as to tobacco or alcohol. This report grew out of studies carried out under the auspices of the La Guardia committee. The AMA *Journal* subsequently published a reasoned, informative editorial on their work, describing it as "a careful study." In reviewing its major findings, the editorial mentioned some possible therapeutic uses for cannabis: symptomatic treatment of depression and anorexia nervosa, and treatment of addiction to opiate derivatives. However, following the *Journal's* publication of letters from H. J. Anslinger (January 1943) and R. J. Bouquet, Expert on the Narcotics Commission of the League of Nations (April 1944), both of whom denounced the La Guardia Report, the American Medical Association made an extraordinary about-face and joined the Federal Bureau of Narcotics in attacking the La Guardia Report. The editorial announcing the change appeared in April 1945:

For many years medical scientists have considered cannabis a dangerous drug. Nevertheless, a book called "Marihuana Problems" by the New York City Mayor's Committee on Marihuana submits an analysis by seventeen doctors of tests on 77 prisoners and, on this narrow and thoroughly unscientific foundation, draws sweeping and inadequate conclusions which minimize the harmfulness of marihuana. Already the book has done harm . . . The book states unqualifiedly to the public that the use of this narcotic does not lead to physical, mental or moral degeneration and that permanent deleterious effects from its continued use were not observed on 77 prisoners. This statement has already done great damage to the cause of law enforcement. Public officials will do well to disregard this unscientific, uncritical study, and continue to regard marihuana as a menace wherever it is purveyed.[38]

With this the *Journal*, in the words of A. S. deRopp: "abandoned its customary restraint and voiced its editorial wrath in scolding tones. So fierce was the editorial that one might suppose that the learned members of the mayor's committee . . . had formed some unhallowed league with the 'tea-pad' proprietors to undermine the city's health by deliberately misrepresenting the facts about marihuana."[39]

Over the past twenty-five years the AMA has steadfastly maintained a position on marihuana closely allied with that of the Federal Bureau of Narcotics. The medical community has become both a victim and an agent of the process of generating misinformation and mythology about marihuana, judging by the published statements of the AMA's Council on Mental Health, and the *Journal of the American Medical Association* apparently discounts as "unscientific" and "uncritical" any study that does not demonstrate marihuana to be a menace. The AMA has completely denied the medical heritage and potential of cannabis; its only interest appears to be in providing quasiscientific support for some of the now widely believed myths about marihuana.

Amphetamine, on the other hand, has for most of its short history enjoyed the unequivocal enthusiasm of the pharmaceutical industry and the medical profession. Only in the past few years has the medical establishment begun to be concerned about the consequences of its romance with this drug. The most important factor in public acceptance of amphetamines was the reception accorded them by the medical profession. As long as the medical community was willing to accept the manufacturers' claims, no one questioned why this new psychoactive "medicine" could be marketed without any proof of safety or efficacy. And the American Medical Association, the Food and Drug Administration, and the Federal Bureau of Narcotics had no authority to deny a drug company the right to sell practically any chemical not specifically forbidden by the Harrison Act of 1914. All the Food and Drug Administration could do was recommend appropriate therapeutic indications; it had absolutely no power to limit or warn against consumer purchase of drugs for which prescriptions were not required. Furthermore, the case of amphetamines clearly demonstrated the ease with which drug manufacturers could expand claims for their products and advertise their usefulness in an unlimited range of areas. Some drug firms obtained patents for amphetamine congeners and combinations on the basis of alleged antidepressant actions, then expanded their advertising claims to include the treatment of conditions as disparate as obesity, alcoholism, and enuresis: others started with the claim that their product was uniquely effective in the treatment of obesity and used the same tactics.

Thus, in the mid-1930s, while marihuana was being brought to the public's attention as a menace capable of wreaking great havoc, amphetamines were introduced and promoted as perhaps the earliest technology-derived drug to provide "better living through chemistry." Amphetamines were products of modern technology; they came from the laboratories of great corporations, and, in the days before the growth of consumer skepticism, this lent them legitimacy; unlike the dangerous foreign weed, they seemed to have reliable, safe, *known* properties. And, of course, they had the backing of medical authority.

Other cultural factors help perpetuate the mirror-image relation of attitudes toward cannabis and amphetamines. Societies tend to sanction for social use those drugs whose psychopharmacological properties accord with their ideas of acceptable behavior and performance. Cannabis has been accepted for centuries among the Brahmins in India, whose cultural background and religious traditions support introspection, meditation, and bodily passivity. This introspective, nonaggressive stereotype is opposed to Western cultural patterns. The West, with its emphasis on achievement, activity, efficiency, speed, and aggressiveness, finds amphetamine more compatible with its values. The psychopharmacological properties fit the American "cultural template" as neatly as those of cannabis fit that of the Indian Brahmins.

Speed in Our Culture

American women in particular suffer from a largely male-imposed need to be energetic, "vitally dynamic," and, above all, thin. Many of the 55,000,000 American women between the ages of fourteen and forty-four have been so strongly influenced by masculine standards of "ideal shape" and "ideal weight" that they want to be thinner than is healthy. At the same time, they are surrounded by psychologically sophisticated appeals to buy and eat food. They often have a good deal of "free time" which they spend in retreat through sleep or other forms of inactivity—or in eating. Current fashion, the system that controls the price of female objects on the sex market place, sets such a high premium on slimness that a woman may not be considered superior in value unless she is nearly emaciated. As Germaine Greer has noted: "That thinnest women either diet because of an imagined grossness somewhere or fret because they are not curvaceous; the curviest worry about the bounciness of their curves, or diet to lose them. The curvy girl who ought to be thin and the thin girl who ought to be curvy are offered more or less dangerous medications to achieve their aims. In each case the woman is tailoring herself to the buyers' market."[40]

This situation is made to order for the appetite-suppressing properties of amphetamines and even for their euphorigenic properties, which may make the woman who uses them *feel* thinner. Amphetamines are also attractive to many women in our society because the artificiality of the ideal imposed on them and its difficulty of attainment cause them to suffer diminished self-confidence. They feel a need for more energy than is naturally available to them. Amphetamines may appear to provide the "extra natural energy" that will enable them to play the role society has provided.

The staggering number of errors the housewife is assured from all directions and through all her media-attuned senses that she will make, has made, or is making, further diminish her sense of value, significance, and capability. Her work seems to have nothing to show for it and is always in need of being done again.

She knows that there is more to life—or could be more—if only she had the energy, if only she did not feel so worn-out, frustrated, trapped, and used. Housewives therefore often have deep feelings of malaise but no medically detectable or organic diseases. It is instructive to read the "advice" columns and see how the media tend to tell American women that their life-situation problems are health problems and their "solutions" visits to the doctor. Consider this letter from a housewife to one such "adviser":

> Maybe mine's more a problem for you, Dr. Meredith, but I'm always bone tired and therefore "bone-idle." And with five children (three at school) you'll guess there's plenty for me to do.
>
> I feel so tired when I wake, I can't think how to cope, let alone start work. I do the minimum of housework, sometimes I don't even get the youngest dressed until just before my husband gets home in the evenings, and only then because he blows his top.
>
> He calls me tired-itis.
>
> How I envy the women who can get up at six and do everything and feel on top of the world. I wish I could do half that they do; now I'm really down and don't feel like trying at all.

This woman received the following unjuistified "advice":

> You're quite right; it's a doctor's case, I'm sure of it. Get down to your doctor, explain everything, the weariness, depression, lassitude; he can help.
>
> And cheer up. Many women with far less to cope with than five children and a quick tongued husband feel worse than you and do less. You're all right, except that you're ill. [41]

She was not advised to see a psychiatrist, although nothing in her letter indicates that what she was suffering from was other than functional. Thus, the current American mythology, which considers her condition a medical (and therefore medically treatable) "illness," is reinforced: amphetamines, if taken on doctor's orders or with his sanction, are "medicines."

The attractiveness of amphetamines to women is only one instance of a far more general and pervasive involvement with speed in our country which derives from social and cultural tensions that developed along with the growth in use of the drug. Amphetamines are especially interesting sociologically because their increasing use and corresponding abuse reflect the characteristic features of our society in two important ways. First, amphetamine use results to a large extent from the pressure many people feel to keep up the increasingly hectic pace of modern life, to cope with a world in which nothing seems predictable but change—constantly accelerating change. On the other hand, the amphetamine abuser, especially the "speed freak" or high-dose intravenous abuser, is a gross caricature of many of the pathological, ultimately destructive features of the society that produced him. To put it quite simply: our culture influences, encourages, and sometimes causes people to use amphetamines; and their behavior under the influence of these drugs often constitutes a caricature of the very society that produced it.

Bibliography, Notes, Index

Selected Bibliography

Aberle, D. F. *The Peyote Religion among the Navajo.* Chicago: Aldine, 1966.

Adlersberg, D., and M. E. Mayer. "Results of prolonged medical treatment of obesity with diet alone, diet and thyroid preparations, and diet and amphetamine," *J. Clin. Endocr.,* 9 (1949), 275-284.

Alles, G. A. "The comparative physiological action of Phenylethanolamine," *J. Pharmacol. Exp. Ther.,* 32 (1928), 121-133.

_____ "Some Relations between Chemical Structure and Physiological Action of Mescaline and Related Compounds," in H. A. Abramson, ed., *Neuropharmacology: Transactions of the Fourth Conference, September 25, 26, and 27, 1957, Princeton, New Jersey.* New York: Josiah Macy, Jr. Foundation, 1959.

American Medical Association Council on Pharmacy and Chemistry. "Present status of Benzedrine sulfate," *J.A.M.A.,* 109 (1937), 2064-2069.

Angrist, B. M., and Samuel Gershon. "Amphetamine abuse in New York City—1966 to 1968," *Semin. Psychiatry,* 1 (1969), 195-207.

Angrist, B. M., J. W. Schweitzer, Samuel Gershon, and A. J. Friedhoff. "Mephentermine psychosis: Misuse of the Wyamine inhaler," *Am. J. Psychiatry,* 126 (1970), 1315-1317.

Askevold, Finn. "The occurrence of paranoid incidents and abstinence delirium in abusers of amphetamine," *Acta Psychiat. et Neurol. Scand.,* 34 (1959), 145-164.

Askew, B. M. "Hyperpyrexia as a contributory factor in the toxicity of amphetamine to aggregated mice," *Br. J. Pharmacol.,* 19 (1962), 245-257.

Ausubel, D. P. "Controversial issues in the management of drug addiction: Legalization, ambulatory treatment and the British system," *Mental Hygiene,* 44 (1960), 535-544.

Ausubel, D. P. *Drug Addiction: Physiological, Psychological, and Sociological Aspects.* New York: Random House, Inc., 1958.

Bahnsen, Poul, Erik Jacobsen, and Harriet Thesleff. "The subjective effect of beta-phenylisopropylaminsulfate on normal adults," *Acta Med. Scand.,* 97 (1938), 89-131.

Barger, G., and H. H. Dale. "Chemical structure and sympathomimetic action of amines," *J. Physiol.,* 41 (1910), 19-59.

Barmack, J. E. "The effect of 10 mg of Benzedrine sulfate on the Otis test scores of college students," *Am. J. Psychiatry,* 97 (1940), 163-166.

_____ "The effects of Benzedrine sulfate (benzyl methyl carbinamine) upon the report of boredom and other factors," *J. Psychol.,* 5 (1938), 125-133.

_____ "Studies on the psychophysiology of boredom: Part 1. The effect of 15 mg of Benzedrine sulfate and 60 mg of ephedrine hydrochloride on blood pressure, report of boredom and other factors," *J. Exp. Psychol.,* 25 (1939), 494-505.

Beamish, P., and L. G. Kiloh. "Psychoses due to amphetamine consumption," *J. Ment. Sci.,* 106 (1960), 337-343.

Bejerot, Nils, with the assistance of C. Maurice-Bejerot. *Addiction and Society.* Springfield, Ill.: Charles C. Thomas, 1970.

Bell, D. S. "Comparison of amphetamine psychosis and schizophrenia," *Br. J. Psychiatry,* 111 (1965), 701-707.

_____ and W. H. Trethowan. "Amphetamine addiction," *J. Nerv. Ment. Dis.,* 133 (1961), 489-496.

295

_____ and W. H. Trethowan. "Amphetamine addiction and disturbed sexuality," *Arch. Gen. Psychiatry*, 4 (1961), 74-78.

Bender, Lauretta, and F. Cottington. "The use of amphetamine sulfate (Benzedrine) in child psychiatry," *Am. J. Psychiatry*, 99 (1942), 116-121.

Bett, W. R. "Benzedrine sulphate in clinical medicine: A survey of the literature," *Postgrad. Med. J.*, 22 (1946), 205-218.

Bloomberg, Wilfred. "End results of use of large doses of amphetamine sulfate over prolonged periods," *New Eng. J. Med.*, 222 (1940), 946-948.

Blum, R. H. and Associates. *Drugs I: Society and Drugs*, San Francisco: Jossey-Bass, 1970.

_____ *Drugs II: Students and Drugs*, San Francisco: Jossey-Bass, 1970.

Blumberg, A. G., M. Cohen, A. M. Heaton, and D. F. Klein. "Covert drug abuse among voluntary hospitalized psychiatric patients," *J.A.M.A.*, 217 (1971), 1659-1661.

Bradley, C. "The behavior of children receiving benzedrine," *Am. J. Psychiatry*, 94 (1937), 577-585.

_____ "Benzedrine and Dexedrine in the treatment of children's behavior disorders," *Pediatrics*, 5 (1950), 24-36.

_____ and M. Bowen. "Amphetamine (Benzedrine) therapy of children's behavior disorders," *Am. J. Orthopsychiatry*, 11 (1941), 92-103.

Bradley, P. B. "The effect of some drugs on the electrical activity of the brain of the conscious cat," *Electroencephalogr. Clin. Neurophysiol.* (1953), suppl. III, 21.

_____ and J. Elkes. "The effect of amphetamine and d-lysergic acid diethylamide (LSD 25) on the electrical activity of the brain of the conscious cat," *J. Physiol.*, 120 (1953), 13P-14P.

_____ and J. Elkes. "The effects of some drugs on the electrical activity of the brain," *Brain*, 80 (1957), 77-117.

_____ and B. J. Key. "The effect of drugs on the arousal responses produced by electrical stimulation of the reticular formation of the brain," *Electroencephalogr. Clin. Neurophysiol.*, 10 (1958), 97-110.

Brecher, Edward M., and the Editors of Consumer Reports. *Licit and Illicit Drugs: The Consumers Union Report on Narcotics, Stimulants, Depressants, Inhalants, Hallucinogens, and Marijuana—Including Caffeine, Nicotine, and Alcohol*. Boston: Little, Brown, 1972.

Breitner, Carl. "The hazard of amphetamine medication," *Psychosomatics*, 6 (1965), 217-219.

Calder, Nigel. *The Mind of Man*. New York: Viking, 1970.

Canadian Government Commission of Inquiry. *Interim Report of the Commission of Inquiry into the Non-Medical Use of Drugs*. Ottawa: Information Canada, 1970.

Carey, J. T., and Jerry Mandel. "A San Francisco Bay area 'speed' scene," *J. Health Soc. Behav.*, 9 (1968), 164-174.

Carr, R. B. "Acute psychotic reaction after inhaling methylamphetamine," *Br. Med. J.*, 1 (1954), 1476.

Chein, Isidor, D. L. Gerard, R. S. Lee, and Eva Rosenfeld. *The Road to H: Narcotics, Delinquency, and Social Policy*. New York: Basic Books, 1964.

Chen, K. K., and C. F. Schmidt. "The action of ephedrine, the active principle of the Chinese drug Ma Huang," *J. Pharmacol. Exp. Ther.*, 24 (1924-1925), 339-357.

_____ "Ephedrine and related substances," *Medicine*, 9 (1930), 1-117.

Cohen, Sidney. *The Drug Dilemma*. New York: McGraw-Hill, 1969.

Cole, J. O., and J. R. Wittenborn. *Drug Abuse: Social and Psychopharmacological Aspects*. Springfield, Ill.: Charles C. Thomas, 1970.

Connell, P. H. *Amphetamine Psychosis.* London: Oxford University Press, 1958.

_____ "Use and abuse of amphetamine," *The Practitioner,* 200 (1968), 234-243.

Conners, C. K. "The effect of dexedrine on rapid discrimination and motor control of hyperkinetic children under mild stress," *J. Nerv. Ment. Dis.,* 142 (1966), 429-433.

_____ "Symposium: Behavior modification by drugs—II. Psychological Effects of stimulant drugs in children with minimal brain dysfunction," *Pediatrics,* 49 (1972), 702-708.

_____ and Leon Eisenberg. "The effects of methylphenidate on symptomatology and learning in disturbed children," *Am. J. Psychiatry,* 120 (1963), 458-463.

_____ Leon Eisenberg, and A. Barcai. "Effect of dextroamphetamine on children: Studies on subjects with learning disabilities and school behavior problems," *Arch. Gen. Psychiatry,* 17 (1967), 478-485.

_____ Leon Eisenberg, and Lawrence Sharpe. "Effects of methylphenidate (Ritalin) on paired-associate learning and Porteus Maze performance in emotionally disturbed children," *J. Consult. Psychol.,* 28 (1964), 14-22.

_____ G. Rothschild, Leon Eisenberg, L. S. Schwartz, and E. Robinson. "Dextroamphetamine sulfate in children with learning disorders: Effects on perception, learning, and achievement," *Arch. Gen. Psychiatry,* 21 (1969), 182-190.

Costa, Erminio, and Silvio Garattini, eds. *International Symposium on Amphetamines and Related Compounds: Proceedings of the Mario Negri Institute for Pharmacological Research, Milan, Italy.* New York: Raven Press, 1970.

Cox, Carole, and R. G. Smart. "The nature and extent of speed use in North America," *Can. Med. Assoc. J.,* 102 (1970), 724-729.

Cutler, M., J. W. Little, and A. A. Strauss. "The effect of Benzedrine on mentally deficient children," *Am. J. Ment. Defic.,* 45 (1940), 59-65.

Davis, D. R. "Psychomotor effects of analeptics and their relation to 'Fatigue' phenomena in air-crew," *Br. Med. Bull.,* 5 (1947), 43-45.

Deno, R. A., T. D. Rowe, and D. C. Brodie. *The Profession of Pharmacy: An Introductory Textbook.* Philadelphia: Lippincott, 1959.

Dowling, Harry F. *Medicines for Man: The Development, Regulation and Use of Prescription Drugs.* New York: Alfred A. Knopf, Inc., 1970.

Durrant, B. W. "Amphetamine addiction," *The Practitioner,* 194 (1965), 649-651.

Edeleano, L. "Uber einige derivate der phenylmethacrylsaure und der phenylisobuttersaure," *Ber. Deutsch. Chem. Ges.,* 20 (1887), 616-622.

Eisenberg, Leon. "Symposium: Behavior modification by drugs—III. The clinical use of stimulant drugs in children," *Pediatrics,* 49 (1972), 709-715.

_____ C. K. Conners, and L. Sharpe. "A controlled study of the differential application of outpatient psychiatric treatment for children," *Jap. J. Child. Psychiatry,* 6 (1965), 125-132.

_____ R. Lachman, P. A. Molling, A. Lockner, J. D. Mizelle, C. K. Conners. "A psychopharmacologic experiment in a training school for delinquent boys," *Am. J. Orthopsychiatry,* 33 (1963), 431-446.

Ellinwood, Everett H., Jr. "Amphetamine psychosis: A multi-dimensional process," *Semin. Psychiatry,* 1 (1969), 208-226.

_____ "Amphetamine psychosis: I. Description of the individuals and process," *J. Nerv. Ment. Dis.,* 144 (1967), 273-283.

_____ "Assault and homicide associated with amphetamine abuse," *Am. J. Psychiatry,* 127 (1971), 1170-1175.

Epstein, L. C., L. Lasagna, C. K. Conners, and A. Rodriguez. "Correlation of Dextroamphetamine excretion and drug response in hyperkinetic children," *J. Nerv. Ment. Dis.,* 146 (1968), 136-146.

Evans, John. "Psychosis and addiction to phenmetrazine (Preludin)," *Lancet,* 2 (1959), 152-155.

Evans, W. O., and R. P. Smith. "Some effects of morphine and amphetamine on intellectual functions and mood," *Psychopharmacologia,* 6 (1964), 49-56.

Eysenck, H. J., S. Casey, and D. S. Trouton. "Drug and personality. II. The effect of stimulant and depressant drugs on continuous work," *J. Ment. Sci.,* 103 (1957), 645-649.

Fazekas, J. F., W. R. Ehrmantraut, K. D. Campbell, and N. C. Negron. "Comparative effectiveness of phenylpropanolamine and dextroamphetamine on weight reduction," *J.A.M.A.,* 170 (1959), 1018-1021.

Fink, Max. "Drugs, EEG, and Behavior," in Perry Black, ed., *Drugs and the Brain: Papers on the Action, Use, and Abuse of Psychotropic Agents.* Baltimore: Johns Hopkins, 1969.

_____ "A selected bibliography of electroencephalography in human psychopharmacology, 1951-1962," *Electroencephalogr. Clin. Neurophysiol.,* supplement 23 (1964).

Fish, B. "The 'One child, one drug' myth of stimulants in hyperkinesis," *Arch. Gen. Psychiatry,* 25 (1971), 193-203.

Flory, C.D., and J. Gilbert. "The effects of Benzedrine sulphate and caffeine citrate on the efficiency of college students," *J. Appl. Psychol.,* 27 (1943), 121-134.

Freed, S. C., and E. E. Hays. "A new nonamphetamine anorectic agent," *Am. J. Med. Sci.,* 238 (1959), 55-59.

Freyhan, F. A. "Craving for Benzedrine," *Del. Med. J.,* 21 (1949), 151-156.

Gaffin, Ben, and Associates. *Attitudes of U.S. Physicians toward the American Pharmaceutical Industry.* Chicago: American Medical Association, 1959.

Garai, P. R. "Advertising and Promotion of Drugs," in Paul Taladay, ed., *Drugs in Our Society.* Baltimore: Johns Hopkins, 1964.

Glatt, M. M. "Abuse of methylamphetamine," *Lancet,* 2 (1968), 215-216.

Goldberg, Leonard. "Drug abuse in Sweden (I)," *U.N. Bull. Narc.,* 20:1 (1968), 1-31.

_____ "Drug abuse in Sweden (II)," *U.N. Bull. Narc.,* 20:2 (1968), 9-36.

Goodman, L. S., and Alfred Gilman. *The Pharmacological Basis of Therapeutics,* 2nd, 3rd, and 4th ed. New York: Macmillan, 1955, 1965, and 1970.

Gottlieb, J. S. "The use of sodium Amytal and Benzedrine sulfate in the symptomatic treatment of depressions," *Dis. Nerv. Syst.,* 10 (1949), 50-52.

_____ F. S. Bobbitt, A. W. Freedinger. "Psychopharmacologic study of schizophrenia and depressions. VI. Differences in response to sodium Amytal and Benzedrine sulfate," *Psychosom. Med.,* 14 (1952), 104-114.

_____ and F. E. Coburn. "Psychopharmacologic study of schizophrenia and depressions: Intravenous administration of sodium Amytal and amphetamine sulfate separately and in various combinations," *Arch. Neurol. Psychiatry,* 51 (1944), 260-263.

Greenberg, L. M., M. A. Deem, and S. McMahon. "Effects of Dextroamphetamine, chlorpromazine, and hydroxyzine on behavior and performance in hyperactive children," *Am. J. Psychiatry,* 129 (1972), 532-539.

Greenberg, H. R., and Noel Lustig. "Misuse of Dristan inhaler," *N. Y. State J. Med.,* 66 (1966), 613-617.

Griffith, John. "A study of illicit amphetamine drug traffic in Oklahoma City," *Am. J. Psychiatry*, 123 (1966), 560-569.

Grinspoon, Lester. *Marihuana Reconsidered*. Cambridge, Mass.: Harvard University Press, 1971. *

Gross, M. L. *The Doctors*. New York: Random House Inc., 1966.

Guttmann, E. "The effect of Benzedrine on depressive states," *J. Ment. Sci.*, 82 (1936), 618-620.

Hare, E. H., J. Dominian, and L. Sharpe. "Phenelzine and Dexamphetamine in depressive illness: A comparative trial," *Br. Med. J.*, 1 (1962), 9-12.

Harris, S. C. "Clinically useful appetite depressants," *Ann. N.Y. Acad. Sci.*, 63 (1955), 121-131.

_____ A. C. Ivy, and L. M. Searle. "The mechanism of amphetamine induced loss of weight," *J.A.M.A.*, 134 (1947), 1468-1475.

Hartmann, E. "The effect of four drugs on sleep patterns in man," *Psychopharmacologia*, 12 (1968), 346-353.

Harvey, J. K., C. W. Todd and J. W. Howard. "Fatality associated with Benzedrine ingestion: A case report," *Del. Med. J.*, 21 (1949), 111-115.

Hecht, R., and S. S. Sargent. "Effects of Benzedrine sulfate on performance in two tests of higher mental functions," *J. Exp. Psychol.*, 28 (1941), 529-533.

Hekimian, L. J., and S. Gershon. "Characteristics of drug abusers admitted to a psychiatric hospital," *J.A.M.A..*, 205 (1968), 125-130.

Hentoff, Nat. "Drug-pushing in the schools: The professionals (I)," *The Village Voice*, May 25, 1972, pp. 20-22.

Himwich, H. E. "Anatomy and physiology of the emotions and their relation to psychoactive drugs," in J. Marks and C. M. B. Pare, eds., *The Scientific Basis of Drug Therapy in Psychiatry (A Symposium at St. Bartholomew's Hospital, London, 7th and 8th September, 1964)*. Elmsford, N.Y.: Pergamon, 1965.

Hunsinger, Susan. "School storm: Drugs for children," *Christian Science Monitor*, October 31, 1970, pp. 1,6.

Hurst, P. M., and M. F. Weidner. *Drug Effects upon Cognitive Performance under Stress*, Report ONR-H-66-3, State College, Penn.: Institute for Research, 1966.

Isbell, H. "Historical Development of Attitudes toward Opiate Addiction in the United States," in S. M. Farber and R. H. L. Wilson, eds., *Man and Civilization: Conflict and Creativity: Part Two of Control of the Mind*. New York: McGraw-Hill, 1963.

James, I. P. "A Methylamphetamine epidemic?" *Lancet*, 1 (1968), 916.

Johnson, John and George Milner. "Psychiatric complications of amphetamine substances," *Acta Psychiatr. Scand.*, 42 (1966), 252-263.

Kahn, E., and L. Cohen. "Organic drivenness: A brain-stem syndrome and an experience," *New Eng. J. Med.*, 210 (1934), 748-756.

Kalant, Harold, and O. J. *Drugs, Society, and Personal Choice*. Don Mills, Ont.: Paperjacks, General Publishing, 1971.

Kalant, O. J. *The Amphetamines: Toxicity and Addiction*. Toronto: University of Toronto Press, 1966.

Kales, Anthony. *Sleep: Physiology and Pathology*. Philadelphia: Lippincott, 1969.

Keniston, Kenneth. "Heads and seekers: Drugs on campus, counter-cultures and American society," *The American Scholar*, 38 (1968-1969), 97-112.

Kiloh, L. G., and S. Brandon. "Habituation and addiction to amphetamines," *Br. Med. J.*, 5296 (1962), 40-43.

Knapp, P. H. "Amphetamine and addiction," *J. Nerv. Ment. Dis.*, 115 (1952), 406-432.

Kornetsky, Conan. "Effects of meprobamate, phenobarbital and dextroamphetamine on reaction time and learning in man," *J. Pharmacol. Exp. Ther.,* 123 (1958), 216-219.

_____ A. F. Mirsky, E. K. Kessler, and J. E. Dorff. "The effects of dextro-amphetamine on behavioral deficits produced by sleep loss in humans," *J. Pharmacol. Exp. Ther.,* 127 (1959), 46-50.

Kramer, J. C., V. S. Fischman, and D. C. Littlefield. "Amphetamine abuse: Pattern and effects of high doses taken intravenously," *J.A.M.A.,* 201 (1967), 305-309.

Ladd, E. T. "Pills for classroom peace?" *Saturday Review,* 53 (November 21, 1970), 66-68, 81-83.

Lasagna, Louis. *The Doctor's Dilemmas.* New York: Harper and Brothers, 1962.

_____ J. M. von Felsinger, and H. K. Beecher. "Drug-induced mood changes in man: 1. Observations on healthy subjects, chronically ill patients, and 'postaddicts,' "*J.A.M.A.,* 157 (1955), 1006-1020.

Laufer, Maurice W. "Long-term management and some follow-up findings on the use of drugs with minimal cerebral syndromes," *J. Learn. Dis.,* 4 (1971), 518-522.

_____ Eric Denhoff, and Gerald Solomons. "Hyperkinetic impulse disorder in children's behavior problems," *Psychosom. Med.,* 19 (1957), 38-49.

Laurie, Peter. *Drugs: Medical, Psychological, and Social Facts.* Baltimore: Penguin Books, 1969.

Leake, C. D. *The Amphetamines: Their Actions and Uses.* Springfield, Ill.: Charles Thomas, 1958.

_____ "The Long Road for a Drug from Idea to Use," in F. J. Ayd, Jr., and Barry Blackwell, eds., *Discoveries in Biological Psychiatry.* Philadelphia: Lippincott, 1970.

Levy, S. "The hyperkinetic child — A forgotten entity, its diagnosis and treatment," *Int. J. Neuropsychiatry,* 2 (1966), 330-336.

Lingeman, R. R. *Drugs from A to Z: A Dictionary.* New York: McGraw-Hill, 1969.

Louria, D. B. *The Drug Scene.* New York: McGraw-Hill, 1968.

Masaki, T. "The amphetamine problem in Japan," *WHO Tech. Rep. Ser.,* 102 (1956), 14-21.

Mattson, R. H., and J. R. Calverly. "Dextroamphetamine sulfate-induced dyskinesias," *J.A.M.A.,* 204 (1968), 400-402.

McConnell, T. R., and R. L. Cromwell. "Studies in activity level: VII. Effects of amphetamine drug administration on the activity level of retarded children," *Am. J. Ment. Defic.,* 68 (1964), 647-653.

McCormick, T. C., Jr. "Toxic reactions to the amphetamines," *Dis. Nerv. Syst.,* 23 (1962), 219-224.

Miller, J. G. "Information input overload and psychopathology," *Am. J. Psychiatry,* 116 (1960), 695-704.

Mintz, Morton. *By Prescription Only.* Boston: Beacon, 1967.

Modell, Walter. "Status and prospect of drugs for overeating," *J.A.M.A.,* 173 (1960), 1131-1136.

_____ and G. G. Reader. "Anorexiants," *Drugs of Choice,* 1970-1971, St. Louis: Mosby, 1970.

Molitch, M., and J. P. Sullivan. "The effect of Benzedrine sulfate on children taking the New Stanford Achievement Test," *Am. J. Orthopsychiatry,* 7 (1937), 519-522.

Monroe, R. R., and H. J. Drell. "Oral use of stimulants obtained from inhalers," *J.A.M.A.*, 135 (1947), 909-914.

Morimoto, K. "The problem of the abuse of amphetamines in Japan," *U.N. Bull. Narc.*, 9 (1957), 8-12.

Myerson, Abraham. "Effect of Benzedrine Sulfate on mood and fatigue in normal and in neurotic persons," *Arch. Neurol. Psychiatry,* 36 (1936), 816-822.

_____ "The reciprocal pharmacologic effects of amphetamine (Benzedrine) sulfate and the barbiturates," *New Eng. J. Med.*, 221 (1939), 561-564.

_____ Julius Loman, and William Dameshek. "Physiologic effects of Benzedrine and its relationship to other drugs affecting the autonomic nervous system," *Am. J. Med. Sci.*, 192 (1936), 560-574.

Nagahama, M. "A review of drug abuse and counter measures in Japan since World War II," *U.N. Bull. Narc.*, 20 (1968), 19-24.

Nathanson, M. H. "The central action of beta-aminopropylbenzene (Benzedrine): Clinical observations," *J.A.M.A.*, 108 (1937), 528-531.

National Academy of Sciences—National Research Council. *Committee on Problems of Drug Dependence.* Report of the 32nd Meeting, February 16, 17, and 18, 1970, Washington: NAS-NRC, 1970.

Norman, J., and J. T. Shea. "Acute hallucinosis as a complication of addiction to amphetamine sulfate," *New Eng. J. Med.*, 233 (1945), 270-271.

Novack, H. S. "An educator's view of medication and classroom behavior," *J. Learn. Dis.*, 4 (1971), 507-508.

O'Donnell, J. A., and J. C. Ball, eds. *Narcotic Addiction.* New York: Harper and Row, 1966.

Oswald, Ian. "Human brain protein, drugs and dreams," *Nature*, 223 (1969), 893-897.

_____ H. S. Jones, and J. E. Mannerheim. "Effects of two slimming drugs on sleep," *Br. Med. J.*, 1 (1968), 796-799.

_____ and V. R. Thacore. "Amphetamine and phenmetrazine addiction: Physiological abnormalities in the abstinence syndrome." *Br. Med. J.*, 2 (1963), 427-431.

Payne, R. B., and G. T. Hauty. "Effect of psychological feedback upon work decrement," *J. Exp. Psychol.*, 50 (1955), 343-351.

_____ "The effects of experimentally induced attitudes upon task proficiency," *J. Exp. Psychol.*, 47 (1954), 265-273.

Peoples, S. A., and E. Guttmann. "Hypertension produced with Benzedrine: Its psychological accompaniments," *Lancet*, 1 (1936), 1107-1109.

Perel, J. M., N. Black, R. N. Wharton, and S. Malitz. "Inhibition of imipramine metabolism by methylphenidate," *Fed. Proc.*, 28 (1969), 418.

Peterson, B. H., and D. M. Somerville. "Excessive use of 'Benzedrine' by a psychopath," *Med. J. Aust.*, 2 (1949), 948-949.

Rand, M. E., J. D. Hammond and P. J. Moscou. "A survey of drug use at Ithaca College," *J. Am. Coll. Heath Ass.*, 17 (1968), 43-51.

Rapoport, R., and S. Repo. "The educator as pusher: Drug control in the classroom," *This Magazine is about Schools,* 5 (1971), 87-112.

Report of the Conference on the Use of Stimulant Drugs in the Treatment of Behaviorally Disturbed Young School Children, Washington: U.S. Office of Child Development and the Office of the Assistant Secretary for Health and Scientific Affairs, Department of Health, Education, and Welfare, 1971, reprinted in *J. Learn Dis.*, 4(1971), 523-530.

Rockwell, D. A., and P. Ostwald. "Amphetamine use and abuse in psychiatric patients," *Arch. Gen. Psychiatry*, 18 (1968), 612-616.

Rubin, R. T. "Acute psychotic reaction following ingestion of phentermine," *Am. J. Psychiatry*, 120 (1964), 1124-1125.

Rumbaugh, C. L., R. T. Bergeron, H. C. H. Fang, and R. McCormick. "Cerebral angiographic changes in the drug abuse patient," *Neuroradiology*, 101 (1971), 335-344.

Rumbaugh, Calvin L., R. Thomas Bergeron, Robert L. Scanlan, James S. Teal, Hervey D. Segall, Harry C. H. Fang, and Ruth McCormick. "Cerebral vascular changes secondary to amphetamine abuse in the experimental animal," *Neuroradiology*, 101 (1971), 345-351.

Russo, J. R. ed. *Amphetamine Abuse*. Springfield, Ill.: Charles C. Thomas, 1968.

Safer, D., R. Allen, and E. Barr. "Depression of growth in hyperactive children on stimulant drugs," *New Eng. J. Med.,* 287 (1972), 217-220.

Sano, I., and H. Nagasaka. "Ueber chronische wechaminsucht in Japan," *Fortsohr. Neurol. Psychiatr.*, 24 (1956), 391-394.

Sargant, W., and J. M. Blackburn. "The effect of Benzedrine on intelligence scores," *Lancet*, 231 (1936), 1385-1387.

Satterfield, J. H., L. I. Lesser, R. E. Saul, and D. P. Cantwell. "EEG aspects in the diagnosis and treatment of minimal brain dysfunction," *Ann. N.Y. Acad. Sci.*, 205 (1973), 274-282.

Scher, Jordan. "Patterns and profiles of addiction and drug abuse," *Arch. Gen. Psychiatry*, 15 (1966), 539-551.

Schildkraut, J. J. "The catecholamine hypothesis of affective disorders: A review of supporting evidence," *Am. J. Psychiatry*, 122 (1965), 509-522.

Schneck, J. M. "Benzedrine psychosis: Report of a case," *Military Surgeon*, 102 (1948), 60-61.

Schube, P. G., M. C. McManamy, C. E. Trapp, and A. Myerson. "The effect of Benzedrine sulphate on certain abnormal mental states," *Am. J. Psychiatry,* 94 (1937), 27-32.

Scott, P. D., and D. R. C. Willcox. "Delinquency and the amphetamines," *Br. J. Psychiatry*, 111 (1965), 865-875.

Seevers, M. K. "Medical perspectives on habituation and addiction," *J.A. M.A.*, 181 (1962), 92-98.

Shapiro, M. J. "Benzedrine in the treatment of narcolepsy," *Minn. Med.*, 20 (1937), 28-31.

Sheehy, Gail. *Speed Is of the Essence*. New York: Pocket Books, 1971.

Shorvon, H. J. "Use of Benzedrine sulphate by psychopaths: The problem of addiction," *Br. Med. J.*, 2 (1945), 285-286.

Sjöqvist, Folke, and Malcolm Tottie, eds. *Abuse of Central Stimulants: Symposium Arranged by the Swedish Committee on International Health Relations, Stockholm, November 25-27, 1968*. New York: Raven Press, 1969.

Smith, D. E., ed., "Speed kills: A review of amphetamine abuse," published as *J. Psychedelic Drugs*, 2:2 (1969).

————— and John Luce. *Love Needs Care*. Boston: Little, Brown, 1971.

Smith, G. M., and H. K. Beecher. "Amphetamine sulfate and athletic performance: I. Objective effects," *J.A.M.A.*, 170 (1959), 542-557.

————— "Amphetamine, secobarbital and athletic performance: II. Subjective evaluations of performances, mood states, and physical states," *J.A.M.A.*, 172 (1960), 1502-1514.

Smith, G. M., M. Weitzner, S. R. Levenson, and H. K. Beecher. "Effects of amphetamine and secobarbital on coding and mathematical performance," *J. Pharmacol. Exp. Ther.*, 141 (1963), 100-104.

Smith, L. H., Jr., M. J. Cline, and H. E. Williams. "Changing drug patterns in the Haight-Ashbury," *Calif. Med.*, 110 (1969), 151-157.

Snyder, S. H. "Catecholamines in the brain as mediators of amphetamine psychosis," *Arch. Gen. Psychiatry*, 27 (1972), 169-179.

Sprague, R. L., K. R. Barnes, and J. S. Werry. "Methylphenidate and Thioridazine: Learning, reaction time, activity, and classroom behavior in disturbed children," *Am. J. Orthopsychiatry*, 40 (1970), 615-628.

Straus, Nathan, III. *Addicts and Drug Abusers: Current Approaches to the Problem.* New York: Twayne, 1971.

Swanke, W. R. "Amphetamine abuse," *The New Physician*, 19 (1970), 591-597.

Sykes, D. H., V. I. Douglas, G. Weiss, and K. K. Minde. "Attention in hyperactive children and the effect of methylphenidate (Ritalin)," *J. Child Psychol. Psychiatry*, 12 (1971), 129-139.

Tinklenberg, J. R., and R. C. Stillman. "Drug use and violence," in D. N. Daniels, M. F. Gilula, F. M. Ochberg, eds. *Violence and the Struggle for Existence.* Boston: Little, Brown, 1970.

U.S. Congress, House of Representatives. *Amphetamines: Fourth Report by the Select Committee on Crime.* 91st Congress, 2d Session, House Report No. 91-1807. Washington: Government Printing Office, 1971.

_____ *Federal Involvement in the Use of Behavior Modification Drugs on Grammar School Children of the Right to Privacy Inquiry: Hearing Before a Subcommittee of the Committee on Government Operations, House of Representatives*, 91st Congress, 2d Session, September 29, 1970. Washington: Government Printing Office, 1970.

U.S. Congress, Senate. *Hearings on Administered Prices: Drugs.* Senate Committee on the Judiciary, Subcommittee on Antitrust and Monopoly, 86th Congress, 2d Session. Washington: Government Printing Office, 1960, parts 14, 16, 18.

_____ *Hearings on Drug Industry Antitrust Act*, Senate Committee on the Judiciary, Subcommittee on Antitrust and Monopoly, 87th Congress, 1st Session. Washington: Government Printing Office, 1961, parts 1 and 2.

_____ *Study of Administered Prices in the Drug Industry.* Senate Committee on the Judiciary, Subcommittee on Antitrust and Monopoly, 87th Congress, 1st Session, Senate Report No. 448. Washington: Government Printing Office, 1961.

Von Felsinger, J. M., Louis Lasagna, and H. K. Beecher. "Drug-induced mood changes in man. 2. Personality and reactions to drugs," *J.A.M.A.*, 157 (1955), 1113-1119.

Waud, S. P. "The effects of toxic doses of benzyl methyl carbinamine (Benzedrine) in man," *J.A.M.A.*, 110 (1938), 206-207.

Wheatley, D. "Amphetamines in general practice: Their use in depression and anxiety," *Semin. Psychiatry.*, 1 (1969), 163-173.

Willey, R. T. "Abuse of methylphenidate (Ritalin)," Letter, *New Eng. J. Med.*, 285 (1971), 464.

Wilson, C. W. M., ed. *The Pharmacological and Epidemiological Aspects of Adolescent Drug Dependence: Proceedings of the Society for the Study of Addiction, London, 1 and 2, September, 1966.* New York: Pergamon, 1968.

Wittenborn, J. R., Jean Paul Smith, and Sarah A. Wittenborn, eds. *Drugs and Youth: Proceedings of the 2nd Rutgers Symposium on Drug Abuse.* Springfield, Ill.: Charles C. Thomas, 1970.

Young, David, and W. B. Scoville. "Paranoid psychosis in narcolepsy and the possible danger of Benzedrine treatment," *Med. Clin. N. Am.*, 22 (1938), 637-646.

Zalis, E. G., and L. F. Parmley, Jr. "Fatal amphetamine poisoning," *Arch. Intern. Med.*, 112 (1963), 822-826.

Zarcone, Vincent. "Narcolepsy," *New Eng. J. Med.*, 288 (1973), 1156-1166.

Zondek, L. "Amphetamine abuse and its relation to other drug addictions," *Psychiatr. Neurol.* (Basel), 135 (1958), 227-246.

Notes

Chapter 1. The Contemporary Amphetamine Scene

1. National Clearinghouse for Drug Abuse Information, National Institute of Mental Health, *A Federal Source Book: Answers to the Most Frequently Asked Questions About Drug Abuse* (Washington: U.S. Government Printing Office, 1970), pp. 17-18.

2. Bett, "Benzedrine sulphate in clinical medicine," pp. 206-215.

3. Rush Loving, Jr., "Putting some limits on 'speed,' " *Fortune*, March 1971, p. 127.

4. "Benzedrine sulfate 'pep pills,' " Editorial *J.A.M.A.*, 108 (1937), 1973-1974.

5. Sheehy, *Speed Is of the Essence*, p. 62.

6. Monroe and Drell, "Oral use of stimulants obtained from inhalers," pp. 910,911.

7. Greenberg and Lustig, "Misuse of Dristan inhaler," p. 613.

8. Ibid., pp. 613, 615, 616-617.

9. Angrist, Schweitzer, Gershon, and Friedhoff, "Mephentermine psychosis: Misuse of the Wyamine inhaler," pp. 1315, 1316.

10. Griffith, "A study of illicit amphetamine drug traffic in Oklahoma City," p. 561.

11. Zondek, "Amphetamine abuse and its relation to other drug addictions," pp. 229-230 (quoting Straub in G. Bonhoff and H. Lewrenz, *Uber Weckamine* [Berlin, 1954]). See also Leake, *The Amphetamines*, p. 115.

12. W. R. Bett, Leonard H. Howells, and A. D. MacDonald, *Amphetamine in Clinical Medicine: Actions and Uses* (London and Edinburgh: E. and S. Livingstone, 1955), p. 4; the authors cite D. N. W. Grant, *Air Force*, Official Service Journal of the U.S. Army Air Force, (Washington: Government Printing Office, 1944), p. 25. Monroe and Drell, "Oral use," p. 911.

13. *Amphetamines: Fourth Report by the Select Committee on Crime*, 91st Congress, 2d Session, House Report No. 91-1807, pp. 7-8.

14. R. L. Ohler, "Heroin use by veterans," Letter, *New Eng. J. Med.,* 285 (1971), 692.

15. G. D. Mellinger, "The psychotherapeutic drug scene in San Francisco," in P. H. Blachly, ed., *Drug Abuse: Data and Debate* (Springfield, Ill. 1970), pp. 226-240; G. D. Mellinger, M. B. Balter, and D. I. Manheimer, "Patterns of psychotherapeutic drug use among adults in San Francisco," *Arch. Gen. Psychiatry*, 25 (1971), 389-392; M. B. Balter and Jerome Levine, "The nature and extent of psychotropic drug usage in the United States," *Psychopharmacol. Bull.*, 5(1969), 6-7.

16. T. C. McCormick, Jr., "Toxic reactions to the amphetamines," *Dis. Nerv. Syst.*, 23 (1962), 220; A. S. Flemming, "Amphetamine drugs," *Public Health Reports*, 75 (1960), 49. G. R. Edison, "Amphetamines: A dangerous illusion," *Ann. Intern. Med.*, 74 (1971), 605-606; Committee on Alcoholism and Addiction and Council on Mental Health of the American Medical Association, "Dependence on amphetamines and other stimulant drugs," *J.A.M.A.*, 197 (1966), p. 1024; *Amphetamines: Fourth Report*, pp. 2, 5, 21. National Clearing-House for Drug Abuse Information, *Federal Source Book*, pp. 17-18. H. M.

Schmeck, "U.S. plans 82% cutback in amphetamines," *New York Times*, Feb. 10, 1972, 1.

17. Allen Geller and Maxwell Boas, *The Drug Beat* (New York: Cowles, 1969), pp. 239-240, 245; J. W. Rawlin, "Street Level Abusage of Amphetamines," in Russo, *Amphetamine Abuse*, pp. 55-56.

18. Committee on Alcoholism and Addiction, "Dependence on amphetamines," p. 1025. J. F. Sadusk, "Symposium: Nonnarcotic addiction: Size and extent of the problem," *J.A.M.A.* 196 (1966), 708. J. Walsh, "Psychotoxic drugs: Dodd bill passes Senate, comes to rest in the House: Critics are sharpening their knives," *Science*, 145 (1964), 1418.

19. Ibid., pp. 1419, 1420.

20. *Amphetamines: Fourth Report*, pp. 22-23; Loving, "Putting some limits on speed," p. 127. H. M. Schmeck, "U.S. acts to block amphetamines from Mexico," *New York Times*, Jan. 19, 1972, p. 16; Boyce Resenberger, "Amphetamine maker will end criticized production in Mexico," *New York Times*, Jan. 23, 1972, p. 22.

21. John Griffith, J. Davis, and J. Oates, "Amphetamines: Addiction to a non-addicting drug," *Pharmakopsychiatrie-Neuro-Psychopharmakologie*, 4 (1971), 60. N. R. Ellis, R. E. Davis, and C. A. Denton, "Use of antibiotics, hormones, tranquilizers, and other chemicals in animal production," *The Nature and Fate of Chemicals Applied to Soils, Plants, and Animals*, Symposium U.S.D.A. Agricultural Research Service, September 1960 (Washington: Government Printing Office, 1960), p. 45; Franklin Bicknell, *Chemicals in Your Food and in Farm Produce: Their Harmful Effects* (New York: Emerson, 1960), p. 74.

22. Rawlin, "Street level abusage," p. 54; R. R. Lingeman, *Drugs from A to Z: A Dictionary* (New York, 1969), p. 226 (referring to H. M. Hughs, ed., *The Fantastic Lodge* [Boston, 1961]); Smith and Luce, *Love Needs Care*, pp. 14-19.

23. Rawlin, "Street level abusage," p. 67. And see Roger C. Smith, "Traffic in amphetamines: Patterns of illegal manufacture and distribution," in D. E. Smith, ed., "Speed Kills," p. 20.

24. Personal communication from a colleague of Owsley who wishes to remain anonymous; Smith and Luce, *Love Needs Care*, pp. 17-18, 173.

25. Smith, "Traffic in amphetamines," p. 21.

26. R. C. Smith, "The world of the Haight-Ashbury speed freak," *J. Psychedelic Drugs*, 2 (1969):2, 78; J. C. Kramer, "Introduction to amphetamine abuse," *J. Psychedelic Drugs*, 2 (1969): 2, p. 9; Smith and Luce, *Love Needs Care*, p. 18; Smith, "Traffic in amphetamines," pp. 22-23. Kramer, Fischman, and Littlefield, "Amphetamine abuse," p. 307.

27. Griffith, "Amphetamine drug traffic," pp. 561-565.

28. D. L. Farnsworth and H. K. Oliver, "The drug problem among young people," *W. Va. Med. J.*, 63 (1967), 433-434; reprinted in *Rhode Island Medical Journal*, 51 (1968), 179.

29. Kenneth Keniston, "Heads and seekers," pp. 97-112.

30. R. H. Blum and Associates, *Drugs II*, pp. 79, 188-190.

31. M. E. Rand, J. D. Hammond, P. J. Moscou, "A survey of drug use at Ithaca College," p. 51.

32. Blum, *Drugs II*, pp. 328, 345, 346; and D. E. Smith, "Speed Kills: High Dose Methamphetamine Abuse," *Los Angeles County Med. Soc. Bull.* (June, 1968).

33. V. A. Gelineau, L. A. Zaks, K. M. Novick, and J. M. Camp, *Report of the Youth Study to the Woburn Community*, Division of Drug Rehabilitation, Department of Mental Health, Boston (April 9, 1971), pp. 2, 4; Henry Wechsler and Denise Thum, *The Extent of Drug Use in the Quincy Public Schools*, Report #1

(Boston: Medical Foundation, 1971), p. 5. Henry Wechsler and Denise Thum, *Drug Usage among School-Age Youth in the City of Quincy,* Research Report 2: *The Social Context of Drug Use* (Boston: Medical Foundation, 1972), p. 5. Henry Wechsler and Denise Thum, *Drug Usage among School-Age Youth in the Town of Brookline; Research Report #1* (Boston: Medical Foundation, 1971), pp. 1-20.

34. J. F. E. Schick, D. E. Smith, and F. H. Meyers, "The use of amphetamine in the Haight-Ashbury subculture," *J. Psychedelic Drugs,* 2 (1969):2, p. 71. See also Blum, *Drugs II,* p. 333; D. B. Louria, *The Drug Scene,* p. 44.

Chapter 2. Development and Pharmacology

1. Pierre Huard and Ming Wong, *Chinese Medicine,* trans. B. Fielding (New York: McGraw-Hill, 1968) pp. 10-11. L. S. Goodman and Alfred Gilman, *The Pharmacological Basis of Therapeutics* (2nd ed., New York: Macmillan, 1955), p. 505.

2. Chen and Schmidt, "The action of ephedrine," pp. 339-357. See also F. Stolz, "Ueber adrenalin und alkylaminoaceto-brenzcatechin," *Ber. Deutsch Chem. Ges.,* 37 (1904), 4149-4154; H. D. Dakin, "The synthesis of a substance allied to adrenalin," *Proc. R. Soc.,* 76 (1905), 491-497.

3. L. Edeleano, "Uber einige derivate der phenylmethacrylsaure und der phenylisobuttersaure," *Ber Deutsch Chem. Ges.,* 20 (1887), 616-622. G. Barger and H. H. Dale, "Chemical structure and sympathomimetic action of amines," *J. Physiol.,* 41 (1910), 19-59.

4. J. H. Biel, "Structure-Activity Relationships of Amphetamine and Derivatives," in Costa and Garattini, *International Symposium,* p. 4; J. W. Daly, C. R. Creveling, and B. Witkop, "The chemorelease of norepinephrine from mouse hearts: structure-activity relationships. I. Sympathomimetic and related amines," *J. Med. Chem.,* 9 (1966), 273-280.

5. E. G. Boring, "Psychological factors in the scientific process," *Am. Sci.,* 42 (4) (1954), 639-645. One of the best articles about the "race for priority" among scientists and writers as well is R. K. Merton, "Behavior patterns of scientists," *Am. Sci.,* 57 (1969), 1-23.

6. Alles, "Comparative physiological action of phenylethanolamine," pp. 121-133.

7. L. W. Jones and E. S. Wallis, "The Beckmann rearrangement involving optically active radicals," *J. Am. Chem. Soc.,* 48 (1926), 169-181. A. Ogata, "Desoxyephedrine—A contribution of the structure of ephedrine," *J. Pharm. Soc. Japan,* 51 (1919), 751-764. H. Emde, "Uber diastereomerie: I. Konfiguration des ephedrins," *Helv. Chim. Acta.,* 12 (1929), 365-376.

8. AMA Council on Pharmacy and Chemistry, "Present status of Benzedrine sulfate," p. 2069.

9. Peoples and Guttmann, "Hypertension produced with Benzedrine: its psychological accompaniments," pp. 1107-1109; A. Myerson and M. Ritvo, "Benzedrine sulfate and its value in spasm of the gastro-intestinal tract," *J.A.M.A.,* 107 (1936), 24-26; Guttmann, "Effect of Benzedrine on depressive states," pp. 618-620; Myerson, "Effect of Benzedrine sulfate on mood and fatigue," pp. 816-822; Nathanson, "Central action of beta-aminopropylbenzene (Benzedrine)," pp. 528-531.

10. D. Legge and H. Steinberg, "Actions of a mixture of amphetamine and a barbiturate in man," *Br. J. Pharmacol.,* 18 (1962), 490-500.

11. E. Davidoff and G. L. Goodstone, "The amphetamine-barbiturate therapy in psychiatric conditions," *Psychiatr. Q.,* 16 (1942), 541-548; V. A. Drill, *Pharmacology in Medicine,* 2nd ed. (New York, 1958), p. 402; Gottlieb, "Use of

sodium Amytal and Benzedrine sulphate," pp. 50-52; Gottlieb and Coburn, "Psychopharmacologic study of schizophrenia and depressions," pp. 260-263; H. V. Grahn, "The depressed patient: Management with the aid of new medication," *Am. Prac. Dig. Tr.*, 1 (1950), 795-797; V. G. Laties, "Modification of affect, social behavior and performance by sleep deprivation and drugs," *J. Psychiatr. Res.*, 1 (1961), 12-25; Myerson, "Reciprocal pharmacologic effects of amphetamine (Benzedrine) sulfate and the barbiturates," pp. 561-564; H. Steinberg, R. Rushton, and C. Tinson, "Modification of the effects of an amphetamine-barbiturate mixture by the past experience of rats," *Nature,* 192 (1961), 533-535.

12. Seymour Fiddle, "The Case of 'Peak User' John," in Russo, *Amphetamine Abuse,* pp. 123-124.

13. *Physicians' Desk Reference to Pharmaceutical Specialties and Biologicals* (Oradell, N. J., 1965), p. 594.

14. G. L. Krueger and W. R. McGrath, "2-Benzylpiperidines and related compounds," in Maxwell Gordon, ed., *Psychopharmacological Agents* (New York: Academic Press, 1964), I, 225-250; K. E. Moore, L. A. Carr, and J. A. Dominic, "Functional Significance of Amphetamine-Induced Release of Brain Catecholamines," in Costa and Garattini, *International Symposium*, pp. 377, 380; R. H. Rech, "Amphetamine-Drug Interactions that Relate Brain Catecholamines to Behavior," in Costa and Garattini, pp. 395, 410; A. Randrup and I. Munkvad, "Biochemical, Anatomical and Psychological Investigations of Stereotyped Behavior Induced by Amphetamines," in Costa and Garattini, p. 697.

15. Biel, "Structure-Activity Relationships," pp. 8-9.

16. J. F. Fazekas, W. R. Ehrmantraut, K. D. Campbell, and M. C. Negron, "Comparative effectiveness of phenylpropanolamine and dextroamphetamine on weight reduction," *J.A.M.A.*, 170 (1959), 1018-1021.

17. McCormick, "Toxic reactions to the amphetamines," p. 222.

18. Biel, "Structure-Activity Relationships," p. 12.

19. A. T. Shulgin, "Psychotomimetic agents related to the catecholamines," *J. Psychedelic Drugs,* 2:2 (1969), 19.

20. Smith and Luce, *Love Needs Care*, pp. 172-175, 239.

21. S. H. Snyder, L. A. Faillace, and L. Hollister, 2,5-Dimethoxy-4-methylamphetamine (STP): A new hallucinogenic drug," *Science,* 158 (1967), 669-670.

22. Shulgin, "Psychotomimetic agents," p. 18.

23. Alles, "Some Relations Between Chemical Structure and Physiological Action of Mescaline and Related Compounds," pp. 196-200.

24. Shulgin, "Psychotomimetic agents," p. 26.

25. *Amphetamines: Fourth Report by the Select Committee on Crime*, p. 2.

Chapter 3. Effect on Mood and Performance

1. Peoples and Guttmann, "Hypertension produced with Benzedrine," pp. 1107-1109. Guttmann, "Effect of Benzedrine on depressive states," p. 620.

2. Myerson, "Effect of Benzedrine sulfate on mood and fatigue," p. 816.

3. Nathanson, "Central action of beta-aminopropylbenzene (Benzedrine)," pp. 530-531.

4. Bahnsen, Jacobsen, and Thesleff, "Subjective effect of beta-phenylisopropylaminsulfate," pp. 91-92, 102-108, 117, 121-122, 126-127, 130-131.

5. Lasagna, von Felsinger, and Beecher, "Drug-induced mood changes in man," pp. 1007-1010, 1017.

6. Ibid., pp. 1008-1009, 1018.

7. J. Olds and P. Milner, "Positive reinforcement produced by electrical stim-

ulation of septal area and other regions of rat brain," *J. Comp. Physiol. Psychol.*, 47 (1954), 425.

8. Calder, *Mind of Man*, p. 50.

9. Technically, the hypothalamus is that portion of the anterior end of the diencephalon lying below the hypothalamic sulcus and in front of the interpeduncular nuclei; it is divided into a number of rather loosely conglomerated and diffuse regions, many of which are interconnected with other brain regions, often through intermediate functional areas and brain regions. Perhaps one of its most important such connections is with the posterior lobe of the pituitary gland. In 1947, C. S. Sherrington, in *The Integrative Action of the Nervous System* (Cambridge University Press) suggested that the hypothalamus be considered the "head ganglion of the autonomic system," but even though electrical stimulation or excision of the hypothalamus does result in definite autonomic changes and responses, there is little evidence that it is directly concerned with any regulation of visceral function. However, it does seem clear that autonomic responses triggered by the hypothalamus are directly related to more complex phenomena such as rage and other emotions. Its functions invariably involve a particular response to a particular stimulus; this pattern of stimulus-integration-response is essential to a consideration of the relation of the hypothalamus to any overt behavior presumed to be the result of CNS-arising "drives" or "needs." Similarly, although stimulation of the superior anterior hypothalamus sometimes results in bladder contraction and hence urination, most authorities agree that the existence of any "parasympathetic center" in the hypothalamus is at best highly dubious. On the other hand, hypothalamic regulation of hunger, thirst, temperature of the body, sexual behavior, fear, rage, and even, at least in a limited sense, general "motivation" has been demonstrated to at least a minimal degree in experimental animals. See W. F. Ganong, *Review of Medical Physiology*, 5th ed. (Los Altos, Calif.: Lange, 1971), pp. 157-180.

10. J. E. P. Toman and J. P. Davis, "The effects of drugs upon the electrical activity of the brain," *Pharmacol. Rev.*, 1 (1949), 428.

11. Fink, "Drugs, EEG, and Behavior," pp. 150, 151; Fink, "Selected Bibliography of Electroencephalography," Max Fink, "EEG and human psychopharmacology (Symposium in conjunction with Third World Congress of Psychiatry, Montreal, Canada, 1961), *Electroencephalogr. Clin. Neurophysiol.*, 15 (1963), 133-137; M. Fink, "Clinical Neurophysiology," in D. Bente and P. Bradley, eds., *Neuro-Psychopharmacology, Collegium International Neuro-Psychopharmacologium Proceedings, Fourth Meeting* (Amsterdam, 1966), pp. 64-69.

12. Bradley and Elkes, "Effect of amphetamine and d-lysergic acid diethylamide," 13P-14P. Leake, *The Amphetamines*, pp. 26-27; Bradley and Key, "Effect of drugs on the arousal responses produced by electrical stimulation of the reticular formation of the brain," 108.

13. I. I. Baryshnikov, "On the question of the effect on the central nervous system of some phenamine derivatives" (Russian), *Fiziol. Zhu.* SSSR, 41 (1955), 660-665. Leake, *The Amphetamines*, pp. 27-28.

14. M. A. Rubin, W. Malamud, and J. M. Hope, "The electroencephalogram and psychopathological manifestations in schizophrenia as influenced by drugs," *Psychosom. Med.*, 4 (1942), 355-361. F. A. Gibbs and G. L. Maltby, "Effect on the electrical activity of the cortex of certain depressant and stimulant drugs—barbiturates, morphine, caffeine, Benzedrine and adrenalin," *J. Pharmacol. Exp. Ther.*, 78 (1943), 1-10. D. B. Lindsley and C. E. Henry, "The effect of drugs on behavior and the electroencephalograms of children with behavior disorders," *Psychosom. Med.* 4 (1942), 140-149.

15. Barmack, "The effects of Benzedrine sulfate upon the report of boredom

and other factors"; Barmack, "Studies on the psychophysiology of boredom," p. 501; H. F. Adler, W. L. Burkhardt, A. C. Ivy, and A. J. Atkinson, "Effect of various drugs on psychomotor performance at ground level and at simulated altitudes of 18,000 feet in a low pressure chamber," *J. Aviat. Med.*, 21 (1950), 221-236. D. P. Cuthbertson and J. A. C. Knox, "The effects of analeptics on the fatigued subject," *J. Physiol.* 106 (1947), 42-58; R. H. Seashore and A. C. Ivy, "Effects of analeptic drugs in relieving fatigue," *Psychol. Monogr.* 67 (no. 15) (1953), 1-16; W. Somerville, "The effect of Benzedrine on mental or physical fatigue in soldiers," *Can. Med. Assoc. J.*, 55 (1946), 470-476; D. B. Tyler, "The effect of amphetamine sulfate and some barbiturates on the fatigue produced by prolonged wakefulness," *Am. J. Physiol.* 150 (1947), 253-262. See also Note 19.

16. Payne and Hauty, "Effects of experimentally induced attitudes upon task proficiency," pp. 267, 268, 272. "Apparatus Tests," in A. E. Melton, ed., *AAF Aviation Psychology Program Research Reports,* Report No. 4 (Washington: U.S. Government Printing Office, 1947). R. B. Payne and G. T. Hauty, "Factors affecting the endurance of psychomotor skill," *J. Aviat. Med.*, 26 (1955), 382-389.

17. G. T. Hauty and R. B. Payne, "Mitigation of work decrement," *J. Exp. Psychol.*, 49 (1955), 60-67.

18. Payne and Hauty, "Effect of psychological feedback upon work decrement."

19. Davis, "Psychomotor effects of analeptics," pp. 43-45. According to Davis, a new approach to "pilot-fatigue" was made possible by the development of the Cambridge Cockpit, an apparatus that provided the means of analyzing the performance of pilots in an instrument flying-exercise.

20. Kornetsky, "Effects of meprobamate, phenobarbital and dextroamphetamine on reaction time and learning in man," pp. 216-219.

21. Kornetsky, Mirsky, Kessler, and Dorff, "Effects of dextroamphetamine on behavioral deficits produced by sleep loss in humans," pp. 46, 48. The findings which produced this study are found in Eysenck, Casey, and Trouton, "Drugs and personality: II. The effect of stimulant and depressant drugs on continuous work." For microsleep, see W. B. Webb, "Twenty-four-Hour Sleep Cycling," in Anthony Kales, ed., *Sleep: Physiology and Pathology: A Symposium* (Philadelphia: Lippincott, 1969), 59; W. T. Liberson, "Problem of sleep and mental disease," *Digest Neurol. Psychiat.*, 13 (1945), 93-108; L. C. Johnson, "Physiological and Psychological Changes Following Total Sleep Deprivation," in Kales, *Sleep*, p. 211; L. C. Johnson, E. S. Slye, and W. Dement, "Electroencephalographic and autonomic activity during and after prolonged sleep deprivation," *Psychosom. Med.*, 27 (1965), 415-423; P. Naitoh, E. J. Kollar, and A. Kales, "The EEG changes after a prolonged sleep loss," *Electroencephalogr. Clin. Neurophysiol.*, 26 (1969), 238.

22. Hurst and Weidner, *Drug Effects Upon Cognitive Performance,* pp. i, 1, 7 (italics in original). J. G. Miller, "Information input overload and psychopathology," *Am. J. Psychiatry*, 116 (1960), 695-704.

23. Miller, J. G., "Information input overload," pp. 695, 696.

24. Hurst and Weidner, *Drug Effects upon Cognitive Performance*, pp. 7-8.

25. Hurst and Weidner, *Drug Effects upon Cognitive Performance*, pp. 14-15. For PSMT, see K. E. Lloyd, L. S. Reid, and J. B. Feallock, "Short-term retention as a function of the average number of items presented," *J. Exp. Psychol.*, 60 (No. 4) (1960), 201-207.

26. Hurst and Weidner, *Drug Effects,* pp. 28 (italics in original), 36.

27. Ibid., pp. 37, 39, 67, 71 (table 14).

28. Ibid., pp. 78-80; A. R. Holliday, "A comparison of benzquinamide with pentobarbital and a placebo in regard to effects on performance of a simple

mental task by fatigued humans," *Proc. West. Pharmacol. Soc.*, 7 (1964), 75-78; A. R. Holliday and J. M. Dille, "The effects of meprobamate, chlorpromazine, pentobarbital, and a placebo on a behavioral task performed under stress conditions," *J. Comp. Physiol. Psychol.*, 51 (no. 6) (1958), 811-815.

29. Hurst and Weidner, pp. 105 (figure 15), 119, 122.

30. Sargant and Blackburn, "Effect of Benzedrine on intelligence scores." Barmack, "Effect of 10 mg of Benzedrine sulfate on the Otis," pp. 163, 165.

31. Hecht and Sargent, "Effects of Benzedrine sulfate on performance in two tests," pp. 529-533; *Benzedrine Sulfate Protocol* (February 1940), published (mimeographed) by Smith, Kline and French Laboratories. G. P. Carl and W. D. Turner, "The effects of Benzedrine sulfate (amphetamine sulfate) on performance in a comprehensive psychometric examination," *J. Psychol.*, 8 (1939), 165-216.

32. Flory and Gilbert, "Effects of Benzedrine sulphate and caffeine citrate on the efficiency of college students," pp. 121-122.

33. Ibid., pp. 122-123.

34. Ibid., pp. 127-129, 132-133.

35. Smith, Weitzner, Levenson, and Beecher, "Effects of amphetamine and secobarbital on coding and mathematical performance," pp. 102, 104, 101.

36. Evans and Smith, "Some effects of morphine and amphetamine on intellectual functions and mood," p. 50. The term was first coined by J. P. Guilford in 1956 and later refined by Guilford and P. R. Merrifield. See J. P. Guilford, "Structure of intellect," *Psychol Bull.*, 53 (1956), 267-293.

37. Evans and Smith, "Some effects of morphine and amphetamine," pp. 50, 51-54.

38. Smith and Beecher, "Amphetamine sulfate and athletic performance: I. Objective effects," pp. 542-557.

39. P. V. Karpovich, "Effect of amphetamine sulfate on athletic performance," *J.A.M.A.*, 170 (1959), 558-561. B. Weiss and V. G. Laties, "Enhancement of human performance by caffeine and the amphetamines," *Pharmacol. Rev.*, 14 (1962), 1-36. J. Haldi and W. Wynn, "Action of drugs on efficiency of swimmers," *Research Quarterly*, 17 (1946), 96-101.

40. F. A. Hellebrandt and P. V.Karpovich, "Fitness, fatigue, and recuperation: Survey of methods used for improving the physical performance of man," *War Medicine*, 1 (1941), 747-748.

41. "Russell used drugs in 2 Celtics games," *Boston Globe*, Feb. 25, 1973.

42. R. Kostelanetz, " 'Nick the Knife,' or, the life of a football doctor," *New York Times Magazine*, Dec. 19, 1971, p. 26.

Chapter 4. Further Psychological Effects

1. Connell, *Amphetamine Psychosis*, pp. 51-52. Institute of Psychiatry Maudsley Monographs No. 5, published for the Institute of Psychiatry by Oxford University Press.

2. Waud, "Effects of toxic doses of benzyl methyl carbinamine," p. 207. P. Schilder, "The psychological effect of Benzedrine sulfate," *J. Nerv. Men. Dis.*, 87 (1938), 584. Knapp, "Amphetamine and addiction," pp. 412, 419; F. H. Wiechman, Letter, "Drug-induced impotence?" *J.A.M.A.* 174 (1960), 2096. E. Guttmann, "Discussion on Benzedrine: Uses and Abuses," *Proc. Roy. Soc. Med.*, 32 (1939), 389.

3. Seymour Fiddle, "The Case of 'Peak User' John," in Russo, *Amphetamine Abuse*, pp. 135-136.

4. W. H. Hampton, "Observed psychiatric reactions following use of amphetamine and amphetamine-like substances," *Bull. N.Y. Acad. Med.*, 37 (1961), 172. Norman and Shea, "Acute hallucinosis as a complication of addic-

tion," p. 270. G. Rylander, "Clinical and Medico-criminological aspects of addiction to Central Stimulating Drugs," in Sjöqvist and Tottie, *Abuse of Central Stimulants*, pp. 255-256.

5. Bell and Trethowan, "Amphetamine addiction," *J. Nerv. Ment. Dis.*, pp. 491-492.

6. Ellinwood, "Amphetamine psychosis: I. Description of individuals and process," p. 278.

7. Cox and Smart, "Nature and extent of speed use in North America," p. 725.

8. Sidney Cohen, "Pot, acid and speed," *Medical Science* (February 1968), p. 35. Angrist and Gershon, "Amphetamine abuse in New York City," p. 201.

9. L. E. A. Berman, "The role of amphetamine in a case of hysteria," *J. Am. Psychoanal. Assoc.*, 20 (1972), 329.

10. Carey and Mandel, "San Francisco Bay area 'speed' scene," p. 167.

11. J. M. Henslin, "Changes in perceptions of sexual experiences of college students while under the influence of drugs," in National Academy of Sciences, *Committee on Problems of Drug Dependence: 1970*, (Washington: 1970), p. 6531.

12. Bell and Trethowan, "Amphetamine addiction and disturbed sexuality," pp. 76-78.

13. Scott and Willcox, "Delinquency and the amphetamines," p. 873.

14. Griffith, "Study of illicit amphetamine drug traffic in Oklahoma City," p. 564.

15. Smith and Luce, *Love Needs Care*, p. 221. Seymour Fiddle, "Circles beyond the Circumference: Some Hunches About Amphetamine Abuse," in Russo, *Amphetamine Abuse*, p. 72.

16. J. D. Griffith, "Psychiatric Implications of Amphetamine Abuse," in Russo, *Amphetamine Abuse*, p. 27.

17. Rylander, "Clinical and medico-criminological aspects," pp. 256-259.

18. Ellinwood, "Amphetamine psychosis: a multi-dimensional process," p. 217.

19. Kramer, Fischman, and Littlefield, "Amphetamine abuse," p. 306.

20. Rylander, "Clinical and medico-criminological aspects," pp. 257-258.

21. Ibid., p. 258. A. Randrup, I. Munkvad, and P. Udsen. "Adrenergic mechanisms and amphetamine-induced abnormal behaviour," *Acta Pharmacol. Toxicol.* (Kbh.), 20 (1963), 145-157.

22. A. Randrup and I. Munkvad, "Biochemical, Anatomical and Psychological Investigations of Stereotyped Behavior Induced by Amphetamines," in Costa and Garattini, *International Symposium*, pp. 695-696, 703-709.

23. A. Randrup and I. Munkvad, "Stereotyped activities produced by amphetamine in several animal species and man," *Psychopharmacologia* (Berlin), 11 (1967), 300-310.

24. Ellinwood, "Amphetamine psychosis: a multi-dimensional process," p. 221. E. H. Ellinwood and O. Escalante, "Behavior and histopathological findings during chronic methedrine intoxication," *Biol. Psychiatry*, 2 (1970), 27-39.

25. Ellinwood, "Amphetamine psychosis: a multi-dimensional process," p. 218.

26. S. Goldstone, W. K. Boardman, and W. T. Lhamon, "Effect of quinalbarbitone, dextro-amphetamine, and placebo on apparent time," *Br. J. Psychol.*, 49 (1958), 324-328.

27. R. C. Smith, "The world of the Haight-Ashbury speed freak," *J. Psychedelic Drugs*, 2:2 (1969), p. 79.

28. Ibid.; Carey and Mandel, "Bay Area 'speed' scene," p. 170.

29. Ellinwood, "Amphetamine psychosis: A multi-dimensional process," p. 216; Ellinwood, "Amphetamine psychosis: I. Description," p. 273-276.

30. Fiddle, "Circles beyond circumference," p. 83, 85.

31. D. McNeill, "An amphetamine apple in psychedelic Eden," *The Village Voice,* Feb. 2, 1967.

32. Carey and Mandel, "Bay Area 'speed' scene," p. 167.

33. Ellinwood, "Amphetamine psychosis: a multi-dimensional process," pp. 210, 217.

Chapter 5. Effects of Short- and Long-Term Use

1. Connell, *Amphetamine Psychosis*, pp. 31 (table 1), 37. Kalant, *The Amphetamines,* pp. 37-38.

2. Young and Scoville, "Paranoid psychosis in narcolepsy and the possible danger of Benzedrine treatment," p. 642.

3. Monroe and Drell, "Oral use of stimulants obtained from inhalers," pp. 909, 913; quotation p. 914.

4. Schneck, "Benzedrine psychosis: report of a case," pp. 60-61.

5. Norman and Shea, "Acute hallucinosis as a complication of addiction to amphetamine sulfate," pp. 270-271.

6. Shorvon, "Use of Benzedrine sulphate by psychopaths," pp. 285-286.

7. P. M. O'Flanagan and R. B. Taylor, "A case of recurrent psychosis associated with amphetamine addiction," *J. Ment. Sci.*, 96 (1950), 1033-1036.

8. Carr, "Acute psychotic reaction after inhaling methylamphetamine," p. 1476.

9. A. H. Chapman, "Paranoid psychosis associated with amphetamine usage: A clinical note," *Am. J. Psychiatry*, 111 (1954), 43.

10. M. Herman and S. H. Nagler, "Psychoses due to amphetamine," *J. Nerv. Ment. Dis.*, 120 (1954), 268-272.

11. Ellinwood, "Amphetamine psychosis: I. Description of the individuals and process," p. 277.

12. Ellinwood, "Amphetamine psychosis: a multi-dimensional process," p. 214.

13. F. A. Freyhan, "Craving for Benzedrine," *Del. Med. J.*, 21 (1949), 151-156. Ellinwood, "Amphetamine psychosis: I. Description," p. 273.

14. R. T. Rubin reports a similar case in "Acute psychotic reaction following ingestion of phentermine," *Am. J. Psychiatry,* 120 (1964), 1124-1125.

15. Johnson and Milner, "Psychiatric complications of amphetamine substances," pp. 252-263.

16. Connell, *Amphetamine Psychosis*, p. 64.

17. Ellinwood, "Amphetamine psychosis: a multi-dimensional process," p. 215; "Amphetamine psychosis: I. Description," pp. 281-282.

18. Kalant, *Amphetamines*, pp. 57, 58.

19. Connell, *Amphetamine Psychosis*, pp. 29, 52.

20. G. G. Wallis, J. F. McHarg, and O. C. A. Scott, "Acute psychosis caused by dextroamphetamine," *Br. Med. J., ii* (1949), 1394. Kalant, *Amphetamines,* p. 23. Connell, *Amphetamine Psychosis*, pp. 42-43. R. Carratala and J. C. Calzetta, and C. Ruiz Ogara cited in Kalant, *Amphetamines*, p. 26.

21. Knapp, "Amphetamine and addiction," p. 406. Hekimian and Gershon, "Characteristics," p. 126.

22. Kalant, *Amphetamines*, p. 69. H. J. Bakst, "Daily use of Benzedrine sulfate over a period of nine years," *U.S. Naval Med. Bull.*, 43 (1944), 1228-1231. Bloomberg, "End results of use of large doses of amphetamine sulfate over prolonged periods."

23. Askevold, "The occurrence of paranoid incidents and abstinence delirium

in abusers of amphetamine," p. 147. W. B. McConnell, "Amphetamine substances in mental illnesses in Northern Ireland," *Br. J. Psychiat.*, 109 (1963), 221. John Johnson and George Milner, "Amphetamine intoxication and dependence in admissions to a psychiatric unit," *Br. J. Psychiatry*, 112 (1966), 617-619. Rockwell and Ostwald, "Amphetamine use," pp. 613-614; amphetamine or methamphetamine was detected in the urine of 15 percent of their random sample.

24. Blumberg, Cohen, Heaton, and Klein, "Covert drug abuse among voluntary hospitalized psychatric patients," pp. 1659, 1660. M. Cohen and D. F. Klein, "Drug abuse in a young psychiatric population," *Am. J. Orthopsychiatry* 40 (1970), 448-455.

25. Kalant, *Amphetamines,* p. 48. See also W. R. Swanke, "Amphetamine abuse," *The New Physician* (July 1970), p. 595.

26. Carl Breitner, "Discussion" on Frederick Lemere's "The danger of amphetamine dependency," *Am. J. Psychiatry*, 123 (1966), 572.

27. Kramer, Fischman, and Littlefield, "Amphetamine abuse," p. 306.

28. J. D. Griffith, J. Cavanaugh, J. Held, and J. Oates, "Experimental psychosis Induced by the Administration of d-amphetamine," in Costa and Garattini, *International Symposium*, pp. 901-902.

29. D. S. Bell, "The experimental reproduction of amphetamine psychosis," *Arch. Gen. Psychiatry* 29 (1973), 35-40.

30. R. O. Pasnua, P. Naitch, S. Stier, and E. J. Kollar, "The psychological effects of 205 hours of sleep deprivation," *Arch. Gen. Psychiatry*, 18 (1968), 496-505.

31. Askevold, "Paranoid incidents," p. 162.

32. G. G. Young, C. B. Simson, and C. E. Frohman, "Clinical and biochemical studies of an amphetamine withdrawal psychosis," *J. Nerv. Ment. Dis.*, 132 (1961), 234-238. S. H. Snyder, "Catecholamines in the brain as mediators of amphetamine psychosis," *Arch Gen. Psychiatry*, 27 (1972), 169-179.

33. S. Tatetsu, "Methamphetamine psychosis," *Folia Psychiatr. Neurol. Jap. Suppl.*, 7 (1963), 377-380.

34. Ellinwood, "Amphetamine psychosis: a multi-dimensional process," p. 223.

35. Bell, "Comparison," p. 706.

36. Alles, "Some Relations between Chemical Structure and Physiological Action of Mescaline and Related Compounds," pp. 205-208.

37. S. H. Snyder, K. M. Taylor, J. T. Coyle, and J. L. Meyerhoff, "The role of brain dopamine in behavioral regulation and the actions of psychotropic drugs," *Am. J. Psychiatry*, 127 (1970), 201. B. M. Angrist and Samuel Gershon, "A pilot study of pathogenic mechanisms in amphetamine psychosis utilizing differentiai effects of d and l amphetamine," *Pharmakopsychiatrie Neuro-Psychopharmakologie* 4:2 (1971), 64-75.

38. The debate continues, however. A. Randrup of Denmark, summarizing many studies including his own, states that the stereotyped behavior caused by amphetamine abuse results from these drugs' influence on dopamine tracts in the corpus striatum, whereas the usual signs of behavioral excitation are manifestations of norepinephrine interactions, and certain bizarre postures in birds as well as head twitches in rats are caused by interference with serotonin levels and availability. Everett H. Ellinwood and Sidney Cohen, "(Meetings:) Amphetamine abuse," *Science*, 171 (1971), 420-421. See also A. Randrup and I. Munkvad, "Biochemical, Anatomical, and Psychological Investigations of Stereotyped Behavior Induced by Amphetamines," in Costa and Garattini, *International Symposium*, pp. 695-713; and E. Costa and A. Groppetti, "Biosynthesis and storage of catecholamines in tissues of rats injected with various doses of

d-amphetamine," in Costa and Garattini, *International Symposium*, pp. 231-255.

39. Kalant, *Amphetamines,* p. 60. Bell and Trethowan, "Amphetamine addiction," p. 492. Breitner, "The hazard of amphetamine medication," p. 218. Durrant, "Amphetamine addiction," pp. 649-651.

40. Robert Watson, Ernest Hartmann, and Joseph J. Schildkraut, "Amphetamine withdrawal: Affective state, sleep patterns, and MHPG excretion," *Am. J. Psychiatry,* 129 (1972), 263-269.

41. L. C. Smith, "Collapse with death following the use of amphetamine sulfate," *J.A.M.A.,* 113 (1939), 1022-1023.

42. A. J. Hertzog, A. E. Karlstrom, and M. J. Bechtel, "Accidental amphetamine sulfate poisoning," *J.A.M.A.,* 121 (1943), 256-257. O. L. Gericke, "Suicide by ingestion of amphetamine sulfate," *J.A.M.A.* 128 (1945), 1098-1099.

43. J. T. A. Lloyd and D. R. H. Walker, "Death after combined Dexamphetamine and Phenelzine," *Br. Med. J.* 2(1965), 168-169. Roger W. Jelliffe, Dennis Hill, Dorothy Tatter, Edward Lewis, Jr., "Death from weight-control pills: A case report with objective postmortem confirmation," *J.A.M.A.,* 208 (1969), 1846.

44. Zalis and Parmley, "Fatal amphetamine poisoning," p. 824.

45. B. H. Ong, "Dextroamphetamine poisoning," *New Eng. J. Med.,* 266 (1962), 1321-1322. Kalant, *Amphetmines,* p. 14. Connell, "Use and abuse of amphetamine," pp. 234-243.

46. Myerson, Loman and Dameshek, "Physiologic effects of Benzedrine and its relationship to other drugs affecting the autonomic nervous system," p. 570. S. L. Simpson, "Correspondence: Benzedrine," *Br. Med. J.,* 1 (1937), 93. J. N. Berry, "Acute myeloblastic leukemia in a Benzedrine addict," *Southern Med. J.,* 59 (1966), 1169-1170.

47. E. Fischer, "An unusual complication resulting from amphetamine sulfate (Benzedrine): A case report," *Med. J. Aust.* 46 (1959), 361.

48. R. H. Mattson and J. R. Calverly, "Dextroamphetamine-sulfate-induced dyskinesias."

49. S. C. Jordan and F. Hampson, "Amphetamine poisoning associated with hyperpyrexia," *Br. Med. J.,* 2 (1960), 844. See also Harvey, Todd, and Howard, "Fatality associated with Benzedrine ingestion," pp. 111-115; Zalis and Parmley, "Fatal amphetamine poisoning," p. 825.

50. Askew, "Hyperpyrexia as a contributory factor in the toxicity of amphetamine to aggregated mice." E. N. Greenblatt and A. C. Osterberg, "Correlations of activating and lethal effects of excitatory drugs in grouped and isolated mice," *J. Pharmacol.* 131 (1961), 115-119. D. I. Peterson, M. G. Hardinge, and B. E. Tilton, "Neuromuscular block as a possible mechanism of death in amphetamine poisoning," *J. Pharmacol. Exp. Ther.* 146 (1964), 175-179.

51. E. W. Anderson and W. C. M. Scott, "Cardiovascular effects of Benzedrine," *Lancet,* 2 (1936), 1461-1462.

52. Myerson, Loman, and Dameshek, "Physiologic effects of Benzedrine," pp. 561-563, 568-569. J. H. Fisher, "Correspondence: Cardiovascular effects of Benzedrine," *Lancet,* 1 (1937), 52.

53. Waud, "Effects of toxic doses of benzyl methyl carbinamine (Benzedrine) in man." G. A. Curry, "Amphetamine poisoning," *J.A.M.A.,* 140 (1949), 850.

54. Jorgen Malmquist, Erik Trell, Alf Torp, and Clas Lindstrom, "A case of drug-induced pulmonary hypertension," *Acta. Med. Scand.* 188 (1970), 271. Rumbaugh, Bergeron, Scanlan, Teal, Segall, Fang, and McCormick, "Cerebral vascular changes secondary to amphetamine abuse in the experimental animal," pp. 345-351.

55. H. H. Hahn, A. I. Schweid, and H. N. Beaty, "Complications of injecting

dissolved methylphenidate tablets," *Arch. Intern. Med.,* 123 (1969), 656-659. G. B. Hopkins and D. G. Taylor, "Pulmonary talc granulomatosis: A complication of drug abuse," *Am. Rev. Respir. Dis.,* 101 (1970), 101. William E. Atlee, Jr., "Talc and cornstarch emboli in eyes of drug abusers," *J.A.M.A.* 219 (1972), 49-51.

56. B. Philip Citron, Mordecai Halpern, Margaret McCarron, George D. Lundberg, Ruth McCormick, Irwin J. Pincus, Dorothy Tatter, and Bernard J. Haverback, "Necrotizing angiitis associated with drug abuse," *New Eng. J. Med.,* 283 (1970), 1003-1011.

57. Rumbaugh, Bergeron, Fang, and McCormick, "Cerebral angiographic changes in the drug abuse patient," pp. 335, 340, 341.

58. Rumbaugh et al., "Cerebral vascular changes," pp. 345-351.

59. S. J. Goodman and D. P. Becker, "Intracranial hemorrhage associated with amphetamine abuse," *J.A.M.A.,* 212 (1970), 480. S. R. Weiss, Robert Raskind, N. L. Morganstern. P. J. Pytlyk, T. C. Baiz, "Intracerebral and subarachnoid hemorrhage following use of methamphetamine ('speed')," *Int. Surg.,* 53 (1970), 124-125.

60. R. W. Bell, R. R. Drucker, and A. B. Woodruff, "The effects of prenatal injections of adrenalin chloride and *d*-amphetamine sulfate on subsequent emotionality and ulcer-proneness of offspring," *Psychon. Sci.,* 2 (1965), 269-270.

61. Editorial, "Drugs Under Suspicion," *Br. Med. J.,* 2 (1962), 1456. P. D. Moss, "Correspondence: Phenmetrazine and foetal abnormalities," *Br. Med. J.,* 2(1962), 1610. P. D. Powell, and J. M. Johnstone, "Correspondence: Phenmetrazine and foetal abnormalities," *Br. Med. J.,* 2 (1962), 1327.

62. J. J. Nora, A. H. Nora, R. J. Sommerville, R. M. Hill, and D. G. McNamara, "Maternal exposure to potential teratogens," *J.A.M.A.,* 202 (1967), 1065-1069.

Chapter 6. Habituation, Dependence, and Addiction

1. A. L. Tatum and M. H. Seevers, "Theories of drug addiction," *Physiol. Rev.,* 11 (1931), p. 108, as quoted in Seevers, "Medical perspectives on habituation and addiction," p. 93.

2. C. K. Himmelsbach and L. F. Small, "Clinical studies of drug addiction: II. 'Rossium' treatment of drug addiction," *Public Health Reports* (suppl. 125; 1937), as quoted in Seevers, p. 93.

3. World Health Organization Expert Committee on Addiction-Producing Drugs, *WHO Tech. Rep. Ser.,* 116 (1957), 9-10.

4. *Report of the Great Britain Interdepartmental Committee on Drug Addiction* ("Brain Report"), Ministry of Health and Department of Health for Scotland (London, Her Majesty's Stationery Office, 1961), p. 8 ¶ 20.

5. Council on Drugs of the American Medical Association, "New drugs and developments in therapeutics," *J.A.M.A.,* 183 (1963), 362-363.

6. World Health Organization, Expert Committee on Addiction-Producing Drugs, *WHO Tech. Rep. Ser.,* 273 (1964), 9, 14-15.

7. Kramer, Fischman, and Littlefield, "Amphetamine abuse," p. 307.

8. Ellis Stungo, "'Addiction' to anorexigenic drugs," *The Medical Press,* 246 (1961), 77-79.

9. J. Haguenau and W. Aubrun, "Intoxication chronique par le sulfate de Benzedrine," *Revue Neurologique,* 79 (1947), 129-131.

10. Kiloh and Brandon, "Habituation and addiction to amphetamines," pp. 40, 42.

11. Askevold, "Occurrence of paranoid incidents and abstinence delirium in abusers of amphetamine"; Lingeman, *Drugs from A to Z,* p. 6; M. H. Seevers, "Use, Misuse, and Abuse of Amphetamine-type Drugs from the Medical Viewpoint," in Russo, *Amphetamine Abuse,* p. 12. Ian Oswald, "Sleep and Dependence on Amphetamine and other Drugs," in Kales, *Sleep,* p. 322; Knapp, "Amphetamine and addiction," pp. 411, 412, 417. Beamish and Kiloh, "Psychoses due to amphetamine consumption"; Carey and Mandel, "San Francisco Bay area 'speed' scene," pp. 169, 170; Smith, Cline, and Williams, "Changing drug patterns in the Haight-Ashbury"; Sheehy, *Speed Is of the Essence,* p. 55; Zondek, "Amphetamine abuse and its relation to other drug addictions," pp. 233, 237; Waud, "Effects of toxic doses of benzyl methyl carbinamine." Carr, "Acute psychotic reaction after inhaling methyl-amphetamine."

12. Personal communication.

13. Laurie, *Drugs,* p. 23; H. W. Elliot, B. M. Tolbert, T. K. Adler, H. H. Anderson, "Excretion of carbon-14 by man after administration of morphine-N-methyl-C-14," *Proc. Soc. Exp. Biol. Med.,* 85 (1954), 77-81. Swanke, "Amphetamine abuse," p. 592; G. A. Alles and B. B. Wisegarver, "Amphetamine excretion studies in man," *Toxic. Appl. Pharmacol.,* 3 (1961), 678-688. H. Isbell and W. M. White, "Clinical characteristics of addictions," *Am. J. Med.,* 14 (1953), 561.

14. Ausubel, *Drug Addiction,* p. 23.

15. Isidor Chein, D. L. Gerard, R. S. Lee, and Elsa Rosenfeld, *Road to H: Narcotics, Delinquency, and Social Policy* (New York: Basic Books, 1964), p. 248.

16. Oswald and Thacore, "Amphetamine and phenmetrazine addiction," pp. 427, 428.

17. R. J. Berger, "The Sleep and Dream Cycle," in Kales, *Sleep,* pp. 17-32. S. R. Clemes and W. C. Dement, "Effect of REM sleep deprivation on psychological functioning," *J. Nerv. Ment. Dis.,* 144 (1967), 485-491.

18. Oswald and Thacore, "Amphetamine and phenmetrazine addiction," pp. 428, 430-431.

19. Oswald, "Sleep and Dependence," in Kales, *Sleep,* p. 325. See also ibid., pp. 320-322, 328, 329; Oswald, Jones, and Mannerheim, "Effects of two slimming drugs on sleep," pp. 797-798. Frederick Baekeland, "The effect of methyl phenidate on the sleep cycle in man," *Psychopharmacologia,* 10 (1966), 179-183. Rubin, "Acute psychotic reaction following ingestion of Phentermine." Hartmann, "Effect of four drugs on sleep patterns in man." M. M. Gross, Donald Goodenough, Michael Tobin, Eugene Halpert, Dominick Lepore, Abraham Perlstein, Milton Sirota, Joseph DiBianco, Ruth Fuller, and Ira Kishner, "Sleep disturbances and hallucinations in the acute alcoholic psychoses," *J. Nerv. Ment. Dis.,* 142 (1966), 493-514; Ramon Greenberg and Chester Pearlman, "Delirium tremens and dreaming," *Am. J. Psychiatry,* 124 (1967), 133-142.

20. A. F. Mirsky, "Some Comments on the Issue of Altered Consciousness in Drug Addiction," in Wittenborn, Smith, and Wittenborn, *Drugs and Youth: Proceedings of the Second Rutgers Symposium on Drug Abuse,* p. 140. And see Bradley and Elkes, "Effects of some drugs on the electrical activity of the brain"; B. K. Lester and R. Guerrero-Figueroa, "Effects of some drugs on electroencephalographic fast activity and dream time," *Psychophysiology,* 2 (1966), 224-236.

21. M. O. Akindele, J. Evans, and Ian Oswald, "Mono-amine oxidase inhibitors, sleep and mood," *Electroencephalogr. Clin. Neurophysiol.,* 29 (1970), 47-56; S. A. Lewis and Ian Oswald, "Overdose of tricyclic anti-depressants and deductions concerning their cerebral action," *Br. J. Psychiatry,* 115 (1969), 1403-1410.

22. H. Utena, T. Ezoe, N. Kato, and H. Hada, "Effects of chronic administration of methamphetamine in enzymic patterns in brain tissue," *J. Neurochem.*, 4 (1959), 161-169. Oswald, "Human brain protein, drugs and dreams"; p. 895 refers to A. Lajtha, "Protein metabolism of the nervous system," *Int. Rev. Neurobiol.*, 6 (1964), 1-98.

23. A. R. Lindesmith, "Basic Problems in the Social Psychology of Addiction and a Theory," in O'Donnell and Ball, eds. *Narcotic Addiction,* pp. 94-95, 100. And see A. Wikler, *Opiate Addiction: Psychological and Neurophysiological Aspects in Relation to Clinical Problems* (Springfield, Ill., 1953); A. Wikler, "Psychologic Bases of Drug Abuse," in *Proceedings: White House Conference on Narcotics and Drug Abuse*, Washington, D.C., September 27 and 28, 1962, pp. 150-151. J. R. Nichols, C. P. Headless, and H. W. Coppock, "Drug addiction I: Addiction by escape training," *J. Am. Pharm. Assoc.* (scientific ed.), 45 (1956), 788-791; J. R. Nichols and W. M. Davis, "Drug addiction II: Variation of addiction," *J. Am. Pharm. Assoc.* (scientific ed.), 48 (1959), 259-262; W. M. Davis and J. R. Nichols, "Physical dependence and sustained opiate-directed behavior in the rat," *Psychopharmacologia*, 3 (1962), 139-145.

24. Bejerot, *Addiction and Society*, pp. 23-24.

25. Oswald and Thacore, "Amphetamine and phenmetrazine addiction," p. 431.

26. Freyhan, "Craving for Benzedrine," p. 153. E. C. Reifenstein, Jr. and Eugene Davidoff, "The treatment of alcoholic psychoses with Benzedrine sulfate: Preliminary report," *J.A.M.A.*, 110 (1938), 1811-1812; S. Friedenberg, "Addiction to amphetamine sulfate," *J.A.M.A.*, 114 (1940), 956; Peterson and Somerville, "Excessive use of 'Benzedrine,' " p. 949; Cox and Smart, "Speed use," pp. 728-729; R. H. Berg, "Why Americans hide behind a chemical curtain," *Look* (Aug. 8, 1967), p. 12; Evans, "Psychosis," p. 154; Berchmans Rioux, "Is Ritalin an addiction-producing drug?" *Dis. Nerv. Syst.*, 21 (1960), 348; Kramer, Fischman, and Littlefield, "Amphetamine abuse," pp. 308-309; Kiloh and Brandon, "Habituation and addiction," pp. 40-42; Oswald and Thacore, "Amphetamine and phenmetrazine addiction," p. 431; J. L. Burn, "Addiction to amphetamines" (Correspondence) *Br. Med. J.*, 2(1962), 481; Knapp, "Amphetamine and addiction," pp. 411, 418. Kalant, *The Amphetamines*, pp. 77-132. Bejerot, *Addiction and Society*, pp. 80-82.

27. Ausubel, *Drug Addiction*, pp. 26-27; Ausubel, "Controversial issues in the management of drug addiction," pp. 535-544; Lingeman, *Drugs from A to Z*, p. 105.

28. Scher, "Patterns and profiles of addiction and drug abuse," p. 543; see also D. P. Ausubel, "The Dole-Nyswander treatment of heroin addiction," *J.A.M.A.*, 195 (1966), 949-950.

29. Chein et al., *Road to H*, p. 243.

30. O'Donnell and Ball, *Narcotic Addiction*, p. 58. The reference is to R. H. Turner, "The quest for universals in sociological research," *American Sociological Review*, 18 (1953), 605.

31. Ausubel, *Drug Addiction*, p. 27.

32. Travis Thompson and Warren Ostlund, Jr., "Susceptibility to readdiction as a function of the addiction and withdrawal environments," *J. Comp. Physiol. Psychol.*, 60 (1965), 388, 392.

33. Scher, "Patterns and profiles," p. 550. C. R. Schuster, W. S. Dockens, and J. H. Woods, "Behavioral variables affecting the development of amphetamine tolerance," *Psychopharmacologia* (Berlin), 9 (1966), 177.

34. Louria, *Drug Scene*, pp. 177-178; L. N. Robins and G. E. Murphy, "Drug use in a normal population of young negro men," *Am. J. Public Health*, 57

(1967), 1580-1596; C. Winick, "Maturing out of narcotic addiction," *UN Bulletin on Narcotics*, 14 (1962), 1-7; Scher, "Patterns and profiles," pp. 539, 550; Jordan Scher, "Group structure and narcotic addiction: Notes for a natural history," *Int. J. Group Psychother.*, 11 (1961), 88-93; Laurie, *Drugs*, pp. 141-148.

35. Ausubel, *Drug Addiction*, pp. 26, 35.

36. Cohen, *Drug Dilemma*, p. 107.

37. Ben Karpman, "Psychopathy in the scheme of human typology," *J. Nerv. Ment. Dis.*, 103 (1946), 276-288. S. B. Maughs, "A concept of psychopathy and psychopathic personality: Its evolution and historical development," *J. Crim. Psychopathol.*, 2 (1941), 329-356, 465-499; J. M. Caldwell, "Neurotic components of psychopathic behavior," *J. Nerv. Ment. Dis.*, 99 (1944), 134-148; I. Kavka, "Between psychosis and psychopathy," *J. Nerv. Ment. Dis.*, 106 (1947), 19-45.

38. Monroe and Drell, "Oral Use," p. 914; *Nomenclature and Method of Recording Diagnosis*, U.S. War Department Technical Bulletin (TB. Med. 203; Washington, Oct. 19, 1945).

39. H. B. Gwynn and W. M. Yater, "A study of the temporary use of therapeutic doses of Benzedrine sulfate in 147 supposedly normal young men (medical students)," *Med. Ann. D.C.*, 6 (1937), 356-359.

40. Blum, *Drugs II*, pp. 126-127.

41. Chein et al., *Road to H*, p. 358: "many addicts . . . continued at their jobs, with sufficient industry and deportment to satisfy their employers. If, however, they were unable to satisfy their self-induced need for drugs before going to work, they might be too restless and irritable (early symptoms of the withdrawal syndrome) to work or be late or absent from work because of many hours spent 'making a connection.' If addicts lose their jobs, it is because they could not regularly obtain drugs, not because the opiates made their work unsatisfactory to their employers."

42. Scher, "Patterns and profiles," p. 545; Melitta Schmideberg, "Socio-Psychological Factors in Drug Dependence," in Wilson, *Adolescent Drug Dependence*, p. 180.

43. C. W. M. Wilson, "The Patterns of Drug Abuse: The Clinical and Social Pharmacology of Drugs of Dependence," in Wilson, *Adolescent Drug Dependence*, pp. 427,428.

44. V. S. Fischmann, "Stimulant users in the California Rehabilitation Center," *Int. J. Addict.*, 3 (1968), 113-130.

45. Von Felsinger, Lasagna, and Beecher, "Drug-induced mood changes in man," pp. 1113-1114, 1118. See also confirmation in P. Hubin and J. Servais, "Etude des effets subjectifs de l'amphetamine chez l'homme en fonction de la personnalité," *Psychopharmacologia* (Berlin), 12 (1968), 239-249; C. M. Idestrom and D. Schalling, "Influence of Personality on Effects of Centrally Stimulating Drugs," in Sjöqvist and Tottie, *Abuse of Central Stimulants*, pp. 61-69.

46. Connell, *Amphetamine Psychosis*, pp. 62-63.

47. M. M. Glatt, letter to the editor, "Abuse of methylamphetamine," *Lancet*, ii (1968), 215. This physician also observed that "the position has changed so much that, though until about a year ago the expression '4 and 4' in addicts' slang meant gr. 4 of heroin and gr. 4 of cocaine it now stands for gr. 4 heroin and 4 ampoules of methylamphetamine."

48. Willey, "Abuse of methylphenidate," p. 464.

49. K. Rohl, "Zur frage der erzeugung von suchten durch 1-phenyl-2-methyl-aminopropanhydroclorid," *Arzneimittel-Forsch.*, 6 (1956), 402-406.

50. O'Donnell and Ball, *Narcotic Addiction*, p. 2; Isbell, "Historical development," pp. 157-158; Henry Brill, "Recurrent Patterns in the History of Drugs of Dependence and Some Interpretations," in Wittenborn, *Drugs and Youth*, pp. 10-13, 16, 21.

Chapter 7. Crime and Violence

1. H. J. Anslinger and C. R. Cooper, "Marijuana: Assassin of youth," *American Magazine*, 124 (July 1937), 150. For a discussion of this myth, see ch. 11, "Crime and Sexual Excess," in Grinspoon, *Marihuana Reconsidered*, pp. 291-322.

2. W. Bromberg, "Marihuana: A psychiatric study," *J.A.M.A.*, 113 (1939), 9, 10.

3. J. F. Siler, W. L. Sheep, L. B. Bates, G. F. Clark, G. W. Cook, and W. A. Smith, "Marijuana smoking in Panama," *The Military Surgeon*, 73 (1933), 279, 280.

4. W. Bromberg and T. C. Rodgers, "Marihuana and aggressive crime," *Am. J. Psychiatry*, 102 (1946), 825, 826.

5. R. N. Chopra and G. S. Chopra, "The present position of hemp drug addiction in India," *Indian Med. Res. Mem.*, 31 (1939), 92.

6. For valuable background material see Isbell, "Historical Development of Attitudes toward Opiate Addiction in the United States," pp. 157-169.

7. Bill Drake, *The Cultivator's Handbook of Marijuana* (Berkeley, 1970), pp. 85-88.

8. Straus, *Addicts and Drug Abusers*, pp. 20-21.

9. Ausubel, "Controversial issues in the management of drug addiction," p. 536.

10. Masaki, "Amphetamine problem in Japan," pp. 15, 19. H. Noda, "Concerning Wake-Amine intoxication" (Japanese), *Kurime Igakki Zasshi*, 13 (1950), 294-298. Nagahama, "Review of drug abuse and counter measures in Japan since World War II," p. 20.

11. *Task Force Report: Narcotics and Drug Abuse*, Task Force on Narcotics and Drug Abuse: The President's Commission on Law Enforcement and Administration of Justice, (Washington, 1967), p. 30. *Amphetamines: Fourth Report by the Select Committee on Crime*, p. 14; Dr. Kramer's quotation on p. 16.

12. Carey and Mandel, "Bay area 'speed' scene," p. 169.

13, Tinklenberg and Stillman, "Drug Use and Violence," p. 333.

14. Carey and Mandel, "Bay area 'speed' scene," p. 169.

15. Griffith, "Study of illicit amphetamine drug traffic in Oklahoma City," p. 565.

16. Angrist and Gershon, "Amphetamine abuse in New York City," p. 204.

17. M. M. O'Connor, "Law Enforcement and the Amphetamines," in Russo, *Amphetamine Abuse*, p. 92.

18. Scott and Willcox, "Delinquency and the amphetamines"; quotations pp. 873, 870-871.

19. E. H. Ellinwood, "Assault and homicide associated with amphetamine abuse," *Am. J. Psychiatry*, 127 (1971), 1170-1175. Copyright 1971, the American Psychiatric Association. Quotations are from pp. 1171, 1170, 1173.

20. Smith and Luce, *Love Needs Care*, pp. 19-21.

21. Smith, Cline and Williams, "Changing drug patterns in the Haight-Ashbury," p. 154.

22. Smith and Luce, *Love Needs Care*, pp. 22-23.

23. Tinklenberg and Stillman, "Drug use," p. 334.

24. Angrist and Gershon, "Amphetamine abuse," p. 205. Bell and Trethowan, "Amphetamine addiction," pp. 493, 495.

25. Ellinwood, "Assault and homicide," p. 1172. Ellinwood, "Amphetamine psychosis," p. 275.

26. Tinklenberg and Stillman, "Drug use," pp. 335-336.

27. *Amphetamines: Fourth Report*, pp. 14-15.

28. O'Connor, "Law enforcement," p. 92.

29. R. C. Smith, "The world of the Haight-Ashbury speed freak," *J. Psychedelic Drugs,* 2 (1969), p. 81.

Chapter 8. The Place of Amphetamines in Medicine

1. Bett, "Benzedrine sulphate in clinical medicine," pp. 205, 216, 217.

2. Fazekas, Ehrmantraut, Campbell, and Negron, "Comparative effectiveness of phenylpropanolamine and dextroamphetamine on weight reduction," p. 1018. Kalant, *The Amphetamines,* p. 66. Harris, "Clinically useful appetite depressants," pp. 128-129. Modell and Reader, "Anorexiants," pp. 287-288.

3. R. H. Williams, W. H. Daughaday, W. F. Rogers, S. P. Asper, B. T. Towery, "Obesity and its treatment, with particular reference to the use of anorexigenic compounds," *Ann. Intern. Med.,* 29 (1948), 512. See also L. J. Cass, "Evaluation of appetite suppressants," *Ann. Intern. Med.,* 51 (1959), 1295.

4. Harris, Ivy, and Searle, "Mechanism of amphetamine induced loss of weight," pp. 1468, 1471-1472. John R. Brobeck, Joy Tepperman, and C. N. H. Long, "Experimental hypothalamic hyperphagia in the albino rat," *Yale J. Biol. Med.,* 15 (1943), 831-853.

5. Bahnsen, Jacobsen, and Thesleff, "Subjective effect of beta-phenylisopropylaminsulfate on normal adults," 89-131. Mark F. Lesses and Abraham Myerson, "Human autonomic pharmacology: XVI. Benzedrine sulfate as an aid in treatment of obesity," *New Eng. J. Med.,* 218 (1938), 119-124; P. Rosenberg, "Clinical use of Benzedrine sulfate (amphetamine) in obesity," *Medical World* (London), 57 (1939), 656.

6. Harris, Ivy, and Searle, "The Mechanism," pp. 1468-1469, 1470.

7. W. Harding LeRiche and A. Csima, "Sustained release appetite suppressant combined with reducing diet," *Applied Therapeutics,* 7 (1965), 226-228.

8. Adlersberg and Mayer, "Results of prolonged medical treatment of obesity with diet alone, diet and thyroid preparations, and diet and amphetamine." E. Philip Gelvin and Thomas H. McGavack, "Dexedrine and weight reduction," *N.Y. State J. Med.,* 49 (1949), 280-282.

9. Harris, Ivy, and Searle, "The Mechanism," pp. 1469-1471.

10. R. P. Shapiro and K. I. Michaile, "The use of a sustained-release d-amphetamine-amobarbital preparation in the treatment of obesity," *International Record of Medicine and General Practice Clinics,* 169 (1956), 638-641; William Drayton, Jr., "Recognition and management of the depressed mental state," *Penn. Med. J.,* 54 (1951), 949-953; Philip Rosenberg, "The use of mood ameliorating agents in the treatment of psychogenic obesity," *Am. Practitioner,* 4 (1953), 818 (quoted). H. Necheles and H. Sorter, "Balanced amphetamine and sedative combination in the treatment of obesity," *Lancet,* i (1957), 215-216. "Anorectics have limited use in treatment of obesity," *F.D.A. Drug Bulletin,* Rockville, Md., U.S. Dept. of Health, Education, and Welfare, 1972.

11. Modell, "Status and prospect of drugs for overeating," p. 1133.

12. I. H. Kupersmith, "Value of ephedrine-ethylenediamine as an appetite depressant: Comparison with d-amphetamine sulfate," *Curr. Ther. Res.* 2 (1960) 39-42.

13. Freed and Hays, "A new nonamphetamine anorectic agent," pp. 57, 59.

14. Ibid, p. 55. Modell, "Status and prospect of drugs for overeating," p. 1135. Modell and Reader, "Anorexiants," p. 289.

15. J. W. Finch, "The overweight obstetric patient with special reference to the use of Dexedrine sulfate," *J. Okla. State Med. Assoc.,* 40 (1947), 119-122.

16. Oswald, Jones, and Mannerheim, "Effects of two slimming drugs on

sleep," p. 796. See also Ian Oswald, "Sleep and Dependence on Amphetamine and Other Drugs," in Kales, *Sleep*, pp. 321, 322, 326; J. C. LeDouarec and C. Neveu, "Pharmacology and Biochemistry of Fenfluramine," in Costa and Garattini, *International Symposium*, pp. 77-83, 89, 91; Edward Woodward, Jr., "Clinical Experience with Fenfluramine in the United States," in Costa and Garattini, pp. 684-691; J. F. Munro, D. A. Seaton, and L. J. P. Duncan, "Treatment of refractory obesity with fenfluramine," *Br. Med. J.*, 2 (1966), 624-625.

17. "Anorectics have limited use," *F.D.A. Drug Bulletin.*

18. Louis Lasagna, "Attitudes toward appetite suppressants: A survey of U.S. physicians," *J.A.M.A.*, 225 (1973), 44-48.

19. *Amphetamines: Fourth Report*, p. 5. Prepared testimony of A. Goldstein, Chairman, Huntington Narcotics Guidance Council before the Subcommittee to Investigate Juvenile Delinquency of the Committee on the Judiciary, United States Senate, 92nd Congress, 1st Session, Feb. 7, 1972, p. 129. Zarcone, "Narcolepsy," p. 1161. R. E. Yoss and D. D. Daly, "Narcolepsy," *Med. Clin. N. Amer.*, 44 (1960), 953-968.

20. Edith Krabbe and Gudmund Magnussen, "On narcolepsy: I. Familial narcolepsy," *Acta Psychiatrica Neurologica*, 17 (1942), 173. D. D. Daly and R. E. Yoss, "A Family with Narcolepsy," *Proceedings of the Staff Meetings of the Mayo Clinic*, 34 (1959), 318.

21. Zarcone, "Narcolepsy."

22. Myron Prinzmetal and Wilfred Bloomberg, "The use of Benzedrine for the treatment of narcolepsy," *J.A.M.A.*, 105 (1935), 2052. H. Ulrich, C. E. Trapp, and B. Vidgoff, "The treatment of narcolepsy with Benzedrine sulphate," *Ann. Intern. Med.*, 9 (1936), 1213-1221. Shapiro, "Benzedrine," p. 31. Bloomberg, "End results of use of large doses of amphetamine sulfate over prolonged periods." D. M. Williamson, "A case of long-standing narcolepsy in a coalminer," *The Practitioner*, 193 (1964), 69-70.

23. A. Rechtschaffen and W. C. Dement, "Narcolepsy and Hypersomnia," in Kales, *Sleep*, p. 126.

24. Wheatley, "Amphetamines in general practice," pp. 163-173; J. E. Overall, L. E. Hollister, M. Johnson, and V. Pennington, "Nosology of depression and differential response to drugs," *J.A.M.A.*, 195 (1966), 846-848; B. J. Goldstein and B. Brauzer, "Pharmacologic considerations in the treatment of anxiety and depression in medical practice," *Med. Clin. N. Am.*, 55 (1971), 485-494.

25. Guttmann, "Effect of Benzedrine on depressive states." Peoples and Guttmann, "Hypertension produced with Benzedrine," p. 1109. E. Guttmann and W. Sargant, "Observations on Benzedrine," *Br. Med. J.*, 1 (1937), 1013-1015.

26. D. L. Wilbur, A. R. MacLean, and E. V. Allen, "Clinical observations and the effect of Benzedrine sulphate," *Proceedings of the Staff Meetings of the Mayo Clinic*, 12 (1937), 97-104.

27. Eugene Davidoff and E. C. Reifenstein, Jr., "The results of eighteen months of Benzedrine sulfate therapy in psychiatry," *Am. J. Psychiatry*, 52 (1939), 945-970. Schube, McManamy, Trapp, and Myerson, "Effect of Benzedrine sulphate on certain abnormal mental states." Nathanson, "Central action of beta-aminopropylbenzene." F. J. Braceland, "Stimulants and tranquilizers: Their use and abuse," *Bull. N.Y. Acad. Med.*, 39 (1963), 661.

28. Bett, "Benzedrine sulfate," pp. 205-218; R. L. Gorrell, "The uses of Benzedrine sulfate in general practice," *J. Iowa State Med. Soc.*, 29 (1939), 451. Leake, *Amphetamines*, pp. 67-69. M. H. Johnson, "Drugs in the management of depression, " *Northwest Medicine*, 69 (1970), 780-784.

29. Erich Lindemann, "The psychopathological effect of sodium Amytal," *Proc. Soc. Exper. Biol. Med.*, 28 (1931), 864-866; E. Lindemann, "Psychological

changes in normal and abnormal individuals under the influence of sodium Amytal," *Am. J. Psychiatry*, 11 (1932), 1083-1091. Myerson, "Reciprocal pharmacologic effects of amphetamine (Benzedrine) sulphate and the barbiturates," p. 562.

30. Gottlieb, "Use of sodium Amytal and Benzedrine sulfate in the symptomatic treatment of depressions," pp. 50-52; Gottlieb and Coburn, "Psychopharmacologic study of schizophrenia and depressions," p. 261; Gottlieb, Bobbitt, and Freidinger, "Psychopharmacologic study of schizophrenia and depressions," pp. 104-114.

31. Breitner, "Hazard of amphetamine medication," p. 218. Wheatley, "Amphetamines in general practice."

32. A. L. Natenshon, "Clinical evaluation of Ritalin," *Dis. Nerv. Syst.*, 17 (1956), 394. A. Jacobson, "The use of Ritalin in psychotherapy of depressions of the aged," *Psychiatr. Q.*, 32 (1958), 474-483. M. E. Landman, R. Preisig, and M. Perlman, "A practical mood stimulant," *J. Med. Soc. N.J.*, 55 (1958), 55-58.

33. F. J. Ayd, Jr., "A clinical evaluation of methyl-phenydilacetate hydrochloride (Ritalin)," *Journal Clinical & Experimental Psychopathology & Quarterly Review of Psychiatry & Neurology*, 18 (1957), 342-346; A. A. Robin and S. Wiseberg, "A controlled trial of methyl phenidate (Ritalin) in the treatment of depressive states," *J. Neurol. Neurosurg. Psychiatry*, 21 (1958), 57. Nathan Thal, "Cumulative index of antidepressant medications," *Dis. Nerv. Syst.*, 20 (1959), 201.

34. Schildkraut, "Catecholamine hypothesis of affective disorders."

35. Thal, "Cumulative Index." Hare, Dominian, and Sharpe, "Phenelzine and Dexamphetamine," p. 11. J. W. L. Doust, D. J. Lewis, A. Miller, D. Sprott, and R. L. D. Wright, "Controlled assessment of antidepressant drugs, including Tofranil," *Can. Psychiatr. Assoc. J.*, 4 (1959), Suppl. 190-194. J. E. Overall, L. E. Hollister, A. D. Pokorny, J. F. Casey, and G. Katz, "Drug therapy in depressions: Controlled evaluation of imipramine, isocarboxazine, dextroamphetamine-amobarbital, and placebo, *Clin. Pharmacol. Ther.*, 3 (1962) pp. 16-21.

36. Harbans Lal, Surendra K. Puri, and George C. Fuller, "Inhibition of hepatic hexobarbital metabolism by dextroamphetamine, *Psychopharmacologia*, 16 (1970), 395-398. See also L. K. Garrettson, J. M. Perel, and P. G. Dayton, "Methylphenidate interaction with both anticonvulsants and ethyl biscoumacetate: A new action of methylphenidate," *J.A.M.A.*, 207 (1969), 2053-2056; J. M. Perel, N. Black, R. N. Wharton, and S. Malitz, "Inhibition of imipramine metabolism by methylphenidate," *Fed. Proc.*, 28 (1969), 418.

37. R. N. Wharton, J. M. Perel, P. G. Dayton, and Sidney Malitz, "A potential clinical use for methylphenidate with tricyclic antidepressants," *Am. J. Psychiatry*, 127 (1971), 1619-1625.

38. Philip Zeidenberg, James M. Perel, Maureen Kanzler, Ralph N. Wharton, and Sidney Malitz, "Clinical and metabolic studies with imipramine in man," *Am. J. Psychiatry*, 127 (1971), 1321-1326.

39. S. Brandon and D. Smith, "Amphetamines in general practice," *Journal of the College of General Practitioners*, 5 (1962), 603-606.

Chapter 9. The Treatment of Hyperkinetic Children

1. "Omaha Pupils Given 'Behavior' Drugs," *Washington Post*, June 29, 1970, pp. 1, 8. *Federal Involvement in the Use of Behavior Modification Drugs on Grammar School Children of the Right to Privacy Inquiry*, pp. 16, 53 (letter from

M. J. Ryan, Director, Office of Legislative Services, Department of Health, Education, and Welfare, Public Health Service, FDA, Aug. 6, 1970, sent to Mr. Ernie Chambers, Omaha, and submitted as testimony); "Treatment for fidgety kids? A story of drug use in Omaha kicks up national fuss with some racial overtones," *National Observer,* July 6, 1970, pp. 1, 5.

2. Hunsinger, "School storm," pp. 1, 6, 10 (testimony of Dr. Ronald Lipman, FDA); Laufer, "Long-term management and some follow-up findings on the use of drugs with minimal cerebral syndromes," pp. 521-522.

3. Hentoff, "Drug-pushing in the schools," p. 21.

4. Quoted material from Hentoff, p. 20, and Hunsinger.

5. Eric Denhoff, "To medicate—to debate—or to validate," editorial, *J. Learn. Dis.,* 4 (1971), 469. Selznick quoted in Sue Miller, "Use of tranquilizers by city pupils reported increasing," Baltimore *Evening Sun,* Oct. 2, 1970, p. c-2. See also Eisenberg, "Symposium: Behavior modification by drugs," p. 710; M. A. Stewart, F. N. Pitts, A. G. Craig, and W. Dierof, "The hyperactive child syndrome," *Am. J. Orthopsychiatry,* 36 (1966), 861; M. A. Stewart, "Hyperactive children," *Sci. Am.* (April 1970), p. 94; H. F. R. Prechtl and C. J. Stemmer, "The choreiform syndrome in children," *Dev. Med. Child Neurol.,* 4 (1962), 119; H. R. Huessey, "Study of the prevalence and therapy of the hyperkinetic syndrome in public school children in rural Vermont," *Acta Paedopsychiatr.,* 34 (1967), p. 130.

6. Bradley, "Behavior of children receiving Benzedrine," pp. 578, 579, 582.

7. Conners, "Effect of Dexedrine on rapid discrimination and motor control of hyperkinetic children under mild stress," p. 432. Bradley, "Benzedrine and Dexedrine in the treatment of children's behavior disorders," p. 35.

8. Molitch and Sullivan, "Effect of Benzedrine sulfate on children taking the New Stanford Achievement Test."

9. Bradley, "Behavior of children receiving Benzedrine," pp. 578, 582. See also Molitch and Sullivan, "Effect of Benzedrine sulfate on children," p. 521.

10. Cutler, Little, and Strauss, "Effect of Benzedrine on mentally deficient children." Bradley and Bowen, "Amphetamine (Benzedrine) therapy of children's behavior disorders."

11. Bender and Cottington, "Use of amphetamine sulfate (Benzedrine) in child psychiatry." S. R. Korey, "The effects of Benzedrine sulfate on the behavior of psychopathic and neurotic juvenile delinquents," *Psychiatr. Q.* 18 (1944), 127-137.

12. Benjamin Pasamanick, "Anticonvulsant drug therapy of behavior problem children with abnormal electroencephalograms," *Arch. Neurol. Psychiatry,* 65 (1951), 763.

13. Kahn and Cohen, "Organic drivenness: A brain-stem syndrome and an experience," pp. 749, 752.

14. Laufer, Denhoff, and Solomons, "Hyperkinetic impulse disorder in children's behavior problems," p. 38. Henri Gastaut, "Combined photic and Metrazol activation of the brain," *Electroencephalogr. Clin. Neurophysiol.,* 2 (1950), 256-258.

15. Gabrielle Weiss, John Werry, Klaus Minde, Virginia Douglas, and Donald Sykes, "Studies on the hyperactive child: V. The effects of Dextroamphetamine and Chlorpromazine on behavior and intellectual functioning," *J. Child Psychol. Psychiatry,* 9 (1968), 148, 150-151, 153.

16. Eisenberg, Conners, and Sharpe, "A controlled study of the differential application of outpatient psychiatric treatment for children."

17. Epstein, Lasagna, Conners, and Rodriguez, "Correlation of dextroamphetamine excretion and drug response in hyperkinetic children," p. 141.

18. Eisenberg, Lachman, Molling, Lockner, Mizelle, and Conners, "A psychopharmacologic experiment in a training school for delinquent boys," pp. 432, 439-441, 443-445.

19. Conners and Eisenberg, "Effects of methylphenidate on symptomatology and learning in disturbed children," pp. 459-461. See also Conners, Eisenberg, and Sharpe, "Effects of methylphenidate (Ritalin) on paired-associate learning and Porteus Maze performance in emotionally disturbed children."

20. Conners, Rothschild, Eisenberg, Schwartz, and Robinson, "Dextroamphetamine sulfate in children with learning disorders: Effects on perception, learning, and achievement," pp. 183, 186-188.

21. Sprague, Barnes, and Werry, "Methylphenidate and Thioridazine: Learning, reaction time, activity, and classroom behavior in disturbed children." J. G. Millichap, F. Aymat, L. H. Sturgis, K. W. Larsen, and R. A. Egan, "Hyperkinetic behavior and learning disorders: III. Battery of neuropsychological tests in controlled trial of Methylphenidate," *Am. J. Dis. Child.*, 116 (1968), 235-244. J. G. Millichap and E. E. Boldrey, "Studies in hyperkinetic behavior: II. Laboratory and clinical evaluations of drug treatments," *Neurology*, 17 (1967), 468-469. McConnell and Cromwell, "Studies in activity level: VII. Effects of amphetamine drug administration on the activity level of retarded children."

22. Conners, Eisenberg, and Barcai, "Effect of dextroamphetamine on children," pp. 478, 483, 484. See also C. K. Conners, Leon Eisenberg, and A. Barcai, "Effect of dextroamphetamine on children: Studies on subjects with learning disabilities and school behavior problems," *Arch. Gen. Psychiatry*, 17 (1967), 482-484; C. K. Conners, "A teacher rating scale for use in drug studies with children," *Am. J. Psychiatry*, 126 (1969), 886-888.

23. A. A. Strauss and N. C. Kephart, *Psychopathology and Education of the Brain-Injured Child.* Vol II. *Progress in Theory and Clinic* (New York: Grune and Stratton, 1955), pp. 135-139. Sykes, Douglas, Weiss, and Minde, "Attention in hyperactive children and the effect of methylphenidate (Ritalin)." H. E. Rosvold, A. F. Mirsky, I. Sarason, E. D. Bransome, and L. H. Beck, "A continuous performance test of brain damage," *J. Consult. Psychol.*, 20 (1956), 343-350.

24. Stimulant-related improvement on the Porteus Maze has been cited as evidence that stimulants potentiate the inhibition of impulsive responding. Since impulsivity is one of the most disturbing elements of the hyperkinetic syndrome, great import has been attributed to this finding. See Sykes, Douglas, Weiss, and Minde, "Attention in hyperactive children," p. 129.

25. Eisenberg, Conners, and Sharpe, "A controlled study of the differential application."

26. Conners, Rothschild, Eisenberg, Schwartz, and Robinson, "Dextroamphetamine sulfate in children with learning disorders."

27. In a group of seventy-six black boys, between the ages of six and a half and eleven, referred to an outpatient clinic for symptoms of hyperactivity, impulsivity, poor attentional span, and poor academic performance, those given dextroamphetamine (average 25 mg per day) did significantly better on the WISC performance IQ than those given placebo. (Greenberg, Deem, and McMahon, "Effects of dextroamphetamine, chlorpromazine, and hydroxyzine," pp. 534-535, table 4.) But in a group of white children of the same age with similar symptoms, there was *no* significant difference between WISC performance IQ scores between dextroamphetamine (maximum 20 mg per day) and placebo groups. (G. Weiss, K. K. Minde, J. S. Werry, V. I. Douglas, and E. Nemeth, "Studies on the hyperactive child: VIII. Five-year follow-up," *Arch. Gen. Psychiatry*, 24 [1971], 145-146.) Results on the Bender-Gestalt Visual-Motor Perceptual tests showed no significant drug effects in either study.

28. Conners, "Symposium: Behavior modification by drugs," p. 708.

29. Laufer, Denhoff, and Solomons, "Hyperkinetic impulse disorder," pp. 45, 47.

30. Bradley, "Effect of some drugs on the electrical activity of the brain of the conscious cat," p. 21. H. W. Magoun, "An ascending reticular activating system in the brain stem," *Arch. Neurol. Psychiatry*, 67 (1952), 145-154.

31. Bradley and Elkes, "Effects of some drugs on the electrical activity of the brain," p. 111; Bradley and Key, "Effect of drugs on arousal responses produced by electrical stimulation of the reticular formation of the brain." Conan Kornetsky, "Psychoactive drugs in the immature organism," *Psychopharmacologia* (Berlin), 17 (1970), 128.

32. G.D. Davis, "Effects of central excitant and depressant drugs on locomotor activity in the monkey," *Am. J. Physiol.*, 188 (1957), 619. R. A. Blum, J. S. Blum, and K. L. Chow, "Production of convulsions by administration of Benzedrine following brain operations in monkeys," *Arch. Neurol. Psychiatry*, 64 (1950), 685; M. W. Adler, "Changes in sensitivity to amphetamine in rats with chronic brain lesions," *J. Pharmacol. Exp. Ther.*, 134 (1961), 214-221.

33. Conners, "Effect of Dexedrine on rapid discrimination and motor control," p. 432.

34. Bradley, "Benzedrine and Dexedrine in the treatment of children's behavior disorders," p. 32. Levy, "The hyperkinetic child—A forgotten entity, its diagnosis and treatment." Mattson and Calverly, "Dextroamphetamine sulfate-induced dyskinesias." H. H. Eveloff, "A case of amphetamine-induced dyskinesia," *J.A.M.A.*, 204 (1968), 933. P. G. Ney, "Psychosis in a child associated with amphetamine administration," *Can. Med. Assoc. J.*, 97 (1967), 1026-1029.

35. A. R. Lucas and M. Weiss, "Methylphenidate hallucinosis," *J.A.M.A.*, 217 (1971), 1079-1081.

36. Harry Bakwin, "Benzedrine in behavior disorders of children," *J. Pediat.*, 32 (1948), 216; Molitch and Sullivan, "Effect of Benzedrine sulfate on children," pp. 519-522; Bradley and Bowen, "Amphetamine (Benzedrine) therapy," p. 100; Bradley, "Benzedrine and Dexedrine in the treatment of children's behavior disorders," p. 32; Levy, "The hyperkinetic child," pp. 330-336. Weiss, "Studies on the hyperactive child," p. 152; Greenberg, Deem, and McMahon, "Effects of dextroamphetamine, chlorpromazine, and hydroxyzine on behavior and performance in hyperactive children," pp. 533-534; Conners et al., "Dextroamphetamine sulfate in children with learning disorders," p. 183; Epstein et al., "Correlation of dextroamphetamine excretion and drug response," p. 142. Greenberg et al., "Effects of dextroamphetamine, chlorpromazine, and hydroxyzine," pp. 533, 536; McConnell and Cromwell, "Studies in activity level," p. 650. A. DiMascio, J. J. Soltys, and R. I. Shader, "Psychotropic Drug Effects in Children," in R. I. Shader and A. DiMascio, eds., *Psychotropic Drug Side Effects,* (Baltimore: Williams and Wilkins, 1970), p. 255.

37. Safer, Allen, and Barr, "Depression of growth in hyperactive children on stimulant drugs," pp. 218-219.

38. Leon Eisenberg, "The hyperkinetic child and stimulant drugs," *New Eng. J. Med.*, 287 (1972), 249.

39. S. D. Clements, *Task Force I: Minimal Brain Dysfunction in Children*, National Institute of Neurological Diseases and Blindness, Monograph no. 3 (Washington: Department of Health, Education and Welfare, 1966), pp. 9-10; italics added.

40. C. J. Weithorn, "Hyperactivity and the CNS: An etiological and diagnostic dilemma," *J. Learn. Dis.*, 6 (1973), 44.

41. Fish, "The 'one child, one drug' myth of stimulants in hyperkinesis," p. 193.

42. Maurice W. Laufer and Eric Denhoff, "Hyperkinetic behavior syndrome in children," *J. Pediatr.*, 50 (1957), p. 470. Bender and Cottington, "Use of amphetamine sulfate," pp. 116-121. Barbara Fish, "Drug therapy in child psychiatry: Pharmacological aspects," *Compr. Psychiatry*, 1 (1960), 219-223.

43. Fish, "'One child, one drug' myth," p. 198. Conners et al., "Dextroamphetamine sulfate in children with learning disorders," p. 188.

44. Conners et al., "Effect of dextroamphetamine on children," pp. 478-485.

45. Satterfield, Lesser, Saul, and Cantwell, "EEG aspects in the diagnosis and treatment of minimal brain dysfunction."

46. J. S. Werry and R. L. Sprague, "Hyperactivity," in C. G. Costello, ed., *Symptoms of Psychopathology* (New York: Wiley, 1970), p. 398. Fish, " 'One child, one drug' myth," pp. 197, 198.

47. Ladd, "Pills for classroom peace?," pp. 66-68, 81-83. Careth Ellingson, "The children with no alternative," *Saturday Review*, 53 (Nov. 21, 1970), 67.

48. Ladd, "Pills for classroom peace?," p. 81.

49. *Report of the Conference on the Use of Stimulant Drugs in the Treatment of Behaviorally Disturbed Young School Children,* p. 529.

50. Letter from Robert Pulliam, Program Director of the Biological Sciences Communication Project, sent to Satu Repo, Oct. 12, 1971; printed in Rapoport and Repo, "The Educator as Pusher," pp. 96, 97, 99.

51. Ibid., p. 97.

52. R. D. Freeman, "Drug effects on learning in children: A selective review of the past thirty years," *Journal of Special Education*, 1 (1966), 17-44 and "Review of medicine in special education: Another look at drugs and behavior," ibid., 4 (1970), 377-384. A. M. Freedman, A. S. Effron, and L. Bender, "Pharmacology in children with psychiatric illness," *J. Nerv. Ment. Dis.*, 122 (1955), 479-486; H. R. Alderton and B. A. Hoddinott, "A controlled study of the use of thioridazine in the treatment of hyperactive and aggressive children in a children's psychiatric hospital," *Can. Psychiatr. Assoc. J.*, 9 (1964), 239-247; J. S. Werry, G. Weiss, V. Douglas, and J. Martin, "Studies on the hyperactive child: III. The effect of chlorpromazine upon behavior and learning ability," *J. Am. Acad. Child Psychiatry*, 5 (1966), 292-312. "Graded imipramine regiment favored in hyperkinetic children," *J.A.M.A.*, 208 (1969), 1613-1614. D. Brown, B. G. Winsberg, I. Bialer, and M. Press, "Imipramine therapy and seizures: Three children treated for hyperactive behavior disorders," *Am. J. Psychiatry*, 130 (1973), 210-212.

53. Novack, "Educator's view of medication and classroom behavior," p. 507.

54. Laufer, "Long-term management and some follow-up findings," pp. 519-522. Weiss et al., "Studies on the hyperactive child," pp. 409-414.

55. W. Mendelson, N. Johnson, and M. A. Stewart, "Hyperactive children as teenagers: A follow-up study," *J. Nerv. Ment. Dis.*, 153 (1971), 273-279.

56. Novack, "Educator's view," p. 508. Werry and Sprague, "Hyperactivity," p. 408.

57. S. G. Doubros and G. J. Daniels, "An experimental approach to the reduction of overactive behavior," *Behav. Res. Ther.*, 4 (1966), 251-258; G. R. Patterson, R. Jones, J. Whittier, and M. A. Wright, "A behavior modification technique for the hyperactive child," *Behav. Res. Ther.*, 2 (1965), 217-226. D. A. Overton, "State-dependent learning produced by depressant and atropine-like drugs," *Psychopharmacology*, 10 (1966), 6-31; N. E. Miller, "Some animal experiments pertinent to the problem of combining psychotherapy with drug therapy," *Compr. Psychiatry*, 7 (1966), 1-12; R. K. Turner and G. C. Young, "CNS stimulant drugs and conditioning treatment of nocturnal enuresis: A long-term follow-up study," *Behav. Res. Ther.*, 4 (1966), 225-228.

Chapter 10. Living With Speed

1. Gross, *The Doctors*, p. 510. Lasagna, *Doctor's Dilemmas*, p. 140. W. B. Bean, "Recent setbacks in medicine," *Northwest Medicine*, 55 (1956), 158.

2. Gaffin, *Attitudes of U.S. Physicians*, p. 20, c-16. Pharmaceutical Manufacturers Association, *Survey of Physicians*, (Washington, 1960), quoted in J. J. Harris, "Survey of medical communication sources available for continuing physician education," *J. Med. Educ.*, 41 (1966), 739.

3. Garai, "Advertising and Promotion of Drugs," in Talalay, *Drugs in our Society*, pp. 191-192, 199.

4. J. L. Goddard, testimony before the House Intergovernmental Relations Subcommittee, House Committee on Government Operations, May 25, 1966, p. 1896; see also Goddard, "Drug establishment," *Esquire*, (March 1969), pp. 117-121, 151-153; these figures are also cited by F. J. Ingelfinger, "Annual discourse—Swinging copy and sober science," *New Eng. J. Med.*, 281 (1969), 527. U.S. Senate, *Study of Administered Prices*, p. 157. Dowling, *Medicines for Man*, p. 122, referring to *Study of Administered Prices*. Richard Burack, *The New Handbook of Prescription Drugs* (New York: Pantheon, 1970), pp. 17-23.

5. "Medical advertising—Sales tools, postgraduate course for M.D.," *Advertising Age* (Jan. 15, 1963), pp. 216-219. Mintz, *By Prescription Only*, pp. 66, 79.

6. Information on finances is from U.S. Senate, *Hearings on Drug Industry Antitrust Act*, part 1, pp. 126-127, 129; part 2, p. 530.

7. For a discussion of the drug evaluation matter see Dowling, *Medicines for Man*, pp. 166-177; quotation p. 177.

8. Mintz, *By Prescription Only*, pp. 79-80, 92a.

9. Gross, *The Doctors*, p. 499. "Apothecaries undismayed," editorial, *New Eng. J. Med.*, 269 (1963), 480-481. Deno, Rowe, and Brodie, *Profession of Pharmacy*, p. 166.

10. U.S. Senate, *Hearings on Administered Prices: Drugs*, part 18, p. 10453.

11. Solomon Garb, "The reaction of medical students to drug advertising," *New Eng. J. Med.* (special article), 259 (1958), 121-122; "The student looks at drug advertising," editorial, *New Eng. J. Med.*, 259 (1958), 143-144; Solomon Garb, "Teaching medical students to evaluate drug advertising," *J. Med. Educ.*, 35 (1960), 729-739.

12. A. H. Robins Company, "Yardley Crabgrass gets 'Nervous Indigestion' over . . ." (advertisement), *Drug Therapy*, 1 (August 1971), 24-25.

13. Robert Seidenberg, "Advertising and abuse of drugs," editorial, *New Eng. J. Med.*, 284 (1971), 789; reprinted by permission.

14. M. Weatherall, "Side-effects," *Br. Med. J.*, 1 (1965), 1174.

15. Gross, *The Doctors*, pp. 500-501.

16. Ingelfinger, "Annual discourse," p. 530.

17. Smith, Kline & French Company, "Dexamyl," in the *1970 Physicians Desk Reference to Pharmaceutical Specialties and Biologicals*, 27th ed. (Oradell, N.J., 1970), p. 1206.

18. *Hearings on Administered Prices: Drugs*, part 16, p. 9034.

19. Gaffin and Associates, *Attitudes*, pp. 20-21, C-16.

20. N. Hawkins, "The detail man and preference behavior," *Southwestern Social Science Quarterly*, 40 (1959), 213-224.

21. The executive, Herman W. Leitzow, Vice President, Schering Corp., was quoted by S. Blackman, in *Hearings on Administered Prices: Drugs*, part 14, p. 8219.

22. Gross, *The Doctors*, p. 492.

23. *Hearings on Administered Prices: Drugs*, part 18, p. 10426.

24. Morton Mintz, *The Therapeutic Nightmare* (Boston: Houghton Mifflin, 1965), pp. 58, 512-525.

25. H. Yockey, "Why medicine is high in public esteem," *Am. Med. News*, (Oct. 9, 1972), p. 4.

26. Henry Wechsler and Denise Thum, *Drug Usage Among School-Age Youth in the Town of Brookline: Research Report #1* (Boston, 1971), pp. 12-17.

27. Brecher, *Licit and Illicit Drugs*, p. 233.

28. R. N. Chopra and G. S. Chopra, "The present position of hemp drug addiction in India," *Indian Med. Res. Mem.*, 31 (1939), 1-119. Blum and Associates, *Drugs I: Society and Drugs*, pp. 35-36, citing K. H. Connell, "Ether drinking in Ulster," *Q. J. Stud. Alcohol*, 26 (1965), 631-632, 641.

29. Personal communication from William E. Doering, Mallinckrodt Professor of Organic Chemistry, Harvard University, Dec. 13, 1972.

30. "G.A.O. says heroin smuggling is too sweeping to halt at borders," *New York Times*, Dec. 13, 1972, p. 31.

31. Bejerot, *Addiction and Society*, pp. 267, 271-279.

32. Brecher, *Licit and Illicit Drugs*, p. 205.

33. Pierre Huard and Ming Wong, *Chinese Medicine* (New York: McGraw-Hill, 1968), trans. B. Fielding, pp. 10-11. W. B. O'Shaughnessy, "On the preparations of the Indian Hemp, or Gunjah (*cannabis indica*): The effects on the animal system in health, and their utility in the treatment of tetanus and other convulsive diseases," *Transactions of the Medical and Physical Society of Calcutta* (Calcutta, 1842), p. 460.

34. Grinspoon, *Marihuana Reconsidered*, pp. 218-230.

35. A. E. Fossier, "The mariahuana menace," *New Orleans Med. Surg. J.*, 84 (1931), 249. See also C. H. Whitebread, II and R. J. Bonnie, *The Marihuana Conviction: A History of Marihuana Prohibition in the United States* (Charlottesville: Univ. Press of Virginia, 1974), pp. 31-52.

36. U.S. Congress, House, Ways and Means Committee, *Taxation of Marihuana, Hearings on HR 6385*, 75th Congress, 1st Session, April 27, 1937, p. 116.

37. Council on Mental Health and Committee on Alcoholism and Drug Dependence, American Medical Association, "Dependence on cannabis (marihuana)," *J.A.M.A.*, 201 (1967), 368-371.

38. S. Allentuck and K. M. Bowman, "The psychiatric aspects of marihuana intoxication," *Am. J. Psychiat.*, 99 (1942), 248-251. Editorial, "Recent investigation of marihuana," *J.A.M.A.*, 120 (1942), 1128-1129. H. J. Anslinger, "The psychiatric aspects of marihuana intoxication," Letter, *J.A.M.A.*, 121 (1943), 212-213; R. J. Bouquet, "Marihuana intoxication," Letter, *J.A.M.A.*, 124 (1944), 1010-1011. "Marihuana problems," Editorial, *J.A.M.A.*, 127 (1945), 1129.

39. R. S. deRopp, *Drugs and the Mind* (New York: Grove, 1957), pp. 108-109.

40. Germaine Greer, *The Female Eunuch* (New York: McGraw-Hill, 1971), pp. 25-26.

41. Ibid., pp. 272-273, quoting "Letter to 'Evelyn Home,'" *Woman*, Aug. 2, 1968.

Index

Abbott Laboratories, 23

Abstinence syndrome: in amphetamine dependence, 153; physiological symptoms of, 160

Achievement, effect of amphetamines on, 231-232, 254

Activity level, and amphetamines, 239

Acute poisoning, by amphetamines, 138-139

Addict: attempts to define, 171-177; amphetamine, 176-177

Addiction: terminology of, 149-153; vs. habituation, 150; basis of, 170

Adler, H. F., 71

Adlersberg, D., 210

Ad-Nil, 46

Adverse effects of amphetamines, 244-246. See also Medicine, amphetamines as

Advertising of drugs, 258-271; volume of, 262; and the AMA, 263-265; slickness of, 265-266; emphasis on expanded use, 266-267; minimization of side effects, 267-269; by detail men, 269-270

Age, and effect of amphetamines, 195

Aggressive behavior: related to amphetamines, 190-198; enhanced by overcrowding, 198-199; and long-term drug use, 200. See also Crime; Homicide

Air Force, U.S., 19

Alcohol: and grades 28; effects of compared to amphetamine, 115, 129, 179-180; in multiple drug use, 123, 197; tolerance for, 154; and REM sleep, 162; prohibition of, 280

Alertonic, 49

Allen, R., 245

Allentuck, S., 286

Alles, Gordon A., 43-44, 56, 61; account of MDA, 57-59; on amphetamine psychosis, 132

Alpha waves, 69, 70

Ambar, 223

American Medical Association, 22; approval of amphetamine tablets by, 45, 189; Council on Drugs, 152; on clinics for addicts, 187, 188; and advertising of drugs, 262-263; on cannabis, 187-189, 285-287

Amines: defined, 41-42; sympathomimetic, 41

Amodex, 46

Amodril, 46

Amphaplex, 46

Amphate, 46

Amphetamine Psychosis (Connell), 191-202

Amphetamines: early uses of, 11-12; misuse of, 12-14, 18-20; ban of, 17; on black market, 21-24; illegal manufacture of, 24-26; student use of, 27-39; basic structure of, 42; first use as medicine, 45; racemic and dextroamphetamine, 46; combinations of, 46-49; derivatives of, 49-51; psychedelic, 51-61; psychological effects of, 62-95; and crime, 189-205; place of in medicine, 206-226; for hyperkinesis, 227-257; advertising of, 258-271; education concerning, 272-274; prohibition of, 274-277; treatment of abusers of, 277-282; attitudes toward marihuana and amphetamines compared, 282-289; as reflection of society, 290-291

Anderson, E. W., 141

Angrist, B. M., 16-17, 99, 134, 200

Animals, effect of amphetamines on, 104-106, 146

Anker, J. L., 33

Anorectic drugs. See Obesity

Anslinger, H. J., 183, 285, 286

Anxiety attacks, 157

Appetite, suppression of, 209-210. See also Obesity

Appetite-inhibitors, 46

Aristotle, 150

Armed Forces, use of amphetamines by, 18-20

Askevold, F., 124, 130

Askew, B. M., 140

Assassins, 183

Atlee, W. E., 143

Attention, effect of amphetamines on, 240-241, 248

Ausubel, D. P., 159, 167